Breast Cancer

Philip K
2016

Breast Cancer

Fundamentals of Evidence-Based Disease Management

I. Craig Henderson, MD

Professor of Medicine
University of California, San Francisco
Helen Diller Family Comprehensive Cancer Center
San Francisco, California

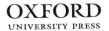

OXFORD
UNIVERSITY PRESS

OXFORD
UNIVERSITY PRESS

Oxford University Press is a department of the University of Oxford.
It furthers the University's objective of excellence in research,
scholarship, and education by publishing worldwide.

Oxford   New York

Auckland   Cape Town   Dar es Salaam   Hong Kong   Karachi
Kuala Lumpur   Madrid   Melbourne   Mexico City   Nairobi
New Delhi   Shanghai   Taipei   Toronto

With offices in

Argentina   Austria   Brazil   Chile   Czech Republic   France   Greece
Guatemala   Hungary   Italy   Japan   Poland   Portugal   Singapore
South Korea   Switzerland   Thailand   Turkey   Ukraine   Vietnam

Oxford is a registered trademark of Oxford University Press
in the UK and certain other countries.

Published in the United States of America by
Oxford University Press
198 Madison Avenue, New York, NY 10016

© Oxford University Press 2015

Library of Congress Cataloging-in-Publication Data
Henderson, I. Craig, author.
Breast cancer: Fundamentals of evidence-based disease management / I. Craig Henderson.
p. ; cm.
Includes bibliographical references and index.
ISBN 978–0–19–991998–7 (alk. paper)
I. Title.
[DNLM: 1. Breast Neoplasms.   2. Breast—pathology.   3. Combined Modality Therapy.
4. Neoplasm Invasiveness.   5. Neoplasm Metastasis. WP 870]
RC280.B8
616.99′449—dc23
2015012272

This material is not intended to be, and should not be considered, a substitute for medical
or other professional advice. Treatment for the conditions described in this material is highly dependent on
the individual circumstances. And, while this material is designed to offer accurate information with respect
to the subject matter covered and to be current as of the time it was written, research and knowledge about
medical and health issues is constantly evolving and dose schedules for medications are being
revised continually, with new side effects recognized and accounted for regularly. Readers must therefore
always check the product information and clinical procedures with the most up-to-date published product
information and data sheets provided by the manufacturers and the most recent codes of conduct and safety
regulation. The publisher and the authors make no representations or warranties to readers, express or
implied, as to the accuracy or completeness of this material. Without limiting the foregoing, the publisher
and the authors make no representations or warranties as to the accuracy or efficacy of the drug dosages
mentioned in the material. The authors and the publisher do not accept, and expressly disclaim, any
responsibility for any liability, loss or risk that may be claimed or incurred as a consequence of the
use and/or application of any of the contents of this material.

1 3 5 7 9 8 6 4 2
Printed in the United States of America
on acid-free paper

To Mary for her unlimited patience whenever I'm caring
for patients or writing about breast cancer.

CONTENTS

PREFACE

The single most important thing to understand about breast cancer is the great variation in its natural history and its responsiveness to therapy from one patient to another.
Prior to diagnosis, the disease may slowly evolve and grow for a few years to decades.
Following diagnosis, the disease may progress rapidly. But many or most patients will
live for years, even after the appearance of distant metastases, and some of those with
the worst prognostic factors at diagnosis (large tumor size, involved regional lymph
nodes, molecular markers suggestive of aggressive disease) may survive for decades
or never recur. Because the patient is terrified by cancer and the physician is afraid of
missing an opportunity for cure, no matter how slim, patients are often over-treated.
Optimal patient management is to provide neither too much nor too little therapy.
The primary aim of this book is to provide the clinician with the tools to do just that.

Throughout the book an emphasis is placed on the biology of the tumor, how
this will vary between patients, and how this should affect the choice of treatments at
each time point in the patient's course. Before any therapy is begun, the clinician and
patient should think realistically and honestly about what will happen if no treatment
is given; for breast cancer patients, the consequences of no treatment will often be sur-
prisingly benign. The choice among therapies should be based primarily on evidence
from properly controlled clinical trials, usually randomized trials of appropriate size,
that have demonstrated measurable and meaningful benefits, such as improved overall, recurrence-free, or progression-free survival, or a net reduction in symptoms from
the disease relative to the toxicity of treatment. In sum, the clinician must integrate an
assessment of the patient's likely course based on clinical and pathological staging and
laboratory studies (e.g., molecular and genetic markers) with objective evidence on
the benefits of therapy. Hopefully this book will enable this.

This book is shorter than most textbooks on the subject and has been written by
a single author, a medical oncologist. It can comfortably be read from beginning to
end by anyone wishing to obtain a comprehensive understanding of and an integrated
approach to the management of the disease. It is anticipated that most readers will
have a limited knowledge of the subject, such as medical oncology fellows or surgical, radiotherapy, and radiology residents early in their training; oncology nurses
not specialized in breast cancer; non-oncology medical professionals in training or
in practice; and basic scientists seeking a clinical context for their research. Medical
terminology has been defined or explained so that sophisticated patients might also
find the book useful. Descriptions of the evolution in our thinking and understanding
of the disease are often given to provide perspective in the interpretation of evidence
from current studies. Recent references to more comprehensive reviews or expanded
data sets have been provided for each subject. To the extent possible, relevant data

are organized in figures and tables rather than text. Outcomes from randomized trials and meta-analyses are the main basis for clinical management recommendations, but in many instances management guidelines are summarized from respected oncology organizations such as the National Cancer Institute, the National Comprehensive Cancer Network, the American Society of Clinical Oncology, the American Joint Committee on Cancer, the American Cancer Society, the American College of Physicians, the American Society of Radiation Oncology, the American College of Surgeons, the American College of Pathologists, the St. Gallen Conference, the US Preventive Services Task Force, and European counterparts to these organizations. Recommendations for management/treatment are based either on evidence or widely accepted practice, but when changes in the near future are anticipated, this is noted. Although the book is not meant to be a manual for the use of all therapeutic modalities, details about commonly used drug regimens, drug dosage, and the expected side effects have been provided in tabular form for easy access by treating clinicians.

ACKNOWLEDGMENTS

Colleagues who have been helpful on one or another subject for this book are Daniel Hayes, Susan Love, William Wood, Robert Carlson, Nicholas Robert, and John Haybittle. Many others have, over time, substantially influenced my understanding of this disease and have contributed to many of my conclusions; these include Samuel Hellman, Emil Frei III, George Canellos, Marvin Zelen, Francis Moore, Maurice Fox, Bernard Fisher, Michael Baum, Gianni Bonadonna, David Page, Jay Harris, Rebecca Gelman, Richard Gelber, Marc Lippman, Kent Osborne, Norman Wolmark, Ian Smith, Mitchell Dowsett, Dennis Slamon, Martine Piccart-Gebhart, Hyman Muss, Laura Esserman, William Goodson, Richard Peto, Donald Berry, Thea Tlsty, and Joe Gray. Finally, I'm very appreciative of the magnificent support, practical assistance, and amazing patience I've received from my editors at Oxford University Press, especially Rebecca Suzan, Andrea Knobloch, and Andrea Seils, and, in my own office, the assistance of Frances Jordan.

1

EPIDEMIOLOGY AND RISK FACTORS
FOR BREAST CANCER

Breast cancer is the most frequently diagnosed cancer in women in 140 out of 184 countries[1,2] (see Table 1.1). It is now the most common cause of cancer death among women worldwide and is second to lung cancer in the United States.

The chance that an American woman will be diagnosed with either an invasive or in situ breast cancer sometime between birth and age 95 is 1 in 7 (14.8%) and with an invasive cancer 1 in 8 (12.3%).[3] However, her chances of dying of breast cancer are much smaller: 1 in 37 (2.2%). The risk of developing breast cancer is higher among white than black women—15.1% versus 13.2%—but the chance of dying of breast cancer is higher among black than white—3.3% versus 2.7%.

These lifetime risks help put in perspective the importance of breast cancer as a national health problem but are often overwhelming to an individual woman considering her personal risk. For this reason, the risk of developing or dying of breast cancer in shorter intervals of 10, 20, or 30 years for women at various ages is shown in Table 1.2. For example, a 40-year-old woman has slightly less than a 4% risk of developing and a 1% risk of dying of breast cancer by the time she is 60. These numbers are for an "average" woman but can be adjusted for an individual depending on her risk relative to the average (see Table 1.2).

RECENT CHANGES IN INCIDENCE AND MORTALITY

Between 2008 to 2012, breast cancer incidence increased worldwide by 20% while mortality decreased by 14%; this is thought to be due to lifestyle changes that increased risk and improved treatment that decreased the death rate.

In the United States, however, both incidence and mortality have decreased in recent years (see Figure 1.1). The relatively steady increase in incidence between 1975 and 2002 is thought to be due to a number of factors, including fewer children, delayed childbearing, increased obesity, the use of postmenopausal hormone replacement, and, probably most important, the increasing use of screening mammography.[4] This trend abruptly reversed in 2002 due to decreased hormone use after the publication of results from Women's Health Initiative Trial (see discussion later in this chapter). In that year there was a 7% decrease in incidence, primarily in white women aged 50+ and in estrogen receptor positive (ER+) tumors.[5] Since 2006 there has again been an increase in the incidence of ER+ tumors matched by a fall in ER− tumors. In situ breast cancer rose most dramatically during the years when mammography use was increasing, but continues to increase now only in women under age 50.

Table 1.1 Incidence of and Mortality from Breast Cancer Worldwide and in the United States American Cancer Society. Breast Cancer Facts & Figures 2013–2014. Atlanta, GA; 2013; GLOBCAN 2012: Estimated cancer incidence, mortality, and prevalence worldwide, 2012. 2014. (Accessed at http://www.iarc.fr/en/media-centre/pr/2013/index.php)

	United States 2014 (Projections)	Worldwide 2012
Incidence		
All breast cancers	297,310	1,670,000
Invasive cancers	232,340	
In situ cancers	64,640	
Prevalence	2,900,000*	6,300,000**
Deaths	39,620	522,000
Male breast cancer		
Incidence	2,240	
Deaths	410	

* Alive in 2012, diagnosed any time

** Alive in 2012, diagnosed in prior 5 years

Table 1.2 Cumulative Risk of Developing and Dying From Breast Cancer Over a Lifetime or in 10-, 20-, or 30-Year Intervals for Any Given Age

Age Now	Risk of Having a Breast Cancer Diagnosis (%)			
	In 10 Yrs	In 20 Yrs	In 30 Yrs	By Age 95
30	0.4	1.9	4.1	12.5
40	1.5	3.7	6.9	12.2
50	2.3	5.6	8.8	11.1
60	3.5	6.9	8.9	9.4
70	3.9	6.2	—	6.7
80	3.1	—	—	3.8
Risk of Dying From Breast Cancer (%)				
30	0.1	0.6	1.2	2.8
40	0.5	1.1	2.0	2.7
50	0.7	1.6	2.6	2.6
60	1.0	2.0	2.6	2.4
70	1.2	1.9	—	2.0
80	—	—	—	1.6

Data From 18 SEER (Surveillance, Epidemiology, and End Results) Sites Covering 28% of US Population During Years 1975–2011 (SEER Cancer Statistics Review, 1975–2011. National Cancer Institute, 2014. (Accessed at http://seer.cancer.gov/csr/1975_2011/, based on November 2013 SEER data submission, posted to the SEER web site, April 2014.))

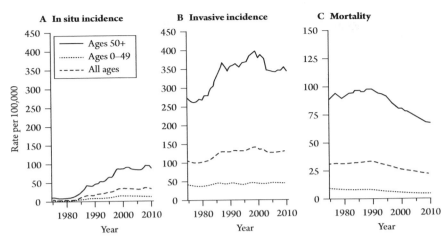

Figure 1.1 Incidence of invasive and in situ breast cancer and breast cancer mortality in the United States, 1975–2010. Rates are age adjusted to the 2000 US standard population within each age group. *Sources:* Surveillance, Epidemiology, and End Results (SEER) Program for incidence data and the National Center for Health Statistics, Centers for Disease Control and Prevention for mortality data. From DeSantis C, Ma J, Bryan L, et al. Breast cancer statistics, 2013. *CA Cancer J Clin.* 2014;64:52–62.

Breast cancer mortality fell by 34% between 1990 and 2010.[4] Among women aged < 50 and those 50+ the decrease was 3.1% and 1.9% per year, respectively. This is thought to be due both to treatment effects, especially the use of adjuvant systemic therapies, and to early detection using screening mammography.[6] Although the mortality of both African-American and white women decreased, breast mortality is consistently higher in African-American than white women. In addition, African-American women have a higher incidence of ER– tumors, are diagnosed on average at a later stage, have a poorer 5-year survival after adjusting for stage, have greater obesity and other comorbidities, and have less access to, compliance with, and response to treatment.[4] This suggests that the differences in breast cancer mortality between whites and African Americans is multifactorial, driven by both intrinsic tumor characteristics and socioeconomic factors.

RISK FACTORS FOR DEVELOPING BREAST CANCER

The list of factors that have been reported in the medical literature and lay press to be associated with an increased risk of breast cancer is almost endless. Most of these risks cannot be confirmed in a second study. Sixty percent of women with breast cancer will have no risk factors. Factors that are clearly associated with different degrees of risk, along with a few that are often cited but are not risk factors, are shown in Table 1.3.

The greatest risk factor is age. In American and European women, risk increases throughout life (Figure 1.2). Only 1 in 68 women will be diagnosed with breast cancer between the ages of 40 and 49, but risk increases more steeply during that decade than after age 50, which is roughly the midpoint for the onset of menses in the United States[7] (see Figure 1.2).

Table 1.3 Risk Factors for Developing Breast Cancer

Relative Risk > 2	Relative Risk 1.2–1.9	Decreased Risk	No Established Risk
Age			
Age ≥ 65 vs. < 50			
Genetic Factors			
Positive family history BRCA1/2 mutations			
Breast Abnormalities			
Dense breasts on mammogram Biopsy: Proliferation with atypia LCIS DCIS Prior invasive breast cancer	Biopsy: Proliferation, no atypia		Biopsy: no increased proliferation Lumpy breast on examination
Reproductive and Menstrual Factors			
	Early menarche	Prolonged breast feeding	Abortion
	Late menopause No or late first pregnancy Hormone replacement therapy	Oophorectomy	Oral contraceptives Fertility drugs
Lifestyle Factors			
	Postmenopausal obesity	Premenopausal obesity	Dietary fat intake
	Alcohol use	Physical activity	Smoking Coffee Aspirin, NSAIDs
Other/Miscellaneous			
Radiotherapy for Hodgkin's Disease			

NSAIDs = non-steroidal anti-inflammatory drugs

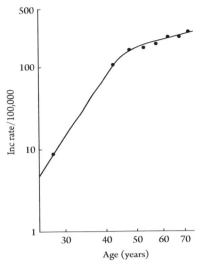

Figure 1.2 Age-specific incidence rates for breast cancer in US white women. Data source: Third National Cancer Survey. The inflection in the curve at about age 50 is called the Clemmesen's Hook and reflects the decrease in the rate of increase after menopause.

Reprinted with permission from Pike MC, Pearce CL. Mammographic density, MRI background parenchymal enhancement and breast cancer risk. *Ann Oncol.* 2013;24 Suppl 8:viii37–viii41.

GENETIC PREDISPOSITION: FAMILY HISTORY AND BRCA1/2

About 10% of breast cancers will occur in women who have a first-degree relative with breast cancer. Five to 10% of breast cancer is associated with an inheritable gene mutation. Women in either of these two groups are among those with the highest risk of developing breast cancer. (These are not mutually exclusive groups, and there is more overlap among younger than older women.)

Having a first- or second-degree relative with breast cancer almost doubles a woman's risk (relative risk [RR] = 1.9; 95% CI, 1.7–2.0.)[8] This is slightly higher if the relative is first degree (mother, sister, daughter with RRs of 2.0, 2.3, and 1.8, respectively). (First-degree relatives also include father, brother, and son; risk is passed through both male and female relatives. However, RR estimates are based primarily on female relatives because breast cancer occurs 100 times more frequently in women than men.) Having two first-degree relatives with breast cancer increases the RR to 3.6 (95% CI, 2.5–5.0); it is not entirely clear that the risk is higher with two sisters than with a mother and sister.[8,9] A woman with a relative whose breast cancer was diagnosed prior to age 50 has a higher risk than if the relative was diagnosed after age 50. This is particularly true for women who are under age 50.[8] Thus a woman aged ≤ 50 with any first-degree relative diagnosed with breast cancer at age < 50 has an RR of 3.3, compared to an RR of 1.8 if her relative was diagnosed at age ≥ 50. A woman aged ≥ 50 with a first-degree relative diagnosed with breast cancer at age < 50 has an RR of 1.8, compared to an RR of 1.7 if her relative was diagnosed at age ≥ 50.

Table 1.4 Cumulative Risk of Developing and Dying From Breast Cancer in Women With a Family History of Breast Cancer

Women's Current Age	Number of Relatives With Breast Cancer					
	None		One		Two	
	Risk of Having a Breast Cancer Diagnosis (%)					
	In 10 Yrs	By Age 80	In 10 Yrs	By Age 80	In 10 Yrs	By Age 80
20	0.04	7.8	0.1	13.3	0.2	21.1
30	0.4	7.7	1.0	13.0	2.0	20.7
40	1.4	7.3	2.5	12.0	5.2	18.9
50	1.9	6.1	3.2	9.8	5.3	14.7
60	2.3	4.5	3.5	7.1	5.6	10.4
70	2.5	2.5	4.2	4.2	5.7	5.7
	Risk of Dying From Breast Cancer (%)					
	By Age 50	By Age 80	By Age 50	By Age 80	By Age 50	By Age 80
20	0.4	2.3	1.0	4.2	1.9	7.6

Results From a Pooled Analysis of 52 Case-Control and Cohort Studies That Included 160,195 Women (58,209 With Breast Cancer) (Familial breast cancer: collaborative reanalysis of individual data from 52 epidemiological studies including 58,209 women with breast cancer and 101,986 women without the disease. Lancet 2001;358:1389–99)

The effect of family history on the cumulative risk of breast cancer is shown in Table 1.4, which is constructed similarly to Table 1.2 so that the two groups can be compared. Risk within 10 years or by age 80 is shown for women of various ages with no, one, or two first-degree relatives with breast cancer.

About 30 genes are known to contribute to breast cancer risk, but collectively these account for only ~30% of the familial risk.[10] Two high-penetrance genes, BRCA1 and BRCA2, account for 16%–20% of the familial risk. Well-defined disease syndromes with known genetic mutations account for a much smaller percentage. These syndromes include Cowden's (PTEN mutation), Peutz-Jeghers (STK11), Li-Fraumeni (TP53), and ataxia-telangiectasia (Louis-Bar syndrome, ATM). A number of low-penetrance susceptibility genes have been found using single nucleotide polymorphisms (SNPs), but these are of uncertain importance as a causal factor for breast cancer. The e-cadherin gene has been shown to suppress the development of lobular breast cancer (see Chapters 3 and 5). Some gene variants are associated with one or another molecular subtype, such as hormone receptor or HER2 positive cancers. In the case of BRCA1/2, BRCA1 tumors are characteristically ER/PR (progesterone receptor) negative with a basal phenotype, while BRCA2 tumors are more often ER/PR positive with a luminal phenotype.[11]

BRCA1/2 are tumor suppressor genes that are active in DNA damage repair pathways. Deletion or mutation (functional loss) of these genes leads to genetic instability and the accumulation of other cancer-promoting genetic mutations.[12] These germline mutations were found through genetic linkage studies of families with early-onset breast cancer and then were further defined using positional cloning. They are autosomal dominant and passaged as Mendelian traits. BRCA1 is on chromosome 17q21 and BRCA2 on 13q12–13. Both are associated with increased risk for cancers other than breast cancer, especially ovarian, pancreatic, and prostate cancer. Men with these mutations are also at increased risk of breast cancer; with BRCA2, risk is increased 100-fold and lifetime cumulative risk is 6%.[12]

One or the other of these genes occur in 0.2%–0.3% of the general population (1 in 300–500 women), 2.1% of Ashkenazi Jewish women, 3% of women with breast cancer, 6% of women whose breast cancer was diagnosed before age 40, and 10% of women with ovarian cancer.[13] The risk is even higher in families with multiple breast and/or ovarian cancers, especially early-onset cancers, where the frequency of gene mutations may be 20%. The prevalence of the gene is 10% among Ashkenazi Jews in these high-risk families. Unique founder mutations have been identified in Ashkenazi Jews, blacks, Hispanics and in some families in the Netherlands, Iceland, Sweden, Hungry, French Canada, and Scotland.

The likelihood that a carrier of one of these mutations will develop breast cancer (i.e., the penetrance) varies, depending on whether the study is retrospective, as most of the early studies were, or prospective, and how large the study or meta-analysis of multiple studies is.

A reasonable estimate of penetrance (i.e., the likelihood that a BRCA1/2 carrier will eventually be diagnosed with breast cancer by age 70) is 60% for BRCA1 and 40% for BRCA2.[14] The risk of developing ovarian cancer is greater for BRCA1 than BRCA2 mutations. By age 75 it is estimated to be 59% and 17%, respectively. Another recent meta-analysis has estimated that the penetrance of breast and ovarian cancer by age 75 in Ashkenazi Jewish women with BRCA1 and BRCA2 mutations is 34% and 21%, respectively.[15]

The effect of BRCA1/2 mutations on the cumulative risk of breast cancer in 10-year intervals, or until age 70, is shown in Table 1.5, which is constructed similarly to Tables 1.2 and 1.4.

Anyone—male or female—at high risk of having a BRCA mutation should be referred to a genetic counselor with expertise in determining who should undergo testing, in selecting the type of test that is most appropriate, and in explaining the results of any test performed. Candidates for testing include breast cancer patients, relatives of a breast cancer patient known to have a BRCA mutation, or anyone with a family history that is typical of BRCA1/2 carriers. The National Comprehensive Cancer Network (NCCN) criteria are among the most commonly used to define patients at high risk of having these mutations (see Box 1.1).[18] A handy score sheet (shown in Figure 1.3) developed to easily identify non-cancer patients who should be referred for genetic counseling was formally evaluated in a cohort of patients undergoing routine mammographic screening.[17] It had a sensitivity of 81.2%, specificity of 91.9%, and discriminatory accuracy of 0.87.

Genetic counselors often use predictive models to calculate the probability that a woman will have a BRCA mutation, and base their decision to test on

Table 1.5 Cumulative Risk of Developing Either Breast Cancer or Ovarian Cancer in Currently Unaffected Women Carrying BRCA1 or BRCA2 Mutations

Age Now	Risk of Having a Breast Cancer Diagnosis (%)				
	In 10 Yrs	In 20 Yrs	In 30 Yrs	In 40 Yrs	By Age 70
BCRA1					
20	1.8	12	29	44	54
30	10	28	44	54	54
40	20	38	49	—	49
50	22	37	—	—	37
60	19	—	—	—	19
BCRA2					
20	1	7.5	21	35	45
30	6.6	20	35	45	45
40	15	30	42	—	42
50	18	32	—	—	32
60	17	—	—	—	17
Risk of Having an Ovarian Cancer Diagnosis (%)					
BCRA1					
20	1	3.2	9.5	23	39
30	2.2	8.7	22	39	39
40	6.7	20	38	—	38
50	15	34	—	—	34
60	22	—	—	—	—
BCRA2					
20	0.2	0.7	2.6	7.5	16
30	0.5	2.4	7.4	16	16
40	1.9	7	16	—	16
50	5.2	14	—	—	14
60	9.8	—	—	—	9.8

Calculations were made using Bayes Mendel risk prediction software and the BRCAPRO prediction tool with data from a meta-analysis of 10 studies that included 18,432 families with 793 BCRA1 and 517 BRCA2 carriers.

Source: Chen S, Parmigiani G. Meta-analysis of BRCA1 and BRCA2 penetrance. *J Clin Oncol.* 2007;25:1329–33.

Box 1.1 NCCN Hereditary Breast and/or Ovarian Cancer Syndrome, Criteria for BRCA1 or BRCA2 Mutation Testing

- Person with a family member known to have a deleterious BRCA1/2 mutation
- Person with breast cancer who has one or more of following:
  - Diagnosed age ≤ 45
  - Diagnosed age ≤ 50 with
    - An additional primary in same or opposite breast
    - ≥ 1 close relative[†] with breast cancer, any age
    - Too few family members to fully assess family history
  - Diagnosed age ≤ 60 with a triple negative breast cancer
  - Diagnosed at any age with
    - ≥ 1 close blood relative[†] with breast cancer diagnosed at age ≤ 50
    - ≥ 2 close blood relatives[†] with breast cancer, any age
    - ≥ 1 close blood relative[†] with epithelial ovarian[††] cancer
    - ≥ 2 close blood relatives with pancreatic cancer and/or prostate cancer (Gleason score ≥ 7) at any age
    - A close male blood relative[†] with breast cancer
    - Ethnicity associated with higher mutation frequency (e.g., Ashkenazi Jew), regardless of family history
- Person with breast cancer who has also had epithelial ovarian cancer[††]
- Male with breast cancer
- Person with breast cancer who has also had pancreatic or prostate cancer (Gleason score ≥ 7) at any age with ≥ 2 close blood relatives[†] with breast and/or ovarian[††] and/or pancreatic or prostate cancer (Gleason score ≥ 7) at any age
- Persons without breast cancer who have a suggestive family history characterized by
  - First- or second-degree relative with any of the characteristics listed above for a person with breast cancer, such as young age, multiple cases of breast cancer on the same side of the family, the occurrence of breast cancer and ovarian,[††] pancreatic, and/or prostatic cancers in the patterns described above, and male breast cancer.
  - Third-degree relative with breast and/or epithelial ovarian cancer with ≥ 2 close blood relatives[†] with breast cancer (at least 1 with breast cancer at age ≤ 50) and/or epithelial ovarian cancer.

[†]*First-, second-, or third-degree relative on same side of the family*
[††]*This category includes fallopian tube and primary peritoneal cancers, including Lynch syndrome.*
Source: NCCN Clinical Practice Guidelines in Oncology (NCCN Guidelines): Genetic/Familial High-Risk Assessment: Breast and Ovarian.

	Breast cancer at or before age 50	Ovarian cancer at any age
Yourself		
Mother		
Sister		
Daughter		
Mother's Side		
Grandmother		
Aunt		
Father's Side		
Grandmother		
Aunt		
Two (2) or more cases of breast cancer (*after age 50*) on <u>same</u> side of the family		
Male breast cancer at *any age* in any relative		
Jewish ancestry		

Figure 1.3 Referral Screening Tool for determining whether to refer a person with any family history of breast or ovarian cancer for genetic counseling and possible BRCA1/2 testing. Any patient with two or more checkmarks should be referred for screening.
Reprinted with permission from Bellcross CA, Lemke AA, Pape LS, et al. Evaluation of a breast/ovarian cancer genetics referral screening tool in a mammography population. *Genet Med.* 2009;11:783–9.

predefined levels of risk calculated with these tools. This is described in greater deal at the end of this chapter.

Although family history of cancer is the most commonly used criteria for determining who should be tested, BRCA mutations are also found in some patients with no family history. The best studied of these are triple negative tumors.

BREAST ABNORMALITIES: DENSITY ON MAMMOGRAMS AND PROLIFERATIVE CHANGES IN BIOPSIES

Breast density has recently emerged as an independent risk factor for developing breast cancer, even though it is closely linked to a number of other modifiable risk factors. As women grow older and/or their BMI increases, fatty tissue increasingly accounts for a larger percentage of the breast.[19] Breast density (BD) is greater in women taking hormone replacement therapy, while it decreases among those taking anti-estrogens. It is also decreased with increased parity. However, twin studies provide strong evidence that BD is heritable, and there is ~ 10% overlap in SNPs associated with breast cancer risk and BD.[20] Because of its growing acceptance as a predictor of future risk, 14 states have now made it mandatory that women be informed of the level of density in their breasts.[19]

The dense areas of the breast are white on a mammogram (Figure 1.4). These areas consist primarily of connective tissue (collagen) and glandular elements, including the

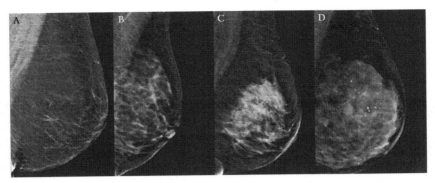

Figure 1.4 Mammograms demonstrating the four levels of breast density used in the Bi-RADS density classification. A: BI-RADS Density 1, almost entirely fat. B: BI-RADS Density 2, scattered areas of fibroglandular tissue. C: BI-RAD Density 3, heterogeneously dense, which could obscure small masses. D: BI-RAD Density 4, extremely dense, which lowers sensitivity of mammography. Reprinted with permission from Wang AT, Vachon CM, Brandt KR, et al. Breast density and breast cancer risk: a practical review. *Mayo Clin Proc.* 2014;89:548–57.

nuclei of breast epithelia (fibroglandular tissue).[7] The causal relationship between BD and breast cancer risk is not established, but one hypothesis is that since dense areas contain many more epithelial cells, women with dense breasts have more breast cells and thus a greater likelihood of mutations leading to breast cancer. Countering this, however, is the fact that there is greater epithelial cell proliferative activity in areas with reduced collagen.[7]

There are a number of classification systems for defining dense breasts. One of these is the BI-RADS density groups (not to be confused with the BI-RADS system for deciding whether a biopsy should be performed, described in Chapter 8).[21-23] The characteristics of each of the classes, an estimate of the percentage of women that will fall into each group, and the relative risk of developing breast cancer are provided in Table 1.6. Characteristic mammograms are shown in Figure 1.4. Although there is agreement that increased density is associated with increased risk of developing breast cancer, this risk needs to be adjusted for patient age, menopausal status, parity, and BMI. A 50% dense breast in a 70-year-old or a woman with a high BMI imparts a greater risk than a 50% dense breast in a younger or smaller woman.[19] At present there are insufficient data to refine risk for these subcategories. In various analyses, the risk of breast cancer in those with the densest breasts (> 75% density) relative to those with fatty breasts (10%–25% fat tissue) is 4–6-fold. However, relative risk of the densest breasts with the "average" breast (see Table 1.6) is only 2-fold, and comparisons within the extremes are even smaller.[21]

As with a number of other risk factors, no association between breast density and the risk of dying of breast cancer has been demonstrated.[25]

Patients with proliferative changes in the breast tissue, especially those with a prior history of invasive or in situ cancers, are at increased risk of developing breast cancer in any remaining breast tissue for the remainder of their lives. There are numerous anecdotes of breast cancers arising in a small pocket of normal tissue after ostensibly complete mastectomy. The relative risk of breast cancer after a biopsy showing hyperplasia

Table 1.6 BI-RADS Density Categories and Relative Risk of Developing Breast Cancer

Group	Appearance of Mammogram[a]	Extent (%) of FGD[b]	Prevalence (%)[b]	Relative Risk vs. D1[c]	vs. "average"[d]
D1	Almost entirely fat	< 25	10	1.0	–
D2	Scattered areas of fibroglandular tissue	25–50	40	2.04	–
	"Average" density*			–	1.0
D3	Heterogeneously dense which could obscure small masses	51–75	40	2.81	1.2
D4	Extremely dense which lowers sensitivity of mammography	> 75	10	4.08	2.1

FGD fibroglandular density.

Prevalence is the frequency with which each of these patterns is expected to be seen on routine mammograms. In practice this will differ for pre- and postmenopausal women.

* Average refers to breasts that are approximately 50% dense or at the threshold between D2 and D3. Relative risk was determined in a meta-analysis comparing breasts with the lowest density (D1) with other densities or comparing "average" density with the two higher risk categories.

[a] D'Orsi CJ, Sickles EA, Mendelson EB, et al., eds. *American College of Radiology Breast Imaging Reporting and Data System BI-RADS*. 5th ed. Reston, VA: American College of Radiology; 2013.

[b] Wang AT, Vachon CM, Brandt KR, et al. Breast density and breast cancer risk: a practical review. *Mayo Clin Proc*. 2014;89:548–57.

[c] McCormack VA, dos Santos Silva I. Breast density and parenchymal patterns as markers of breast cancer risk: a meta-analysis. *Cancer Epidemiol Biomarkers Prev*. 2006;15:1159–69.

[d] Sickles EA. The use of breast imaging to screen women at high risk for cancer. *Radiol Clin North Am*. 2010;48:859–78.

without atypia is < 2.0, but it is increased more than 5-fold if atypia is present and 11-fold with atypia and a family history.[26] This is covered in more detail in Chapter 3.

Many women are told that they have "fibrocystic" disease, either because of lumpy breasts noted on physical examination (a normal finding) or as a result of a biopsy. This is no longer a recognized disease category, and it has no implications regarding a woman's risk of subsequently developing breast cancer.

MENSTRUAL FACTORS, REPRODUCTIVE HISTORY, AND EXOGENOUS HORMONE USE

The relationship between estrogen or progesterone exposure and the risk of developing breast cancer is complex and poorly understood. There is no comprehensive model that integrates all the known interactions. These hormones increase the rate of normal breast cell proliferation. Since cellular mutation rates are usually proportional to the frequency of cell division, this effect alone might account for some of the increased risk. Dividing cells are also more susceptible to the effect of non-hormonal carcinogens. Estrogen and progesterone may induce some dormant breast *cancer* cells to divide or may stimulate slowly proliferating cells to grow faster, and in this way increase the likelihood they will become clinically relevant (see Chapter 4).

The risk of developing breast cancer is increased with higher levels of circulating estrogens (and androgens, as well, in premenopausal women). Women with increased bone density, which correlates with increased estrogen levels, are also at increased risk of breast cancer.[27]

The longer a woman is exposed to premenopausal levels of estrogen and has regular ovulatory cycles, the higher her risk of breast cancer.[27] The key intervals are menarche to pregnancy, which can be increased either by earlier onset of menses or late first pregnancy, and the duration of menses before menopause.

- Menarche: for each year younger that a woman has menarche, her risk of developing breast cancer increases by 5% (RR = 1.05, $p < 0.0001$)[28] (Figure 1.5A). However, if her ovulatory cycles become regular within 1 year of menarche, her risk is double that of a woman whose ovulatory cycles continue only intermittently for the first 5 years.[29] The average age of menarche has steadily decreased over the last century and is continuing to decrease.[30] In the United States it was age > 14 in 1877 and had decreased to 12.4 years in the early 1990s. The timing of this change has varied from one country to another and seems to be related to the adoption of a more Western diet and lifestyle; as the age of menarche decreased, the incidence of breast cancer generally increased in parallel in each country. The increased risk from having menarche 1 year earlier is significantly greater than the risk from undergoing menopause 1 year later.[28] This suggests that these changes

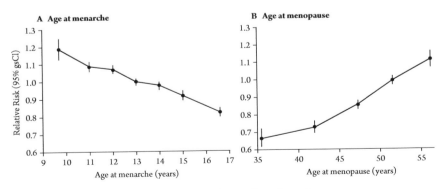

Figure 1.5 Relative risk of breast cancer by age of menarche and age of menopause.
From Collaborative Group on Hormonal Factors in Breast Cancer. Menarche, menopause, and breast cancer risk: individual participant meta-analysis, including 118 964 women with breast cancer from 117 epidemiological studies. *Lancet Oncol.* 2012;13:1141–51.

in risk may not be only the effect of a longer duration of exposure to estrogen and progesterone.

- Parity: There is a transient increase in breast cancer risk during and for 10–15 years after each pregnancy, but then breast cancer risk decreases for the remainder of the woman's life.[31] (There is a small attenuation of this protective effect during the late menopausal years.) During pregnancy the number of hormone-sensitive luminal cells decreases. Following pregnancy, there is a prolonged reduction in circulating prolactin and estrogen levels and an increase in sex hormone–binding globulin.[30] However, the relationship between parity and breast cancer risk is complex:
  - Nulliparous women have a higher risk than those who have a first pregnancy in their twenties but a *lower* risk than women who have a first pregnancy after age 35. For a woman in her fifties, the risk of breast cancer will be ~ 30% less if she has had three pregnancies than if she had none.[32] For a woman in her seventies, the difference in risk between these two groups is only 15%. For a parous woman in her fifties, the risk will be ~ 60% greater if her first pregnancy was after age 30 than if it was between ages 20 and 24. This difference is only 12% for a woman in her seventies.
  - Parous women who develop breast cancer will do so at a younger age than nulliparous women, even though nulliparous women will ultimately have more cancers than parous women.[31] This is related to the transient increased risk of breast cancer in the decade following pregnancy.
  - This transient increased risk following pregnancy is of shorter duration or nonexistent for a woman with two or more pregnancies.[31]
  - The age of a second pregnancy is also important. Compared to a second pregnancy at age 30, a second pregnancy when a woman is in her twenties will decrease risk and > age 35 will increase risk.[31]
  - A pregnancy not carried to full term, either because of a spontaneous or induced abortion, has no impact on risk.
- Breastfeeding: The relative risk of developing breast cancer is reduced by 4.3% per year of breast feeding.[33] This is in addition to a 7% reduction in risk with each birth. Since ovulation is suppressed during breastfeeding, this observation is consistent with the hypothesis that breast cancer risk is closely related to the total number of ovulatory cycles a woman has over her lifetime. This also accounts for much of the difference in the incidence of and mortality from breast cancer in developed and undeveloped countries.[33]
- Menopause: Each year that menopause is delayed increases the risk of developing breast cancer by ~ 3%. (RR = 1.029, $p < 0.0001$)[28] (Figure 1.5B). The mean age of natural menopause worldwide is 49.3 years, with 15% of women having menopause before age 45 and 10% after age 55. A premenopausal woman in the perimenopausal years (age 45–54) has a 43% greater likelihood of developing breast cancer than a woman of the same age who is postmenopausal. The decrease in the risk of breast cancer after menopause is much smaller in heavy than lean women, probably reflecting the fact that postmenopausal women with a high BMI have higher levels of circulating estrogens.[28] Women who have oophorectomy for any reason have a lower risk of developing breast cancer, but the risk of breast cancer

is the same for women who have oophorectomy or a natural menopause at the same age.[28]

EXOGENOUS HORMONES: POSTMENOPAUSAL HORMONE REPLACEMENT AND ORAL CONTRACEPTIVES

Cohort and case-control studies have repeatedly demonstrated that the administration of estrogens (E) or estrogens plus progestins (E + P) increases the risk of breast cancer, with the combination carrying a higher risk that is manifest after a shorter duration of treatment. Nonetheless, 6 million American women, about 17% of all those 50–74 years old, once took some form of hormone replacement therapy (HRT).[34] This was because many of the same studies demonstrated a net decrease in mortality from all causes, decreased mortality from heart disease and osteoporosis, decreased dementia, and improved quality of life due to relief from menopausal symptoms. This changed when the results of the Women's Health Initiative trial became available in 2002. This study randomized 27,347 women who were free of breast cancer in two studies. Those who had an intact uterus received either E + P or placebo. Those who previously had a hysterectomy were randomized to E alone or placebo.[35]

E + P increased the incidence of invasive cancer by 25%[35] (Figure 1.6). While the patients were receiving HRT, the HR for coronary heart disease, stroke, and pulmonary embolus increased significantly by 29%, 41%, and 113%, respectively. During treatment, the HR for endometrial cancer, colorectal cancer, and hip fracture decreased significantly by 17%, 44%, and 34%. The increase in ER+ and PR+ tumors was greater than ER– and PR–, but there was a doubling in the HR for HER2+ tumors and a 78% (not statistically significant) increase in triple negative breast cancers. The effect of E + P on breast cancer risk was greater when therapy was initiated closer to the time of menopause: < 5 versus ≥ 5 years, HRs of 1.41 and 1.15 (p for trend = 0.08). E + P made it more difficult to detect breast cancers on mammograms. There was a rapid fall in the HR for breast cancer immediately after the cessation of E + P, and there was no evidence of increased risk 2.5 years later. The risk of death due to breast cancer was almost doubled (HR 1.96, p = 0.049), but there was no difference in deaths from all causes (HR = 1.04; 95% CI, 0.91–1.18).

In contrast, E alone *reduced* the incidence of invasive cancer by 23%[35] (Figure 1.6). E alone reduced coronary heart disease by 9% and increased colorectal cancer by 15%, but these effects were not statistically significant. Other effects of E alone were in the same direction as E + P but not statistically significant.

Although the effects of E + P on breast cancer incidence were consistent with the results of many prior observational studies, the lack of benefit in reducing heart disease and all-cause mortality was unexpected. This was widely reported in the press and led to a dramatic fall in the use of HRT. The use of Prempro® (a combination of estrogen and progestin) fell by 66% and Premarin® (estrogen alone) by 33% in the year following the first report.[34] The incidence of invasive breast cancer also fell quite suddenly and dramatically, and this was documented in a number of registries both in the United States and other countries (see Figure 1.1B). Between 2001 and 2003 there was a 7% overall decrease in invasive breast cancer and a 12% decrease in the incidence

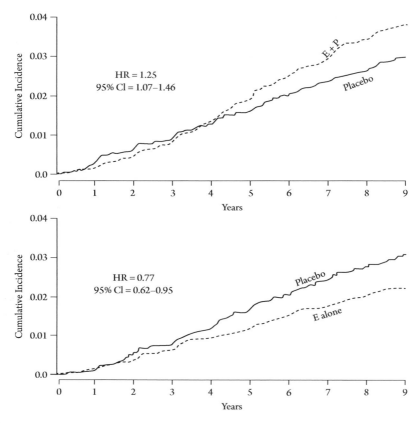

Figure 1.6 Effect of postmenopausal hormone replacement therapy on the incidence of invasive breast cancer: results of the Women's Health Initiative randomized trail. Between 1993 and 1998, 16,808 women with an intact uterus were randomized to E (conjugated equine estrogen, 0.625 mg/day) plus P (medroxyprogesterone acetate 2.5 mg/day) or placebo, and 10,739 women with a prior hysterectomy were randomized to E alone or a placebo.
HR = hazard ratio; CI = confidence interval.
Reprinted with permission from Chlebowski RT, Anderson GL. Changing concepts: Menopausal hormone therapy and breast cancer. *J Nat Cancer Inst.* 2012;104:517–27.

of ER+/PR+ cancers among women aged 50–69 (SEER database).[34] The rapid onset of effect with initiation and rapid fall after discontinuation of E + P suggest that much of the effect might have been due to promotion of subclinical disease present prior to the start of the trial.

The results of E alone were reported more recently and should be interpreted cautiously. Observational studies have shown that the time to the appearance of breast cancer after E alone is nearly twice as long as after E + P.[27] The mean duration of follow-up for the E-alone arm of WHI is only 7.1 years. Duration of exposure is clearly an important factor. In a meta-analysis of 51 observational studies (161,116 women, 80% of whom had E alone), women taking HRT currently or within the last 4 years had an increased breast cancer risk of –1% and 8% (not significant) for durations of

< 1 year or 1–4 years, and 31%, 24%, and 56% for durations of 5–9, 10–14, and ≥ 15 years, respectively.[36] In these studies, however, the women who did develop breast cancer generally had a less advanced stage, and it was not possible to demonstrate an impact on survival.

Almost all the evidence on breast cancer risk and the use of oral contraceptives (OC) is based on their use 30+ years ago. Since then, the ethinyl estradiol doses have decreased from 150 µg to 60 µg, and it very uncertain whether those older data are relevant to today's patient.[37] In a meta-analysis of 54 of these early trials, there was a 24% increase in breast cancer risk while patients were taking OCs and in the 10 years after stopping, but none thereafter.[38] There was no association with the age of first use and duration of use. Since breast cancer is uncommon during the ages when most women take OCs, the estimated number of additional cancers while taking OCs or in the 10 years after stopping was 0.5 (95% CI, 0.3–0.7), 1.5 (CI 0.7–2.3), and 4.7 (CI 2.7–6.7) per 10,000 women aged 16–19, 20–24, or 25–29, respectively, while taking the OCs. A more recent case-control study of 9,257 women in the United States showed absolutely no increase in risk.[39] The effects of OCs, if any, appear to be the same in high-risk women, such as those with BRCA1/2 tumors, as the general population.[40]

Although some studies suggest an increased risk of breast cancer among women exposed to fertility drugs, these associations have generally not reached statistical significance. Very few patients in these studies have reached the age when breast cancer incidence increases. At this time, only very cautious reassurance can be given about the relationship of these treatments to subsequent breast cancer risk.

LIFESTYLE AND ENVIRONMENTAL FACTORS

In the past, Asian women have generally had a much lower incidence of breast cancer, but daughters born to them after they migrated to Hawaii and California had a much higher incidence, equal to that of the American population.[30] This suggests that there are environmental factors that affect breast cancer risk and that these factors may be operative primarily when a woman is young—even prepubertal. Many specific aspects of lifestyle, especially diet, have been posited as being important, but most of them have not been reproducibly shown to be an important cause of risk. A woman's weight and alcohol intake are the exceptions.

Obese postmenopausal women are at increased risk of developing breast cancer. In a cohort study involving almost 200,000 postmenopausal women, the risk of developing breast cancer was 39% greater for those with a BMI ≥ 35 and 22% greater with BMI 30–34.9 compared to those with a BMI of 18.5–24.9.[32] Other studies have shown a similar trend of varying size.[41] An increase in body weight during adulthood may carry a bigger risk than a person's absolute weight. In one study it was observed that there was a 6% increase in risk for every 5 kg of weight gained after age 20.[42]

Adiposity is either not correlated or inversely correlated with premenopausal breast cancer. Several studies have demonstrated that adiposity in late adolescence (age 18–20) results in decreased premenopausal breast cancer risk, possibly due to lasting effects on hormone levels or insulin pathways.[30] The difference in the effects of adiposity on pre- and postmenopausal women is thought to be due to the fact that the main source of estrogen in postmenopausal women is fatty tissue where androgens are

Table 1.7 Models Incorporating Risk Factors to Calculate Risk of Developing Breast Cancer or Having a BRCA Gene Mutation

	Model[a]						
	BCRAT	Claus	IBIS	Rosner-Colditz	BCSC	BOAD-ICEA	BRCA-PRO
Age	Y	Y	Y	Y	Y	Y	Y
Ethnicity	—	—	—	—	Y	—	—
Family History							
Any family history of BC	—	—	—	Y	—	—	—
First-degree with BC	Y	Y	Y	—	Y	Y	Y
Second-degree with BC	—	Y	Y	—	—	Y	Y
Third-degree with BC	—	—	—	—	—	Y	—
Age of onset of BC in a relative	—	Y	Y	—	—	Y	Y
Bilateral BC in a relative	—	—	Y	—	—	Y	Y
Ovarian cancer in a relative	—	—	Y	—	—	Y	Y
Male BC	—	—	—	—	—	Y	Y
Breast Abnormalities							
Breast biopsies	Y	—	Y	(Y)	Y	—	—
Atypical ductal hyperplasia	(Y)	—	Y	Y	—	—	—
Lobular carcinoma in situ	—	—	Y	—	—	—	—
Breast density	—	—	—	—	Y	—	—
Menstrual/Hormonal Factors							
Age at menarche	Y	—	Y	Y	—	—	—
Age at first full-term birth	Y	—	Y	Y	—	—	—
Parity	—	—	(Y)	Y	—	—	—
Birth index	—	—	—	(Y)	—	—	—
Age at menopause	—	—	Y	Y	—	—	—
Oophorectomy	—	—	—	(Y)	—	—	—
Hormone replacement therapy	—	—	Y	(Y)	—	—	—
Oral contraceptive use	—	—	—	Y	—	—	—
Lifestyle Factors							
Body mass index	—	—	Y	Y	—	—	—
Height	—	—	—	Y	—	—	—
Alcohol Intake	—	—	—	(Y)	—	—	—

BC = breast cancer. ( ) = risk factor that was used in some but not other versions of the model.
[a] See text for further definition of models.

Sources: Amir E, Freedman OC, Seruga B, et al. Assessing women at high risk of breast cancer: a review of risk assessment models. *J Nat Cancer Inst.* 2010;102:680–91; Meads C, Ahmed I, Riley RD. A systematic review of breast cancer incidence risk prediction models with meta-analysis of their performance. *Br Cancer Res Treat.* 2012;132:365–77.

converted to estrogens by aromatases. In premenopausal women the ovary is the main source of estrogens.

Increased physical activity, especially during adolescence and young adulthood, is associated with a reduction in both pre- and postmenopausal breast cancer.[30] In a large cohort study, exercise equivalent to brisk walking 10 hours per week reduced breast cancer risk by 21% in all women and 38% in premenopausal women.[42] In another analysis, even exercise after age 50 had some benefit, reducing risk by about 17%.

There is a consistent correlation between alcohol intake and breast cancer risk across multiple studies, but the periods of life when this is most important are not well established. One drink per day increases the risk by 4%.[43] Three drinks per day will increase it by 40%–50%. The mechanisms through which alcohol increases breast cancer risk are not clearly understood. Alcohol increases circulating estrogen levels, and its use increases the incidence of ER+ more than ER– cancers. However, alcohol metabolites are also known carcinogens. Alcohol use during adolescence and early adulthood may have a greater effect on breast cancer incidence than use later in life, but it increases postmenopausal rather than premenopausal breast cancer. Possibly the most important measure is cumulative alcohol consumption.[44] There is no evidence of a difference in risk related to the type of alcohol consumed.

The only large randomized trial evaluating dietary restrictions failed to demonstrate an advantage for reduction of dietary fat.[45] Almost 50,000 women were randomized to either a diet that reduced fat intake by 20% or a regular diet. In actuality, the difference between the groups in change from baseline was 10.7% during year 1 and lower after that. A nonsignificant trend toward reduced breast cancer incidence while patients were on the trial was counterbalanced by a trend in the opposite direction after the trial was discontinued. It is possible that a subset of patients who had a particularly high fat intake at baseline may have benefited from the reduced fat diet.

CALCULATING A WOMAN'S RISK OF DEVELOPING BREAST CANCER

Numerous models have been developed using algorithms to incorporate multiple risk factors into a single risk estimate.[47, 48] Some of those used most often, with the risk factors they have incorporated, are shown in Table 1.7. In these examples, the number of risk factors ranged from 4 to 15. Some are based primarily on family history, while others include menstrual and hormonal factors. The only factors common to all the models is patient age and whether the patient has some family history of breast cancer. None uses the results of BRCA testing, and only one includes breast density. Only the BCRAT (Gail), Rosner-Colditz, and IBIS models have been independently validated. The models are often updated with the inclusion of additional risk factors, so in some cases several variations of the model are in use, sometimes with slight variations of the name (e.g., Gail and Gail-2). Some caveats about the individual models:

- BCRAT (Gail Model) This is one of the oldest models and may underestimate risk because the baseline incidence of breast cancer has increased since it was developed. It places less emphasis on family history and is of limited value in selecting possible

BRCA mutation carriers. The risk calculator can be accessed online at http://www.cancer.gov/bcrisktool/. For African-American women, access at http://dceg.cancer.gov/tools/risk-assessment/care. For Asian Pacific Islander American women, access at http://dceg.cancer.gov/tools/risk-assessment/apa.

- Claus Model: Limited to family history, this model is also based on earlier population data that may lead to an underestimation of risk today. One version of the model has tables, and there may be a difference in outcome between the versions.[46,47]
- IBIS (International Breast Cancer Intervention, Tyrer-Cuzick Model): Based on a Bayesian statistical analysis, this includes more risk factors than any other and in some analyses has been found to be the "most accurate." Access online (but no risk calculator) at http://www.ibis-trials.org/.
- Rosner-Colditz (Disease Risk Index): Although this model includes a long list of risk factors, it is lighter than others on family history and gives more weight to menstrual and lifetime factors. Access online at http://www.diseaseriskindex.harvard.edu/update/.
- BCSC (Breast Cancer Risk Consortium, Tice): This is the only risk calculator that includes breast density, one of the highest risk factors. Access online at https://tools.bcsc-scc.org/BC5yearRisk/.
- BOADICEA (Breast and Ovarian Analysis of Disease Incidence and Carrier Estimation): This was originally developed to determine the likelihood of being a BRCA1/2 carrier, but it is often used more broadly for risk estimation, even though risk factors are limited to family history. Access online at https://vpn.ucsf.edu/boadicea/, DanaInfo = ccge.medschl.cam.ac.uk+.
- BRCAPRO: Also developed primarily to determine the likelihood of carrying a BRCA1/2 mutation, it incorporates the Claus model, uses Bayesian statistics, and calculates both breast and ovarian cancer risk independently in three different populations. In includes no information on risk factors other than family history. It can be downloaded at www4.utsouthwestern.edu/breasthealth/cagene/.

These models are used primarily to determine whether a woman should receive tamoxifen or raloxifene as prophylaxis (see Chapter 2), have genetic testing for BRCA mutations (see earlier discussion in this chapter), or have more intense screening for breast cancer (see Chapter 2). They are particularly useful in generating practice guidelines.

Most of the models provide estimates of lifetime, 10-, or 20-year risk of developing breast cancer, but the value of these numbers in counseling an individual woman is uncertain. The estimate for most women will depend on which model is used. For example, the lifetime risk (LTR) of breast cancer was determined using seven models for two hypothetical patients, each with six different family history pedigrees.[46] Depending on the pedigree, the differences in LTR estimates ranged from 6.1% to 25%. In all but one of the six pedigrees, the different models placed women in different risk categories; for one pedigree the calculated LTR was average with two models (14% and 16%), moderate with four (20%, 21%, 23%, and 27%), and high risk with one (39%).

REFERENCES

1. American Cancer Society. *Breast Cancer Facts & Figures 2013–2014*. Atlanta, GA: American Cancer Society; 2013.
2. *GLOBCAN 2012: Estimated cancer incidence, mortality, and prevalence worldwide, 2012*. 2014. (Accessed at http://www.iarc.fr/en/media-centre/pr/2013/index.php.)
3. *SEER Cancer Statistics Review, 1975–2011*. National Cancer Institute, 2014. (Accessed at http://seer.cancer.gov/csr/1975_2011/, based on November 2013 SEER data submission, posted to the SEER website, April 2014.)
4. DeSantis C, Ma J, Bryan L, et al. Breast cancer statistics, 2013. *CA Cancer J Clin.* 2014;64:52–62.
5. Ravdin PM, Cronin KA, Howlader N, et al. The decrease in breast-cancer incidence in 2003 in the United States. *N Engl J Med.* 2007;356:1670–4.
6. Berry DA, Cronin KA, Plevritis SK, et al. Effect of screening and adjuvant therapy on mortality from breast cancer. *N Engl J Med.* 2005;353:1784–92.
7. Pike MC, Pearce CL. Mammographic density, MRI background parenchymal enhancement and breast cancer risk. *Ann Oncol.* 2013;24 Suppl 8:viii37–viii41.
8. Pharoah PD, Day NE, Duffy S, et al. Family history and the risk of breast cancer: a systematic review and meta-analysis. *Int J Cancer.* 1997;71:800–9.
9. Familial breast cancer: collaborative reanalysis of individual data from 52 epidemiological studies including 58,209 women with breast cancer and 101,986 women without the disease. *Lancet.* 2001;358:1389–99.
10. Collins A, Politopoulos I. The genetics of breast cancer: risk factors for disease. *Appl Clin Genet.* 2011;4:11–9.
11. Pruthi S, Gostout BS, Lindor NM. Identification and management of women with BRCA mutations or hereditary predisposition for breast and ovarian cancer. *Mayo Clin Proc.* 2010;85:1111–20.
12. Martin AM, Weber BL. Genetic and hormonal risk factors in breast cancer. *J Nat Cancer Inst.* 2000;92:1126–35.
13. Nelson HD, Fu R, Goddard K, et al. In: *Risk Assessment, Genetic Counseling, and Genetic Testing for BRCA-Related Cancer: Systematic Review to Update the US Preventive Services Task Force Recommendation*. Rockville, MD: Agency for Healthcare Research and Quality; 2013.
14. Foulkes WD. BRCA1 and BRCA2—update and implications on the genetics of breast cancer: a clinical perspective. *Clin Genet.* 2014;85:1–4.
15. Nelson HD, Fu R, Goddard K, et al. *Risk Assessment, Genetic Counseling, and Genetic Testing for BRCA-Related Cancer: Systematic Review to Update the U.S. Preventive Services Task Force Recommendation*. Evidence synthesis No. 101. AHRQ Publication No 12-05164-EF-1. Rockville, MD: Agency for Healthcare Research and Quality; 2013.
16. Chen S, Parmigiani G. Meta-analysis of BRCA1 and BRCA2 penetrance. *J Clin Oncol.* 2007;25:1329–33.
17. Bellcross CA, Lemke AA, Pape LS, et al. Evaluation of a breast/ovarian cancer genetics referral screening tool in a mammography population. *Genet Med.* 2009;11:783–9.
18. National Comprehensive Cancer Network. *NCCN Clinical Practice Guidelines in Oncology (NCCN Guidelines): Genetic/Familial High-Risk Assessment: Breast and Ovarian*. Version 2.2014. (Accessed September 27, 2014, at http://www.nccn.org/professionals/physician_gls/pdf/genetics_screening.pdf.)

19. Assi V, Warwick J, Cuzick J, et al. Clinical and epidemiological issues in mammographic density. *Nature Rev Clin Oncol.* 2012;9:33–40.

20. Huo CW, Chew GL, Britt KL, et al. Mammographic density-a review on the current understanding of its association with breast cancer. *Br Cancer Res Treat.* 2014;144:479–502.

21. Sickles EA. The use of breast imaging to screen women at high risk for cancer. *Radiol Clin North Am.* 2010;48:859–78.

22. D'Orsi CJ, Sickles EA, Mendelson EB, et al., eds. *American College of Radiology Breast Imaging Reporting and Data System BI-RADS.* 5th ed. Reston, VA: American College of Radiology; 2013.

23. Wang AT, Vachon CM, Brandt KR, et al. Breast density and breast cancer risk: a practical review. *Mayo Clin Proc.* 2014;89:548–57.

24. McCormack VA, dos Santos Silva I. Breast density and parenchymal patterns as markers of breast cancer risk: a meta-analysis. *Cancer Epidemiol Biomarkers Prev.* 2006;15:1159–69.

25. Gierach GL, Ichikawa L, Kerlikowske K, et al. Relationship between mammographic density and breast cancer death in the Breast Cancer Surveillance Consortium. *J Nat Cancer Inst.* 2012;104:1218–27.

26. Singletary SE. Rating the risk factors for breast cancer. *Ann Surg.* 2003;237:474–82.

27. Chen WY. Exogenous and endogenous hormones and breast cancer. *Best Pract Res Clin Endocrinol Metab.* 2008;22:573–85.

28. Collaborative Group on Hormonal Factors in Breast Cancer. Menarche, menopause, and breast cancer risk: individual participant meta-analysis, including 118 964 women with breast cancer from 117 epidemiological studies. *Lancet Oncol.* 2012;13:1141–51.

29. Henderson BE, Ross R, Bernstein L. Estrogens as a cause of human cancer: The Richard and Hinda Rosenthal Foundation Award Lecture. *Cancer Res.* 1988;48:246–53.

30. Colditz GA, Bohlke K, Berkey CS. Breast cancer risk accumulation starts early: prevention must also. *Br Cancer Res Treat.* 2014;145:567–79.

31. Lambe M, Hsieh C, Trichopoulos D, et al. Transient increase in the risk of breast cancer after giving birth. *N Engl J Med.* 1994;331:5–9.

32. Brinton LA, Smith L, Gierach GL, et al. Breast cancer risk in older women: results from the NIH-AARP Diet and Health Study. *Cancer Causes Control.* 2014;25:843–57.

33. Breast cancer and breastfeeding: collaborative reanalysis of individual data from 47 epidemiological studies in 30 countries, including 50302 women with breast cancer and 96973 women without the disease. *Lancet.* 2002;360:187–95.

34. Clarke CA, Glaser SL. Declines in breast cancer after the WHI: apparent impact of hormone therapy. *Cancer Causes Control.* 2007;18:847–52.

35. Chlebowski RT, Anderson GL. Changing concepts: menopausal hormone therapy and breast cancer. *J Nat Cancer Inst.* 2012;104:517–27.

36. Collaborative Group on Hormonal Factors in Breast Cancer. Breast cancer and hormone replacement therapy: collaborative reanalysis of data from 51 epidemiological studies of 52,705 women with breast cancer and 108,411 women without breast cancer. *Lancet.* 1997;350:1047–59.

37. Casey PM, Cerhan JR, Pruthi S. Oral contraceptive use and risk of breast cancer. Mayo Clin Proc 2008;83:86–90.

38. Collaborative Group on Hormonal Factors in Breast Cancer. Breast cancer and hormonal contraceptives: collaborative reanalysis of individual data on 53 297 women with breast cancer and 100 239 women without breast cancer from 54 epidemiological studies. *Lancet.* 1996;347:1713–27.

39. Marchbanks PA, McDonald JA, Wilson HG, et al. Oral contraceptives and the risk of breast cancer. *N Engl J Med.* 2002;346:2025–32.

40. Moorman PG, Havrilesky LJ, Gierisch JM, et al. Oral contraceptives and risk of ovarian cancer and breast cancer among high-risk women: a systematic review and meta-analysis. *J Clin Oncol.* 2013;31:4188–98.

41. Cheraghi Z, Poorolajal J, Hashem T, et al. Effect of body mass index on breast cancer during premenopausal and postmenopausal periods: a meta-analysis. *PLoS One.* 2012;7:e51446.

42. Catsburg C, Kirsh VA, Soskolne CL, et al. Associations between anthropometric characteristics, physical activity, and breast cancer risk in a Canadian cohort. *Br Cancer Res Treat.* 2014;145:545–52.

43. Seitz HK, Pelucchi C, Bagnardi V, et al. Epidemiology and pathophysiology of alcohol and breast cancer: update 2012. *Alcohol and Alcoholism.* 2012;47:204–12.

44. Chen WY, Rosner B, Hankinson SE, et al. Moderate alcohol consumption during adult life, drinking patterns, and breast cancer risk. *JAMA.* 2011;306:1884–90.

45. Thomson CA, Van Horn L, Caan BJ, et al. Cancer incidence and mortality during the intervention and post intervention periods of the Women's Health Initiative Dietary Modification Trial. *Cancer Epidemiol Biomarkers Prev.* 2014;23:2924–35.

46. Jacobi CE, de Bock GH, Siegerink B, et al. Differences and similarities in breast cancer risk assessment models in clinical practice: which model to choose? *Br Cancer Res Treat.* 2009;115:381–90.

47. Amir E, Freedman OC, Seruga B, et al. Assessing women at high risk of breast cancer: a review of risk assessment models. *J Nat Cancer Inst.* 2010;102:680–91.

48. Meads C, Ahmed I, Riley RD. A systematic review of breast cancer incidence risk prediction models with meta-analysis of their performance. *Br Cancer Res Treat.* 2012;132:365–77.

2

PRIMARY AND SECONDARY PREVENTION
OF BREAST CANCER

Breast cancer is an excellent target for both primary and secondary prevention strategies. Many of the factors that impart risk, such as hormones and lifestyle, can be modified, and it has been shown convincingly that targeting at least one or more of these will substantially delay and possibly prevent the onset of breast cancer (primary prevention). Various radiologic techniques can detect breast cancer long before the appearance of a mass in the breast or other symptoms of the disease, and massive randomized trials have shown that routine screening mammography in asymptomatic women will reduce breast cancer mortality in at least some populations (secondary prevention).

SCREENING MAMMOGRAPHY

The first randomized trial evaluating this strategy was initiated in the early 1960s, when mammographic technique was still crude by today's standards. This study, in which women were randomized without their consent or knowledge (which would be considered unethical today), still provides the most compelling evidence that routine mammographic evaluation of asymptomatic women will decrease breast cancer mortality. Subsequently, another eight trials have been completed. In all, 616,327 women have been randomized, and after 13 years of follow-up, 2,355 deaths in these studies were attributable to breast cancer.[1] As seen in Figure 2.1A, the results from the individual trials are highly variable, with some showing no reduction in breast cancer mortality in the screened population, while in others there was a substantial decrease. This was statistically significant in only four studies. In a pooled result that included all age groups, the mortality reduction was 19% (RR = 0.81; 95% CI, 0.74–0.87).

Although most of these studies were not designed and had insufficient power to determine the effectiveness of screening in subsets defined by age, many such analyses have been performed post hoc. Several studies, including Canada 1980b and the UK Age Trial, limited enrollment to women aged < 50. Reductions in breast cancer mortality for this age group were not statistically significant in any single trial, but in a meta-analysis of women aged < 50 in all the trials there was a 16% reduction in breast cancer mortality (RR = 0.84; 95% CI, 0.73, 0.96) (Figure 2.1B). In women 50+ the reduction in mortality was 23% (RR = 0.77; 95% CI, 0.69, 0.86). There are relatively few data on the value of screening mammograms in women 70+. In another meta-analysis there was not much difference in the benefit for women 40–59 and 50–59, but substantially greater benefit for those 60–69.[2]

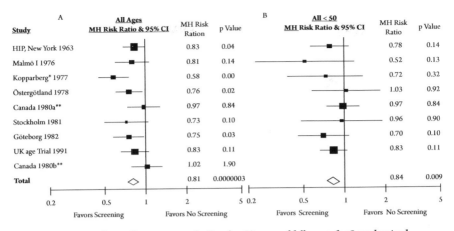

Figure 2.1 Meta-analysis of breast cancer deaths after 13 years of follow-up for 9 randomized screening mammography trials. A: Meta-analysis of all women enrolled in study without regard to age. B: Meta-analysis limited to a subset of women aged < 50.

MH + Mantel-Haenszel method of determining a weighted risk ratio; CI = confidence interval.
* Swedish Two County trial ** Canada trial 1980a enrolled ages 40–49, 1980b ages 50–59; both studies are shown in A and only 1980a in B.
Source: Gotzsche PC, Jorgensen KJ. Screening for breast cancer with mammography. *Cochrane Database Syst Rev.* 2013;6:CD001877.

Even though screening younger women is effective, the harms of a screening program in younger women are considerably higher. This is primarily because the disease is less common in younger women, so the number of women that must be screened to prevent one death is substantially greater[2] (see Table 2.1).

Table 2.1 Number of Women by Age Group That Need to Be Invited to a Screening Mammography Program to Prevent One Death

Age Group	Number Needed to Invite (95% Confidence Interval)
39–49	1,904 (929–6,378)
50–59	1,339 (322–7,455)
60–69	377 (230–1,050)

Based on a meta-analysis of 8 randomized screening mammography trials.
Source: Nelson HD, Tyne K, Naik A, et al. Screening for breast cancer: an update for the U.S. Preventive Services Task Force. *Ann Intern Med.* 2009;151:727–37, W237–42.

HARMS FROM SCREENING: EXCESS BIOPSIES, FALSE POSITIVES, OVERDIAGNOSIS

Many patients have considerable anxiety anticipating their mammogram and waiting for the results. Most have some discomfort during the procedure, and it is painful—sometimes unacceptably painful—for many. Fortunately, these are the most common "harms" associated with mammography, and they are time-limited.

Not infrequently, the initial mammogram is not definitive and the woman must be called back for additional views. It is natural for many of those recalled to assume the worst, and this may generate long-lasting anxiety—even an intense cancer phobia in some—even if subsequent mammograms and/or biopsy show there is no cancer (i.e., that this was a false positive). In a study of 169,456 women undergoing repeated screening mammography, 16.3% had false positive mammograms on their first and 9.6% on a subsequent routine exam.[3] A breast biopsy that demonstrated no evidence of cancer was recommended in 2.5% at an initial and 1% at a subsequent mammogram. If previous mammograms were available to compare with the current study, the false-positive rate was halved. With annual mammograms, the cumulative probability of a false positive mammogram or false biopsy between ages 40–49 was 61.3% and 7.0%, respectively. With biennial mammograms these rates were 41.6% and 4.8%. It was about the same for ages 50–59.

The balance between benefit and risks is illustrated in Figure 2.2, where outcomes are shown from screening 1,000 women for 10 years starting at different ages.[4,5] For younger women the likelihood of having a false-positive mammogram is higher because, among other reasons, it is more difficult to evaluate mammograms in those with denser breasts. The incidence of breast cancer is less in younger women. The net effect is that screening will contribute to the cure of a smaller number of younger women. If 1,000 40-year-old women are screened annually, 615 will be recalled but found to have no cancer, 79 will have a biopsy but found to have no cancer, 5 will be told they have DCIS and receive extensive treatment even though DCIS is unlikely to be fatal (see Chapter 4on Natural History) and only 1 will be cured as a result of having the screening mammogram. For 1,000 60-year old women, these numbers are 400, 80, 9, and 5, respectively. Although the balance sheet clearly favors screening older compared with younger women, the absolute benefits seem small. Some patients will feel this is clearly worth it because for each patient it is "all or none," while others will weigh the effect of the harms on their quality of life and conclude that the benefit is too small.

In addition to the harms of false-positive results, there is a substantial potential for overdiagnosis. This occurs because the preclinical growth (lead-time) of breast cancer is often measured in years, or even decades (see Chapter 4 on Natural History). Many breast cancers grow very slowly. In fact, some cancers grow so slowly that they might not have been detected or have caused any problems during a woman's lifetime if mammography had not been performed. These cancers are referred to as "overdiagnosed" because finding them imparts no benefit to the patient. It is not certain how many breast cancers are in this group, but it may be as high as 31%.[6] This means that 1.3 million women may have been diagnosed with breast cancer in the past 30 years who would not have ever had this diagnosis without screening mammography.

These characteristics of the natural history of breast cancer result in lead-time and length bias in uncontrolled (i.e., non-randomized) trials of mammography.[7] Lead-time bias occurs because screening mammography may detect a cancer 5 years earlier than it would have been detected without the mammogram, while the patient still dies of

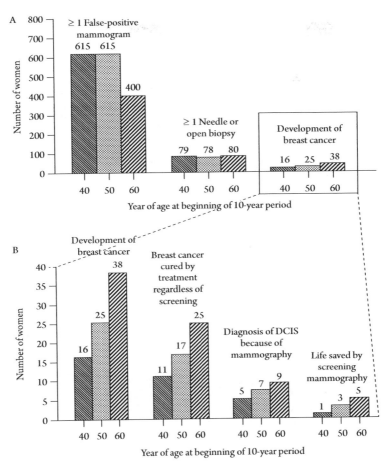

Figure 2.2 Possible outcomes in 1,000 women undergoing screening mammography annually for 10 years starting at age 40, 50, or 60. A: For each age group, the numbers likely to have at least one false-positive mammogram requiring recall, to have at least one biopsy, or to develop breast cancer during 10 years are shown. B: Among those who develop breast cancer, the numbers who would have been cured without having had the screening mammogram, who will have a diagnosis of DCIS, or who are cured because they had the mammogram are shown.

DCIS = ductal carcinoma in situ.

Sources: Fletcher SW, Elmore JG. Clinical practice. Mammographic screening for breast cancer. *N Engl J Med.* 2003;348:1672–80 and updated from Fletcher SW. Screening for breast cancer: Strategies and recommendations. In: Post TW, ed. *UpToDate*. Waltham, MA; 2014.

breast cancer exactly when she would have if the cancer had not been detected earlier. Thus the duration of her life with cancer is prolonged, but her actual life span is unchanged. Length bias occurs because slowly growing cancers have a longer duration in which they can be detected. Comparing the difference in outcome between these slowly growing cancers and those detected without mammography may suggest that screening improved outcome when, in fact, it has merely increased the number of non-lethal cancers that are treated. Data from non-randomized early detection trials have very limited value.

The interval between screening mammograms varied from 1 to 3 years in the randomized trials shown in Figure 2.1, and no direct comparisons of screening interval have been undertaken. Indirect comparisons suggest either that there is no difference in outcome, or that at least 81% of the benefit from screening mammography is obtained with biennial compared with annual exams.[8,9] This may be less true for women aged 40–49 or those with very dense breasts, where the frequency of late-stage cancers is higher among those biennially compared with annually screened.[8] As noted earlier, the incidence of false positives increases with increased screening frequency.

It is also unclear how long routine mammography should be continued, and there are few data from which to draw conclusions. Mathematical models suggest there is an advantage for continuing screening beyond age 70, but the frequency of overdiagnosis is also higher in the older age groups.[9]

RECOMMENDATIONS FOR USING SCREENING MAMMOGRAPHY

Both patients and professionals differ substantially in the way they assess the balance between the harms and benefits from screening mammography. Among women who were aware of the harms/benefit ratios illustrated in Figure 2.2, only 38% felt that the harms should be taken into consideration when deciding on whether to undergo routine screening.[10] All guidelines generated by physicians either for government agencies or professional societies agree that women aged 50–59 should be routinely screened, but there is considerable difference in the recommended frequency (Table 2.2).[11,12] There is generally agreement that some women aged 40–49 should be screened, but differences exist on whether this should be all women or only those at high risk for breast cancer based on family/genetic history or breast density. Almost all recommend screening for some years beyond age 70, but it is not as clear that women who have been regularly screened in the years before age 70 benefit from screening after that age.

SCREENING METHODS OTHER THAN MAMMOGRAPHY

The only screening methodology that has been proven to reduce breast cancer mortality is mammography. Other radiological techniques are more sensitive in detecting breast cancers, but this does not necessarily mean that if used instead of or in addition to mammography they will further reduce mortality or even be as effective. This is because the additional breast cancers being detected by these modalities may not have the same natural history as those being detected by mammograms (see Chapter 4 on Natural History and discussion in this chapter on Harms from Screening). Nearly half of non-palpable malignancies detected on mammograms are found because of microcalcifications. It is plausible that these are among those cancers that most benefit from screening. MRI is less able to detect calcifications than mammograms.[13]

Breast cancers are more difficult to detect in dense breasts (see Chapter 1 on Epidemiology and Risk Factors) and in those with BRCA1 or BRCA2 mutations.[14] It is plausible that using both mammography and MRI in these women and others at particularly high risk would be more effective than mammography alone. This strategy has *not* been tested in randomized trials, but the findings of 10 prospective studies in which

Table 2.2 Recommendations by Various Government and Professional Groups for Screening Asymptomatic Women of Different Ages With Mammography

Agency or Medical Society	Interval (years)**	Age (years) to Screen		
		40–49	50–69	≥ 70
American				
• US Preventive Services Task Force	2	Individualize*	All	To age 75
• American College of Physicians	1–2	Individualize*	All	To age 74
• American Academy of Family Physicians	2	Individualize*	All	To age 74
• US National Cancer Institute	1–2	All without regard to risk	All	No age limit
• American Cancer Society	1	All without regard to risk	All	No age limit
• American College of Radiology	1	All without regard to risk	All	No age limit
• National Comprehensive Cancer Network	1	All without regard to risk	All	No age limit
Non-US				
• Canadian Task Force on Preventive Health Care	2–3	None	All	To age 74
• UK National Health Service	3	Beginning age 47	All	To age 73

* Individualize: screening recommended only for women at higher than average risk or for those who wish mammography after having been informed about the benefits and risks for their specific age group.
** Internal between mammograms.
Data from Warner E. Clinical practice: breast-cancer screening. *N Engl J Med.* 2011;365:1025–32; Tria Tirona M. Breast cancer screening update. *Am Fam Physician.* 2013;87:274–8.

breasts were evaluated using both modalities, usually on the same day but always within 90 days of each other, were included in a meta-analysis.[15] The sensitivities of mammography, MRI alone, or MRI added to mammography were 32%, 75%, and 84%, respectively. The sensitivity of mammography alone is substantially less than in most other mammography trials and likely reflects the unique characteristics of these patients who were primarily young (presumably with denser than average breasts), often BRCA1 or BRCA2 positive, and generally not DCIS positive. The specificity is lower and the call-back and biopsy rates were higher for MRI than mammography in these studies.[14]

In spite of the lack of evidence of superior clinical outcomes, breast MRI is often used in high-risk populations. The American Cancer Society recommends that all patients with a lifetime risk > 20% have both MRI and mammography (see Box 2.1).[16] The National Comprehensive Cancer Network (NCCN) recommends that patients with Hereditary Breast and/or Ovarian Cancer Syndrome (characteristics defined in

---

Box 2.1   American Cancer Society Recommendations for Using MRI in Addition to Mammography in Screening Women With a High Risk of Breast Cancer

MRI recommended along with mammogram, annually, for those are

- BRCA1 or BRCA2 mutation carriers
- First-degree relatives of a BRCA carrier
- Have a lifetime breast cancer risk of 20%–25% based on BRCAPRO or similar models that are based primarily on family history (see Chapter 1)
- History of radiation to their chest between ages 10 and 30
- Li-Fraumeni syndrome or first-degree relatives of those with this syndrome
- Cowden and Bannayan-Riley-Ruvalcaba syndromes and first-degree relatives.

MRI not recommended even though at higher than average risk because of lack of evidence or consensus opinion for those with

- Lobular carcinoma in situ and atypical lobular hyperplasia
- Atypical ductal hyperplasia
- Heterogeneously or extremely dense breast tissue on mammogram
- Breast cancer, including those with DCIS
- A calculated lifetime breast cancer risk of 15%–20%.

Women who should not have an MRI as a screening test for cancer

- Those with a calculated breast cancer risk < 15%.

Source: Saslow D, Boetes C, Burke W, et al. American Cancer Society guidelines for breast screening with MRI as an adjunct to mammography. CA Cancer J Clin. 2007;57:75–89.

Box 1.1 in Chapter 1) have an annual screening with MRI alone between age 25 and 29 and with both mammogram and MRI from age > 30 to 75.[17]

Full-field digital mammography machines now account for > 70% of all accredited mammography machines in the United States.[18] In general, digital mammography has not been shown to be more sensitive, but it may have an advantage in some groups, such as those with *extremely* dense breasts (sensitivity for digital and conventional mammography, respectively, 84% and 68%, $p = 0.051$) and pre- or perimenopausal women (sensitivities 87% and 82%, $p = 0.057$).[18]

The value of routine clinical breast exams (CBE) by a medical professional has not been shown to reduce breast cancer mortality, and no randomized trial has been undertaken to compare CBE plus mammography to mammography alone.[11] Breast self-examination (BSE) trials have also shown no benefit. In spite of the lack of evidence, some groups, including the American Cancer Society and the American College of Obstetrics and Gynecology, recommend regular CBE in addition to mammography, but none now recommends regular BSE.[5]

CHEMOPREVENTION

Exposure to hormones, especially estrogens, is at the very least an important promotional factor in the development of breast cancer (see Chapter 1 on Epidemiology and

Risk Factors and Chapter 8 on Diagnosis, Workup, and Follow-up). It makes sense, then, that hormone perturbation might reduce the risk of developing breast cancer. In adjuvant tamoxifen but not adjuvant chemotherapy trials, there was a significant reduction in the incidence of contralateral breast cancer, providing additional impetus for formally studying this agent as a way of preventing or, at least, substantially delaying the onset of breast cancer.

Eight large randomized trials that together enrolled nearly 71,000 women compared a SERM (selective estrogen-receptor modulator) to a placebo with the primary endpoint being the incidence of breast cancer.[19] The SERMs included were tamoxifen (44% of patients enrolled), raloxifene (28%), arzoxifene (14%), and lasofoxifene (15%). The four tamoxifen trials had substantially longer follow-up with a median of 172 months. There was only one trial each of lasofoxifene and arzoxifene and the median follow-up of these studies was 60 months and 54 months, respectively. Most of the women in the tamoxifen trials were at high risk (projected 5-year risk of 1.66%–2.0%), but the other studies were performed in women unselected for risk factors. Tamoxifen was the only agent evaluated in premenopausal women. Only 59 breast cancer deaths occurred in the 28,193 women randomized in four trials comparing tamoxifen with placebo; fewer or no deaths were reported in the other studies.

In a meta-analysis of these trials, the reduction in total breast cancer incidence (including ductal *carcinoma* in situ) over 10 years of follow-up was 38% ($p < 0.001$).[19] The absolute difference was 2.1% (6.3% in the control and 4.2% in the SERM groups) (see Figure 2.3A). The effect of treatment was smaller but still apparent in years 5–10, when most women had discontinued treatment (see Figure 2.3B). Estrogen receptor positive (ER+) invasive cancers were reduced by 51% (absolute difference 1.9%, from 4.0 to 2.1%, $p < 0.0001$). This means that 53 women had to be treated to prevent one invasive, ER+ tumor in 10 years. The incidence of ER– invasive cancers was increased by 14%, but this difference was not statistically significant.

Tamoxifen and arzoxifene but not raloxifene treatment was associated with a significant increase in the incidence of endometrial cancer while the women were receiving the drug, but not after discontinuing therapy.[17] With tamoxifen the hazard rate (HR) for endometrial cancer was 2.18 (1.39–3.42, $p = 0.001$) and with arzoxifene it was 2.26 (0.70–7.32, $p = 0.2$). There were too few observations to draw conclusions about lasofoxifene. All four agents caused an increase in venous thromboembolic events (OR = 1.73, 1.47–2.05, $p < 0.0001$); the odds ratio was higher for arzoxifene and lasofoxifene than for tamoxifen and raloxifene, which were about the same. There was a significant reduction in the incidence of fractures, especially vertebral fractures, when all the trials are considered together (OR = 0.85, $p < 0.001$), but this effect was not seen in the tamoxifen trials. There was a small but non-significant reduction in ovarian cancer and no effect on colon cancer incidence.

Lasofoxifene is a relatively new agent. The number of patients studied and the length of follow-up is shorter than for tamoxifen and raloxifene, but it is of particular interest because a daily dose of 0.5 mg resulted in a 79% reduction in breast cancer incidence (83% reduction in ER+ invasive cancers), a significant reduction in strokes (OR = 0.67, 0.48–0.92), a decreased frequency of cardiac events and vertebral fractures, and has not been observed to increase endometrial cancer.[19]

The effects of tamoxifen on reducing breast cancer incidence is the same or greater in premenopausal than postmenopausal women.[2,20]

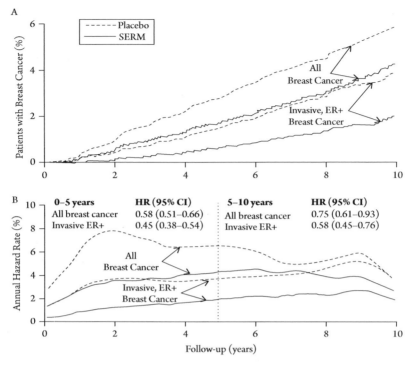

Figure 2.3 Meta-analysis of 8 chemoprevention trials in which almost 71,000 women were randomized to either a SERM or placebo for 4–5 years. Two trials extended the duration of treatment to 8 years. A: Cumulative incidence of either all breast cancers (invasive and ductal in situ) or invasive, ER+ cancers. B: Annual hazard rate of recurrence in years 0–5 and 5–10 for either all breast cancers or only invasive ER+ cancers.
SERM = selective estrogen-receptor modulator; ER+ = tumors with an estrogen receptor.
Source: Cuzick J, Sestak I, Bonanni B, et al. Selective oestrogen receptor modulators in prevention of breast cancer: an updated meta-analysis of individual participant data. Lancet 2013;381:1827–34.

In the only direct comparison between chemopreventive agents 19,490 postmenopausal women with a 5-year breast cancer risk > 1.6% were randomized to 5 years of either tamoxifen or raloxifene. Raloxifene was 19% *less* effective than tamoxifen in preventing all types of breast cancer and 17% less effective in preventing invasive, ER+ cancers.[19] However, it was also less toxic, especially in the frequency of endometrial cancers.

In more recent trials, two aromatase inhibitors (AI), exemestane and anastrozole, have been shown to reduce breast cancer incidence in postmenopausal women. Most of the patients in these studies were at increased risk. The reduction in the incidence of all cancers (invasive and in situ) was 53% in both studies. The reduction in invasive, ER+ tumors was larger and, as with the SERM trials, there was no significant reduction in invasive ER– cancers. The most important side effects that differed significantly between those receiving an AI and placebo were hot flashes and arthralgias/myalgias. There were no significant differences in the frequency of osteoporosis, skeletal fracture, cardiovascular events, endometrial cancer, thromboembolic events, or strokes.

Table 2.3 Aromatase Inhibitors (AIs) as Chemopreventive Agents: Results of Randomized Trials

Agent	Incidence of Breast Cancer			
	Exemestane (25 mg)		Anastrozole (1 mg)	
Trial Characteristics				
Number of patients	4,560		3,864	
Number of invasive cancers	64		125	
Number of breast cancer deaths	1		2	
Median follow-up (Months)	35		60	
Median Gail Risk Score	2.3		2.3	
Results: Endpoint	HR	*p value*	HR	*p value*
Invasive + DCIS cancers	0.47	0.004	0.47	< 0.0001
Invasive, ER+ cancers	0.27	< 0.001	0.42	0.001
Invasive, ER- cancers	0.80	0.74	0.78	0.538

DCIS = ductal carcinoma in situ; ER+ = estrogen receptor positive tumors.

*Women received treatment daily at the dose indicated for 5 years.

Source: Goss PE, Ingle JN, Ales-Martinez JE, et al. Exemestane for breast-cancer prevention in postmenopausal women. N Engl J Med 2011;364:2381–91; Cuzick J, Sestak I, Forbes JF, et al. Anastrozole for prevention of breast cancer in high-risk postmenopausal women (IBIS-II): an international, double-blind, randomised placebo-controlled trial. Lancet 2014;383:1041–8.

There is no evidence in individual trials or meta-analyses of these trials that chemoprevention with SERMs or AIs reduces breast cancer mortality (Table 2.3).[21,22] This is because too few deaths have been observed, with only 10 years of follow-up. However, since the reduction in incidence is substantial, it is plausible that small or modest reductions in mortality will be observed if these patients are followed for 2–4 decades.

RECOMMENDATIONS FOR CHEMOPREVENTION WITH SERMS OR AIS

Patients at increased risk of developing breast cancer should receive one of the agents of proven value to reduce breast cancer risk (see Box 2.2). Most of the patients in clinical studies were treated for 5 years. Even though benefits of treatment continue after 5 years, they are more limited than in the first 5 years (see Figure 2.3B). The use of raloxifene for women with osteoporosis is an exception. It is tempting to continue these treatments for longer periods, especially as this is done now in the adjuvant setting (see Chapter 10 on Adjuvant Therapy), but most experts recommend that this be done only in the context of formal clinical trials because long-term toxicities, especially endometrial cancer with tamoxifen, may outweigh the benefits in a population of otherwise healthy women.

The use of an AI rather than a SERM might be preferable for postmenopausal women since the effect size appears to be larger. The reduction in risk of invasive ER+

Box 2.2 Candidates for Chemoprevention and Possible Agents to Use for Prevention of ER+ Tumors, Based on Recommendations by the American Society of Clinical Oncology (ASCO) With Modifications as Noted

Candidates for chemoprevention

- Age ≥ 60
- Age ≥ 35 with increased risk of breast cancer defined by one of the following:
  - Five-year breast cancer risk ≥ 1.66% using NCI Breast Cancer Risk Assessment Tool or an equivalent measure (see http://www.cancer.gov/bcrisktool/; described in Chapter 1 under BCRAT and Gail Model)
  - Lobular carcinoma in situ (LCIS)
  - Atypical hyperplasia (based on exemestane trials)
  - Patients/families with genetic predisposition of uncertain value; see text.

Agents

- Tamoxifen: 20 mg daily for 5 years
  - Only agent suitable for pre- and postmenopausal women
  - Should not be used in women with history of deep vein thrombosis, pulmonary embolus, stroke or transient ischemic attack, during prolonged immobilization, or in those who are or might become pregnant, while nursing, or in conjunction with the use of any form of hormone therapy
  - Patient should be worked up promptly for abnormal vaginal bleeding.
- Raloxifene: 60 mg daily for 5 years
  - Only in postmenopausal women; has not been evaluated in premenopausal women
  - Although recommended by ASCO, may be inferior to tamoxifen based on most recent analysis of STAR trial data cited in text. However, in postmenopausal women with an intact uterus raloxifene may have a better risk-benefit ratio than tamoxifen.
  - Most often used in women with osteoporosis as the main indication for use; in these patients treatment may exceed 5 years
  - Contraindication same as for tamoxifen.
- Exemestane: 25 mg daily for 5 years
  - Only in postmenopausal women; contraindicated in premenopausal women
  - Should probably not be used in women with severe osteoporosis.
- Anastrozole: 1 mg daily for 5 years
  - Only in postmenopausal women; contraindicated in premenopausal women
  - Should not be used in women with severe osteoporosis.

Only tamoxifen and raloxifene have been approved by the FDA for chemoprevention of breast cancer. Arzoxifene and lasofoxifene have not been approved by the FDA for any indication and for this reason are not listed in recommendations.

Sources: Visvanathan K, Hurley P, Bantug E, et al. Use of pharmacologic interventions for breast cancer risk reduction: American Society of Clinical Oncology clinical practice guideline. J Clin Oncol. 2013;31:2942–62.

Goss PE, Ingle JN, Ales-Martinez JE, et al. Exemestane for breast-cancer prevention in postmenopausal women. N Engl J Med. 2011;364:2381–91.

Cuzick J, Sestak I, Forbes JF, et al. Anastrozole for prevention of breast cancer in high-risk postmenopausal women (IBIS-II): an international, double-blind, randomised placebo-controlled trial. Lancet. 2014;383:1041–8.

tumors over 10 years was 44% and 56% for tamoxifen and raloxifene, respectively, and 73% and 58% for exemestane and anastrozole.[19,21,22] However, there are no direct comparison of these agents, and in the absence of such data, no recommendations have been made by government or specialty groups.

While the evidence that the use of SERMs and AIs will affect the onset of breast cancer is incontrovertible, it is not entirely clear what is happening biologically. Do these agents truly prevent potentially life-threatening breast cancers such that at least some patients will never experience or die of the disease who would have otherwise? Or is this only suppression of tumor growth while treatment is administered so that the onset of disease is delayed but not prevented? The fact that these anti-hormone treatments seem to affect primarily or exclusively ER+ tumors is most compatible with the latter hypothesis.[23]

This uncertainty regarding the nature of the benefit from chemoprevention agents may be one element in their lack of use for this indication. The side effects, although limited, are another important consideration. It has been estimated that more than 2 million American women meet the risk criteria of women in the chemoprevention trials. However, among women who meet these criteria, only 25% say they are "interested" or "willing to take" chemoprevention outside the trial.[24] The actual use in practice appears to be < 15% of high risk women.

A number of other agents are under study, including many non-hormonal agents that might reduce the frequency of ER– tumors. These include agents known to be effective in the treatment of breast cancer, such as the anti-HER2 or anti-EGFR agents, PARP and mTOR inhibitors, and agents found to have anti-tumor effects in preclinical mouse models, such as COX-2 inhibitors, metformin, and retinoids.[25] Most of these agents have not been formally evaluated in the kind of large phase III trials that were used for SERMs and AIs. Aspirin has been shown in trials to cause a very small reduction in breast cancer after prolonged (> 20 years) use, but the effect size is insufficient to recommend its use.[26] Celecoxib is under evaluation in a trial involving 2,590 breast cancer patients. A trial in stage I patients demonstrated a reduction in the risk of new ipsilateral or contralateral breast cancer from the use of fenretinide, but this was significant only in premenopausal women.[25,26] It is now being studied in additional trials. Metformin is associated with reduced risk in epidemiology studies of diabetes patients and has been shown to reduce Ki-67 levels in "window of opportunity" trials[25] (see Chapter 12 on Management of Metastatic Disease). It is being evaluated in a randomized trial of 3,582 patients with early breast cancer. The results of preclinical and clinical studies of statins are inconsistent, but they were not effective in reducing recurrence rates in a randomized trial of patients with early breast cancer.[25] Cohort studies of bisphosphonates suggest they might reduce breast cancer incidence by as much as 30%, but they are not recommended for this indication in the absence of rigorous, prospective trials.[26]

LIFESTYLE CHANGES

The evidence that lifestyle and environment affect breast cancer risk is quite substantial (see Chapter 1 on Epidemiology and Risk Factors). Prospective randomized trials evaluating the effect of lifestyle changes on this risk are almost nonexistent, but observational studies, especially cohort studies, strongly suggest that maintaining healthy body weight, being physically active, and moderating alcohol intake are likely to be beneficial.

Exercise and diet affect endocrine functions that are associated with breast cancer, such as time of menarche or menopause, and studies on international differences in breast cancer incidence suggest that fat intake might be associated with risk (see Chapter 1 on Epidemiology and Risk Factors). The role of dietary fat was evaluated in two trials that randomized postmenopausal women to regular or fat reduced diets and obtained similar results.[27] The largest of these studies, the Women's Health Initiative (WHI), enrolled 48,835 women aged 50–79, most of whom were overweight or obese at entry. The goal for the low fat group was to have < 20% of their energy from fat calories. In actuality they achieved 37.6%. After 7 years of follow-up, there was no difference in the body mass index (BMI) of the two groups. There was no significant difference in the incidence of breast cancer in the two groups (HR = 1.08; 95% CI, 0.94–1.24), but there may have been some reduction in the incidence of invasive breast cancer, especially ER+ tumors, during the years of intervention that disappeared during the post-study follow-up period. There was no effect on breast cancer mortality.

Weight itself may be more important than dietary fat in affecting risk. This is suggested by the observation in the Nurses' Health Study, a large cohort study, that postmenopausal women who had never used hormones and who lost 10 kg or more and kept it off had a greater than 50% reduction in breast cancer risk.[28]

The very compelling evidence that exercise, especially in adolescent girls, will decrease breast cancer risk by as much as 20%–25% is derived entirely from observational studies.[28,29] One prospective cohort study was performed with 74,171 postmenopausal women in the WHI trial.[30] At study entry, recreation activity was assessed by asking participants how many hours and at what speed they walked each week and how many hours they spent in high-, moderate-, or low-intensity non-walking physical activity. Women whose weekly physical activity equaled 1.25–2.5 hours of *brisk* walking subsequently had an 18% reduction in breast cancer incidence compared to those who were inactive. More prolonged periods of physical activity further reduced breast cancer risk, but the benefit of exercise was limited primarily to those who were in the lowest and, to a less extent, middle tertiles of BMI. Similar results were obtained for premenopausal cancers in 64,777 women enrolled in the Nurses' Health Study.[31] Total recreation physical activity equivalent to 3.25 hours/week running or 13 hours/week walking lowered the risk of premenopausal breast cancer by 23%.

Even light alcohol intake increases the risk of breast cancer, and it was shown in the Nurses' Health Study that 10 g/day of alcohol consumed between menarche and first pregnancy increased the subsequent risk of breast cancer by 11%. (A typical drink in the US contains ~ 14 g of alcohol.)[28,32] As with other lifestyle factors, it is not possible to randomize women to different levels of alcohol consumption to assess the effect of changes in lifestyle.

Based on the evidence from the epidemiological data, the American Cancer Society (ACS) has generated lifestyle guidelines (Table 2.4), and the potential value of following these guidelines was assessed in a cohort defined prospectively from the WHI.[33,34] Each of 65,838 women was assigned a score between 0 and 2 for their BMI, level of physical activity, diet (servings of fruit and vegetables, choice of grains, and consumption of red meat), and number of drinks/day based on the responses to questionnaires given upon enrollment in the study. The best score a patient could receive

Table 2.4 American Cancer Society (ACS) Guidelines on Nutrition and Physical Activity

ACS Recommendation	Caveats
1. Maintain a healthy weight throughout life	• Ideal BMI < 25 kg/m^2 after age 18 • For those overweight, lose weight
2. Adopt a physically active lifestyle	• Adults: at least 150 min moderate or 75 min intense, spread throughout week • Children/adolescents: at least 1hour moderate daily and intense activity at least 3 times/week
3. Consume healthy diet with emphasis on plant food	• Eat at least 2.5 cups of fruit and vegetables daily • Choose whole grains instead of refined grains • Limit consumption of processed and red meats
4. Limit alcoholic beverages	• No more than 1 drink per day

Sources: Kushi LH, Doyle C, McCullough M, et al. American Cancer Society Guidelines on nutrition and physical activity for cancer prevention: reducing the risk of cancer with healthy food choices and physical activity. *CA Cancer J Clin.* 2012;62:30–67; Thomson CA, McCullough ML, Wertheim BC, et al. Nutrition and physical activity cancer prevention guidelines, cancer risk, and mortality in the women's health initiative. *Cancer Prev Res.* 2014;7:42–53.

was 8. Twenty percent of the women had scores of 6–8. The incidence of breast cancer in the group with scores of 7–8 was 22% less than that of those with scores of 0–2.

The problem with observational studies is that it is difficult to assess one factor independently from all others. For example, in the WHI cohort study that assessed the impact of following the ACS guidelines, the women with the highest scores also were more likely to be non-Hispanic white, well educated, never-smokers, and to use multivitamins, estrogens, and/or progestins.[34] It is not likely that these lifestyle factors will ever be fully evaluated in prospective randomized trials. The evidence from the observations trials is robust. In this context, the ACS guidelines constitute reasonable advice to a woman who is concerned about her breast cancer risk.

Parity, the age of first pregnancy, and the duration of breast feeding have a major impact on breast cancer risk (see Chapter 1 on Epidemiology and Risk Factors) but also have a greater and less welcome impact on lifestyle than the factors included in the ACS guidelines. Although it is unlikely that modern women will return to patterns of childbearing and breastfeeding that were common around the world a century ago, even modest changes in the timing of pregnancy and duration of breastfeeding are of sufficient importance in determining risk that they should be considered.[35] It has been estimated that if women were to breastfeed each child an additional 6 months, it would reduce breast cancer incidence by 5%, and an additional 12 months, by 11%.

Although the results from various epidemiology studies have varied, the preponderance of evidence fails to demonstrate a benefit from the use of supplemental vitamins, including vitamin A, beta-carotene, the B-group vitamins, folic acid, vitamin C, vitamin D, vitamin E, and multivitamins.[36] Large randomized trials with prolonged administration and follow-up have demonstrated no reduction in breast cancer risk from the use of vitamins C, E, beta-carotene, B$_6$, B$_{12}$, or folic acid.[37,38] The rationale for vitamin D supplementation is strong. Data from preclinical studies are supportive, and the results from some epidemiology studies are suggestive of benefit.[39] Because of this, 25,000 persons have very recently been randomized in a factorial design trial of vitamin D3, omega-3 fatty acid, and placebo.[40] This may provide a conclusive answer on the value of vitamin D, but in the absence of results from this study, vitamin D is not recommended for breast cancer risk reduction.

MODIFYING RISK FROM HEREDITARY BREAST AND OVARIAN CANCER (HBOC) SYNDROME

There are few data from prospective trials of any type to evaluate strategies for reducing breast cancer risk in women (or men) with BRCA1/2 mutations (HBOC syndrome). This is because the discovery of these genes is relatively recent and the number of affected persons is relatively small.

The recommendations of the NCCN are summarized in Table 2.5; other professional groups have generated similar guidelines. Screening is usually started earlier, and MRI is often recommended because of the relative insensitivity of mammography in these patients (see earlier discussion in this chapter). Screening for both breast cancer and ovarian cancer are sometimes begun 5–10 years before the earliest age that either of these was diagnosed in a family member.[16,41] Regular CBEs are recommended by many experts, but there are no data demonstrating that they are any more

Table 2.5 NCCN Recommendations for Management of Persons With Hereditary Breast and Ovarian Cancer (HBOC) Syndrome

Age to Start (Years)		Action
Women	Men	
18	35	Become aware of risk and methods for monitoring
25	35	Start clinical breast exam every 6–12 months
25		Annual MRI (preferred) *or* mammogram
30		Annual mammogram *and* MRI
	40	Baseline mammogram; annual thereafter for gynecomastia or if there is breast density on baseline study
*		Consider bilateral risk-reduction mastectomy
35–40		Recommend risk-reducing salpingo-oophorectomy (RRSO)**
30		If RRSO declined, transvaginal ultrasound and CA-125 every 6 months, earlier if first diagnosis in family is earlier***
35		Consider chemoprevention with tamoxifen (see text)
	40	Recommend prostate screening for BRCA2, consider for BRCA1

* No age specified in guidelines by NCCN (or other groups).

** After completion of childbearing or if family history of early onset ovarian cancer, consider earlier age.

*** If family history of early onset ovarian cancer, begin 5–10 years before first diagnosis in family.

Source: National Comprehensive Cancer Network. NCCN Clinical Practice Guidelines in Oncology (NCCN Guidelines): Genetic/familial high-risk assessment: breast and ovarian. Version 2.2014.

effective in reducing breast cancer mortality in this group than any other (see earlier discussion).

A case-controlled and a large cohort trial demonstrated that prophylactic mastectomy, which does not necessarily remove all breast tissues and does not include node dissection, may reduce breast cancer incidence in 90%–95% of BRCA1 and BRCA2 carriers.[41] It is not clear at what age this should be considered. Bilateral prophylactic salpingo-oophorectomy (RRSO) reduces the risk of ovarian cancer by 80%–90% and the risk of breast cancer by 40%–50%.[41] In those with BRCA2 mutations, the breast cancer risk reduction may be as high as 73%. The benefit of RRSO is less in late than in early premenopausal years. Case-control studies suggest that short-term hormone replacement therapy can be given after RRSO without compromising breast cancer risk reduction. The percentage of mutation carriers who elect RRSO is almost twice that of those who elect prophylactic mastectomy.

There are no results from randomized trials designed to assess the benefits from chemoprevention in BRCA1/2 carriers. In the NSABP chemoprevention trial comparing tamoxifen with placebo, 288 breast cancers were diagnosed; 8 had a BRCA1 and 11 a BRCA2 mutation. A retrospective analysis demonstrated a 62% *reduction* of risk in the BRCA2 and a 67% *increase* in risk in the BRCA1 patients randomized to the tamoxifen arm. Neither of these effects was statistically significant. However, the results are consistent with the known biology of these mutations. Breast cancers in BRCA2 carriers are more often ER+ and might reasonably be suppressed by a SERM, while BRCA1 carriers usually have ER– tumors. However, these data must be balanced with the observations from cohort studies evaluating the effect of adjuvant tamoxifen on contralateral breast cancer (CBC) incidence in BRCA carriers.[42] In a pooled analysis of three studies that included 1,583 BRCA1 and 881 BRCA2 carriers who together developed 520 CBCs, tamoxifen significantly reduced the risk of CBC by 62% and 67% in the BRCA1 and BRCA2 patients, respectively. In the absence of more definitive results, it is difficult to know how to advise mutation carriers regarding the use of chemopreventive agents. Randomized trials evaluating letrozole, exemestane, and fenretinide in these women are underway. In the meantime, tamoxifen seems to be a reasonable recommendation for BRCA2 carriers, at least, and possibly for BRCA1 carriers as well.

REFERENCES

1. Gotzsche PC, Jorgensen KJ. Screening for breast cancer with mammography. *Cochrane Database Syst Rev.* 2013;6:CD001877.
2. Nelson HD, Tyne K, Naik A, et al. Screening for breast cancer: an update for the U.S. Preventive Services Task Force. *Ann Intern Med.* 2009;151:727–37, W237–42.
3. Hubbard RA, Kerlikowske K, Flowers CI, et al. Cumulative probability of false-positive recall or biopsy recommendation after 10 years of screening mammography: a cohort study. *Ann Intern Med.* 2011;155:481–92.
4. Fletcher SW, Elmore JG. Clinical practice: mammographic screening for breast cancer. *N Engl J Med.* 2003;348:1672–80.
5. Fletcher SW. Screening for breast cancer: strategies and recommendations. In: Post TW, ed. *UpToDate.* Waltham, MA (Accessed on October 8, 2014).

6. Bleyer A, Welch HG. Effect of three decades of screening mammography on breast-cancer incidence. *N Engl J Med.* 2012;367:1998–2005.

7. Berry DA. Breast cancer screening: controversy of impact. *Breast.* 2013;22 Suppl 2:S73–6.

8. Kerlikowske K, Zhu W, Hubbard RA, et al. Outcomes of screening mammography by frequency, breast density, and postmenopausal hormone therapy. *JAMA Intern Med.* 2013;173:807–16.

9. Mandelblatt JS, Cronin KA, Berry DA, et al. Modeling the impact of population screening on breast cancer mortality in the United States. *Breast.* 2011;20 Suppl 3:S75–81.

10. Rosenbaum L. Invisible risks, emotional choices—mammography and medical decision making. *N Engl J Med.* 2014;371:1549–52.

11. Warner E. Clinical practice: breast-cancer screening. *N Engl J Med.* 2011;365:1025–32.

12. Tria Tirona M. Breast cancer screening update. *Am Fam Physician.* 2013;87:274–8.

13. Sickles EA. The use of breast imaging to screen women at high risk for cancer. *Radiol Clin North Am.* 2010;48:859–78.

14. McLaughlin S, Mittendorf EA, Bleicher RJ, et al. The 2013 Society of Surgical Oncology Susan G. Komen for the Cure Symposium: MRI in breast cancer: where are we now? *Ann Surg Oncol.* 2014;21:28–36.

15. Warner E, Messersmith H, Causer P, et al. Systematic review: using magnetic resonance imaging to screen women at high risk for breast cancer. *Ann Intern Med.* 2008;148:671–9.

16. Saslow D, Boetes C, Burke W, et al. American Cancer Society guidelines for breast screening with MRI as an adjunct to mammography. *CA Cancer J Clin.* 2007;57:75–89.

17. National Comprehensive Cancer Network. NCCN Clinical Practice Guidelines in Oncology (NCCN Guidelines): Genetic/familial high-risk assessment: breast and ovarian. Version 2.2014. (Accessed September 27, 2014, at http://www.nccn.org/professionals/physician_gls/pdf/genetics_screening.pdf.)

18. Kerlikowske K, Hubbard RA, Miglioretti DL, et al. Comparative effectiveness of digital versus film-screen mammography in community practice in the United States: a cohort study. *Ann Intern Med.* 2011;155:493–502.

19. Cuzick J, Sestak I, Bonanni B, et al. Selective oestrogen receptor modulators in prevention of breast cancer: an updated meta-analysis of individual participant data. *Lancet.* 2013;381:1827–34.

20. Visvanathan K, Hurley P, Bantug E, et al. Use of pharmacologic interventions for breast cancer risk reduction: American Society of Clinical Oncology clinical practice guideline. *J Clin Oncol.* 2013;31:2942–62.

21. Goss PE, Ingle JN, Ales-Martinez JE, et al. Exemestane for breast-cancer prevention in postmenopausal women. *N Engl J Med.* 2011;364:2381–91.

22. Cuzick J, Sestak I, Forbes JF, et al. Anastrozole for prevention of breast cancer in high-risk postmenopausal women (IBIS-II): an international, double-blind, randomised placebo-controlled trial. *Lancet.* 2014;383:1041–8.

23. Cameron DA. Breast cancer chemoprevention: little progress in practice? *Lancet.* 2014;383:1018–20.

24. Ropka ME, Keim J, Philbrick JT. Patient decisions about breast cancer chemoprevention: a systematic review and meta-analysis. *J Clin Oncol.* 2010;28:3090–5.

25. Litzenburger BC, Brown PH. Advances in preventive therapy for estrogen-receptor-negative breast cancer. *Curr Breast Cancer Rep.* 2014;6:96–109.

26. Cuzick J, DeCensi A, Arun B, et al. Preventive therapy for breast cancer: a consensus statement. *Lancet Oncol.* 2011;12:496–503.

27. Thomson CA, Van Horn L, Caan BJ, et al. Cancer incidence and mortality during the intervention and post intervention periods of the Women's Health Initiative Dietary Modification Trial. *Cancer Epidemiol Biomarkers Prev.* 2014;23:2924–35.

28. Colditz GA, Bohlke K. Priorities for the primary prevention of breast cancer. *CA Cancer J Clin.* 2014;64:186–94.

29. Lynch BM, Neilson HK, Friedenreich CM. Physical activity and breast cancer prevention. *Recent Results Cancer Res.* 2011;186:13–42.

30. McTiernan A, Kooperberg C, White E, et al. Recreational physical activity and the risk of breast cancer in postmenopausal women: the Women's Health Initiative Cohort Study. *JAMA.* 2003;290:1331–6.

31. Maruti SS, Willett WC, Feskanich D, et al. A prospective study of age-specific physical activity and premenopausal breast cancer. *J Nat Cancer Inst.* 2008;100:728–37.

32. Liu Y, Colditz GA, Rosner B, et al. Alcohol intake between menarche and first pregnancy: a prospective study of breast cancer risk. *J Nat Cancer Inst.* 2013;105:1571–8.

33. Kushi LH, Doyle C, McCullough M, et al. American Cancer Society Guidelines on nutrition and physical activity for cancer prevention: reducing the risk of cancer with healthy food choices and physical activity. *CA Cancer J Clin.* 2012;62:30–67.

34. Thomson CA, McCullough ML, Wertheim BC, et al. Nutrition and physical activity cancer prevention guidelines, cancer risk, and mortality in the women's health initiative. *Cancer Prev Res.* 2014;7:42–53.

35. Breast cancer and breastfeeding: collaborative reanalysis of individual data from 47 epidemiological studies in 30 countries, including 50302 women with breast cancer and 96973 women without the disease. *Lancet.* 2002;360:187–95.

36. Misotti AM, Gnagnarella P. Vitamin supplement consumption and breast cancer risk: a review. *Ecancermedicalscience.* 2013;7:365.

37. Lin J, Cook NR, Albert C, et al. Vitamins C and E and beta carotene supplementation and cancer risk: a randomized controlled trial. *J Nat Cancer Inst.* 2009;101:14–23.

38. Zhang SM, Cook NR, Albert CM, et al. Effect of combined folic acid, vitamin B6, and vitamin B12 on cancer risk in women: a randomized trial. *JAMA.* 2008;300:2012–21.

39. Manson JE, Mayne ST, Clinton SK. Vitamin D and prevention of cancer—ready for prime time? *N Engl J Med.* 2011;364:1385–7.

40. Manson JE, Bassuk SS, Lee IM, et al. The VITamin D and OmegA-3 TriaL (VITAL): rationale and design of a large randomized controlled trial of vitamin D and marine omega-3 fatty acid supplements for the primary prevention of cancer and cardiovascular disease. *Contemp Clin Trials.* 2012;33:159–71.

41. Pruthi S, Gostout BS, Lindor NM. Identification and management of women with BRCA mutations or hereditary predisposition for breast and ovarian cancer. *Mayo Clin Proc.* 2010;85:1111–20.

42. Phillips KA, Milne RL, Rookus MA, et al. Tamoxifen and risk of contralateral breast cancer for BRCA1 and BRCA2 mutation carriers. *J Clin Oncol.* 2013;31:3091–9.

3

PREMALIGNANT CHANGES AND
IN SITU CARCINOMA

The study of precancerous changes in the breast is a relatively new subject. Ductal and lobular carcinomas in situ (DCIS and LCIS) were first described in the 1940s. At that time these were rare lesions, and DCIS presented primarily as a mass in the breast. Today DCIS constitutes 20%–25% of all cancers and only rarely is found on physical examination. It is uncertain that observations made on patients with palpable masses are applicable to the DCIS diagnosed today with mammography or magnetic resonance imaging (MRI).

EARLIEST CHANGES AND THEORIES
OF DEVELOPMENT

There is a well-established association between non-malignant, proliferative changes in the breast and subsequent risk of either DCIS or invasive breast cancer (IBC), but the biological relationship between these early lesions and cancer is very controversial and a subject of intense study. The oldest and most widely held theory is that increased proliferation in the normal terminal duct lobular unit (UDH, CCH/HELU; see Figure 3.1 and Table 3.1) increases the chance of random mutations that are manifest by small foci of atypical hyperplasia (ADH, ALH).[1-9] These may undergo further mutations to become foci of DCIS or LCIS, which in turn mutate to become an IBC. In this scheme, none of the steps prior to IBC is obligate.[1,2] A number of mutant clones may exist within the DCIS, one or more of which may progress to IBC.[3] An alternative hypothesis regarding the relationship between DCIS and IBC is that both are derived from a common precursor, such as a mutated breast cancer stem cell, and that the DCIS and IBC develop alongside each other, and IBC is not derived from a prior DCIS.[4,5] This suggests that early changes in the breast, including DCIS, are indicators of a breast at risk of developing cancer, but are not really precursors. This makes the argument to surgically remove precursor lesions less compelling. In each of these scenarios, the microenvironment appears to play a critical role in determining not only the type of cancer but also its potential for distant metastases and specific metastatic sites.

LOBULAR NEOPLASIA (LN) OR LOBULAR
CARCINOMA IN SITU (LCIS)

Lobular neoplasia is usually classified and treated as a premalignant disease rather than as an early cancer. Classically its histologic appearance is distinctly different

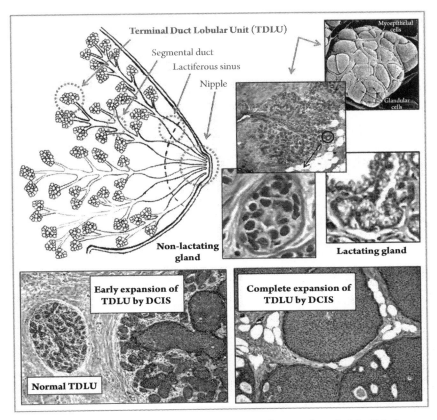

Figure 3.1 Anatomy of the normal breast with sections from the normal terminal duct lobular unit (TDLU) where both ductal and lobular cancers arise, the non-lactating and lactating breast, and DCIS.
Reprinted with permission from Allred DC. Ductal carcinoma in situ: terminology, classification, and natural history. J Natl Cancer Inst Monographs 2010;41:134–8.

from DCIS, but it may be difficult to distinguish from low-grade DCIS.[8] (Table 3.1) There is a loss of e-cadherin expression in LCIS and an increase in DCIS. At one time LCIS and DCIS were thought to arise from different parts of the normal duct, but current evidence suggests that they both arise from the terminal duct lobular unit. Like ADH and other premalignant lesions, LCIS is found incidentally, cannot be detected on mammography, and tends to be scattered throughout both breasts. It is found in 0.5%–3.8% of breasts with benign lesions on biopsy. Often these biopsies have been performed because of suspicious microcalcifications associated with other lesions, such as DCIS, but microcalcifications are not characteristics of LCIS lesions. More than 80% of LCIS is diagnosed in premenopausal women, and the mean age at diagnosis is in the forties. The incidence has increased significantly over the past several decades, especially in postmenopausal women, tracking with increased use of screening mammography. When LCIS is found on a core needle biopsy, it is recommended that a wider excision be performed because of the high

Table 3.1 Non-invasive Proliferative and Non-proliferative Lesions in the Breast, Some of Which Have Been Associated With Increased Risk of Invasive Breast Cancer in Subsequent Years

Lesion	Description[2-4]	Molecular Changes[1]	Risk of Subsequent DCIS or IBC in Either Breast
UDH: Usual ductal hyperplasia*	Increased glandular and myoepithelial cells with loss of contact and usual gland architecture	None	Little (maximum 1.5 X) or none, variable with study
CCH/HELU*: Hyperplastic enlarged lobular units or columnar cell hyperplasia	Terminal ducts lined with hyperplastic columnar epithelial cells, sometimes with atypia. Often associated with ADH.	↑ERα, ↑ EGF, AREG No ↑ in HER2 receptors	Little (maximum 1.5 X) or none, variable with study; as likely to be in contralateral breast
ADH: Atypical ductal hyperplasia	Well differentiated monomorphic cells, numerous enough to distend acini, usually unifocal and very small (<1–2 mm), halfway between UDH and low-grade DCIS. High inter-observer variability.	100% ER/PR+, No ↑ in HER2 or p53 mutations	Increased 4 X (range in studies, 1.47–4.88); 10-year risk 17%
FEA: Flat epithelial atypia	CCH with low-grade nuclear atypia, usually found in biopsy for microcalcifications.		~5% after a long latent period. Usually low-grade IBC, often tubular.
Radial scar	Area of central sclerosis with radiating proliferating cells of various types. Most often incidental, but may present as mass or as a spiculated lesion on mammogram.		Increased 2 X
Papillary lesions	Proliferative changes with apocrine changes, sometimes with atypia.		Increased 1.2–2.4 X

(continued)

Table 3.1 Continued

Lesion	Description[2-4]	Molecular Changes[1]	Risk of Subsequent DCIS or IBC in Either Breast
ALH: Atypical lobular hyperplasia	Similar to DCIS with acini less filled and fewer acini involved.	Same as ADH + loss of 16q, e-cadherin	Increased > 4 X (range in studies 4.21–5.71)[10], 10-year risk 21%
DCIS: Ductal carcinoma in situ	Heterogeneous lesions confined to a ductal lobular tree; low, intermediate, and high grade related to size of nuclei, number of mitotic figures, and amount of necrosis.	Varies with tumor grade within lesions.[1] 44% luminal, 28% HER2+, > 30% p53+; > 65% ER+	Cumulative incidence after 10 years 38%, after 15 years 45%.[5] Higher in younger than older women.
LCIS: Lobular neoplasia	Small round, polygonal or cuboidal cells that completely fill and distend acini. Clear vacuoles in some cells. Usually multifocal and often bilateral	ER/PR+, rare HER2 or p53 mutations. Same as DCIS + loss of e-cadherin	Highly variable with study, range from 3.0–8.0X; 10-year risk 24% (range 7%–24%)[6]

* Most pathologists would not classify this as a "precursor" lesion.

AREG = amphiregullin

[1] Allred DC, Wu Y, Mao S, et al. Ductal carcinoma in situ and the emergence of diversity during breast cancer evolution. *Clin Cancer Res.* 2008;14:370–8.

[2] Boecker W, ed. *Preneoplasia of the Breast: A New Conceptual Approach to Proliferative Breast Disease.* Munich: Elsevier GmbH; 2006.

[3] Allred. *Diseases of the Breast.* 4th ed. Philadelphia: Wolters Kluwer and Lippincott Williams & Wilkins; 2010:321–2.

[4] Simpson. *Diseases of the Breast.* 4th ed. Philadelphia: Wolters Kluwer and Lippincott Williams & Wilkins; 2010:333–40.

[5] Wapnir IL, Dignam JJ, Fisher B, et al. Long-term outcomes of invasive ipsilateral breast tumor recurrences after lumpectomy in NSABP B-17 and B-24 randomized clinical trials for DCIS. *J Nat Cancer Inst.* 2011;103:478–88.

[6] Coopey SB, Mazzola E, Buckley JM, et al. The role of chemoprevention in modifying the risk of breast cancer in women with atypical breast lesions. *Br Cancer Res Treat.* 2012;136:627–33.

Table 3.2 Characteristics of a Recurrent Lesion Found in the Breast After Excision and Diagnosis of a Premalignant Lesion or in Situ Cancer

Premalignant Lesion	ADH	Severe ADH	ALH[a]	LCIS or LN [a]	DCIS
	Frequency (%) of Second Lesions				
Histology of recurrent lesion					
Invasive	36	57	69	71	60
IDC	26	43	39	29	–
ILC	11	0	18	31	–
In situ					
DCIS	51	43	30	27	40
Laterality of recurrent lesion					
Ipsilateral [b]	60	48	61	56	82
Contralateral	39	43	38	38	18
Bilateral	2	5	0	4	–

Data for ADH, severe ADH, ALH, and LCIS were taken from an observational series. Data for DCIS were taken from the lumpectomy only arm of a randomized trial.

[a] The lobular histologies (ALH and LCIS) are significantly ($p = 0.016$) more likely to be invasive than ADH or severe ADH.

[b] ADH, severe ADH, ALH and LCIS are significantly ($p = 0.0047$) more often ipsilateral than contralateral.

ADH = atypical ductal hyperplasia; ALH = atypical lobular hyperplasia; LCIS = lobular carcinoma in situ; LN = lobular neoplasia; DCIS = ductal carcinoma in situ;

IDC = invasive ductal carcinoma; ILC = invasive lobular carcinoma

Sources: Coopey SB, Mazzola E, Buckley JM, et al. The role of chemoprevention in modifying the risk of breast cancer in women with atypical breast lesions. *Br Cancer Res Treat.* 2012;136:627–33.

Wapnir IL, Dignam JJ, Fisher B, et al. Long-term outcomes of invasive ipsilateral breast tumor recurrences after lumpectomy in NSABP B-17 and B-24 randomized clinical trials for DCIS. *J Nat Cancer Inst.* 2011;103:478–88.

likelihood that an occult invasive breast cancer may be nearby that may not be identified on the small specimen. Following a diagnosis of LCIS, a patient has a lifetime increased risk of developing another cancer. More frequently, the subsequent cancer will be invasive rather than in situ, and among the invasive lesions the histology is equally likely to be ductal or lobular (Table 3.2). About 40% of the recurrent tumors will be in the ipsilateral breast, and this has frequently been used as the justification for bilateral mastectomy. However, most patients (83%) today are treated with only biopsy or wide excision; only 5% receive bilateral mastectomy. Tamoxifen and raloxifene have also been shown to decrease the likelihood of a second tumor (see Chapter 2).

DUCTAL CARCINOMA IN SITU (DCIS)

The incidence of DCIS has increased steadily over the last 35 years as the use of screening mammography has increased. Today it accounts for about 25% of all breast cancer diagnosed in the United States. In contrast to LN, a woman's risk of DCIS increases with age.

Although called a "cancer" and generally treated as one, DCIS alone has few or no lethal consequences if left untreated. In many cases, the biopsy that leads to a diagnosis removes most or all of the lesion (see later discussion in this chapter regarding surgical margins). Subsequently a woman has an increased lifetime risk of having either another DCIS or IBC in either the same or the opposite breast (Tables 3.1 and 3.2). In contrast to LN, only about 20% will appear in the contralateral breast. Since each recurrence is associated with considerable psychological trauma and may be more life-threatening than the original tumor, the initial DCIS is treated in order to reduce that risk. Regardless of treatment, the long-term mortality from these secondary breast cancers is only 2.5%–5%.

About 80% of DCIS cases are diagnosed by a biopsy of suspicious microcalcifications on a mammogram; 68% of cancers found in mammograms with microcalcifications and no palpable lesion are DCIS, and in 73% of these there is evidence of necrosis, presumably as a result of DCIS involution.[10] DCIS also accompanies invasive breast cancer, and its presence is considered evidence that a lesion is a primary breast cancer rather than a metastatic lesion.

PREDICTING WHICH PATIENTS WITH BENIGN OR IN SITU LESIONS WILL RECUR AFTER BIOPSY

The lesions described in Table 3.1 rarely cause symptoms, so the only rationale for treatment is to reduce the risk of developing an invasive breast cancer at some later time. Non-proliferative lesions and hyperplasia without atypia are generally not treated because they do not increase risk appreciably. In the past, cysts (fluid-filled masses) found on physical examination or mammography were considered a risk factor, and the presence of multiple cysts was often used as a justification for prophylactic mastectomy. It is now clear that cystic lesions are associated with an increased risk of breast cancer *only* if a high-risk proliferative lesion is found in the wall of the cyst. A fluid-filled cyst can be distinguished from a more worrisome solid mass using ultrasound. The cystic fluid is often aspirated, especially if the cysts cause pain, but there is little or no value in examining the cyst fluid for cancer cells. An exception to this rule is a cyst that either has bloody fluid or that recurs rapidly (e.g., within 6 weeks) after an aspiration. These cysts should be surgically removed, the fluid should be evaluated for cancer cells, and tissue should be submitted for histological evaluation.

The lesions most often associated with a high risk of developing a subsequent in situ or invasive cancer and the patterns of recurrence are shown in Table 3.2.[9,11] ADH, severe ADH, and LN are associated with an increased risk of cancer but are usually diffuse or scattered throughout both breasts. Surgical excision would require bilateral mastectomy, but this is uncommonly performed because the treatment seems draconian relative to the magnitude of the risk. Tamoxifen, raloxifene, and aromatase inhibitors have all been shown to decrease risk associated with these lesions (see Chapter 2).

In contrast, DCIS can usually be fully excised without a mastectomy. Because the risk of recurrence is very small and the risk of death negligible for many DCIS lesions, histological classifications have been developed to identify those who require no treatment beyond simple excision. The oldest schema has two groups: comedo, which refers to the presence of varying amounts of necrotic cell debris in the duct and has the worse prognosis, and non-comedo. ("Comedo" was used because when DCIS presented as a mass it was possible to squeeze out necrotic material, similar to squeezing acne lesions.) Non-comedo DCIS includes cribriform, solid, papillary, and micropapillary histologic patterns. A more meaningful classification divides DCIS into low- (well differentiated, best prognosis), intermediate-, and high-grade (least differentiated, worst prognosis) groups, using criteria similar to those used to grade invasive breast cancers[2] (see Chapter 5). Another system, the Van Nuys index, combines four factors to create three prognostic categories. The factors are size ($\leq$ 15, 16–40, $\geq$ 41 mm), width of surgical margin ($\geq$ 10, 1–9, $\leq$ 1 mm), pathologic classification (non-high grade or nuclear grades 1–2 without necrosis, non-high grade or nuclear grades 1–2 with necrosis, high grade or nuclear grade 3 with or without necrosis), and age (> 60, 40–60, < 40 years).[12] For each factor, the best factor is given a score of 1 and the worst a score of 3. The scores for the four factors are added. Thus the lowest possible Van Nuys score (and best prognostic group) is a 4, which is a lesion $\leq$ 15 mm in size with $\geq$ 10 mm surgical margin, a nuclear grade 1–2 without necrosis, and patient age > 60.

Table 3.3 Predictive Factors for an Ipsilateral Breast Cancer Event (DCIS or IBC) After a Biopsy Showing DCIS

Factor	Comparison	Sample Size	Risk Estimate	95% CI
Comedonecrosis	Present or absent	9,332	1.71	1.36–2.16
Multifocality	Multi vs. unifocal	3,895	1.95	1.59–2.40
Surgical margin	Involved vs. not	12,086	2.25	1.77–2.85
Method of detection	Symptoms vs. not*	9,442	1.35	1.12–1.62
Grade	High vs. low	10,526	1.81	1.52–2.13
	Intermediate vs. low	NA	1.79	1.40–2.28
Tumor size	Large v small**	7,097	1.63	1.30–2.06
Estrogen receptor	Positive vs. negative	555	0.39	0.18–0.86
Progesterone receptor	Positive vs. negative	182	0.56	0.25–1.24
HER2	Positive vs. negative	182	3.07	1.32–7.12

Data were taken from a meta-analysis of 5 randomized trials and 36 observational studies in which patients were treated with lumpectomy alone or with either radiation therapy or tamoxifen.

* "not" means found on mammogram only

** Variable definitions, but small usually $\leq$ 2 cm and large > 2 cm

NA = not available

The degree to which these tumor characteristics predict an ipsilateral breast event (IBE, recurrence either as DCIS or IBC) has been evaluated in a meta-analysis[13] (see Table 3.3).

Among the conventional factors, the most predictive was surgical margin, but all of the other criteria that have been used for decades were validated in this large study. (For this study, an "involved" surgical margin was any evidence of tumor cells at the tumor margin of the surgical specimen. Surgeons differ on what they consider an optimal margin. If DCIS is excised and no radiotherapy given, most would obtain a margin > 1 cm, but if radiotherapy is given most would settle for ≤ 5 mm.[14]) The data on hormone receptors, HER2, p53, Ki-67 (or P21), loss of BCL-2, and HER4 suggest that these are predictive and likely to be useful in the future, but the number of observations and follow-up is still limited.

Age was not included in Table 3.3, but it is clearly prognostic as well. Women diagnosed with DCIS under age 45 have a twofold higher risk than women over 45 of developing an invasive cancer in subsequent years.[9]

A major focus of ongoing research on DCIS is to find new ways to combine both the traditional factors and newer biological criteria into an algorithm that will better identify patients who can get by with little or no treatment,[15] but none has been yet been accepted for general use.[16] Results have recently been published for a 12-gene recurrence score (RS) developed for DCIS, based on the 21-gene assay currently in common use for invasive breast cancer[17] (see Chapter 7). In addition to the reference genes, the DCIS assay includes all of the proliferative genes, the progesterone receptor gene, and GSTMI (estrogen related) from the 21-recurrence score set. Using the DCIS RS, 327 patients with 46 IBEs were placed into low-, intermediate-, and high-risk groups. The IBE rates at 10 years for these groups were 10.6%, 26.7%, and 25.9% ($p = 0.006$), respectively. The rates for an *invasive* IBE were 3.7%, 12.3%, and 19.2% ($p = 0.003$). These results suggest that this may become an important tool for defining DCIS risk groups, but the findings are limited by the small sample size, lack of a confirmatory study, and a paucity of patients with ER-negative or HER2-positive tumors.

TREATMENT OF DCIS: SURGERY, RADIOTHERAPY, AND/OR TAMOXIFEN

No treatment has been shown to significantly reduce further the very low mortality from DCIS.

Mastectomy, unilateral or bilateral, has never been shown to have an advantage over any other treatment. As late as 1980, 80%–90% of DCIS patients in the United States were treated with mastectomy. That gradually changed as the incidence of DCIS increased with widespread mammographic screening, but mastectomy still accounts for 24%–26% of DCIS surgeries.[18,19] Contralateral prophylactic mastectomy has increased from 2.1%–5.2% of all DCIS patients and especially among those who choose ipsilateral mastectomy, 18.4% of whom choose to have the other breast removed as well. (This trend has also been seen among patients with invasive disease.) Those more likely to be treated with mastectomy are younger, have larger lesions, are white, and have LCIS in addition to DCIS.

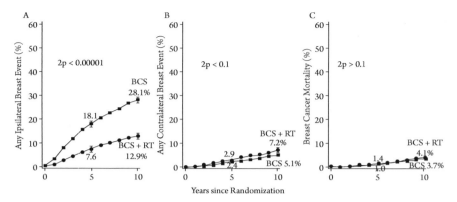

Figure 3.2 Value of adding radiotherapy to surgical excision of DCIS. Meta-analysis of four trials in which 3,729 patients with DCIS were randomized to either breast-conserving therapy (BCS, wide excision only) or the same therapy with whole-breast radiotherapy (BCS + RT) between 1985 and 1990. A: Any ipsilateral DCIS or invasive cancer (IBE); DCIS recurrences accounted for 52% of IBEs in both groups. B: Any contralateral DCIS or invasive cancer. C: Overall survival. There were 924 events (684 ipsilateral, 186 contralateral, 54 regional or distant), and median follow-up was 8.9 woman-years. Women < 50 years were 24% of the population, 15% received tamoxifen (equally divided between the randomized trial arms), and 76% could be detected only on mammography. Only 13% of the tumors were > 2 cm in size (pathological); 26% were high, 25% intermediate, and 50% low grade. Tumor margins were positive in 11%, and 29% were multifocal.
BCS = Breast-conserving surgery; RT = radiotherapy.
Reprinted with permission from Early Breast Cancer Trialists' Collaborative Group, EBCTCG. Overview of the randomized trials of radiotherapy in ductal carcinoma in situ of the breast. *J Natl Cancer Inst Monographs*. 2010;41:162–77.

In contrast, the use of whole breast radiotherapy after complete excision (breast-conserving surgery, BCS) has been evaluated in four large randomized trials, and a meta-analysis of the studies shows that it significantly decreases the chance of a recurrence[20] (Figure 3.2). The addition of radiotherapy to BCS reduced the odds of an additional event (DCIS or invasive breast cancer) in the ipsilateral breast by 54% ($2p < 0.0000$) with the absolute difference in IBEs at 10 years being 15.2%. The proportional reduction in DCIS and invasive cancers was nearly identical. There was a significant benefit in women younger and older than age 50 (although the effect size appeared to be greater among the older women), those with limited or larger excisions, and those who did or did not receive tamoxifen. A significant reduction in recurrences was also seen in those detected by mammography as well as those with clinical symptoms, those with involved and clear margins, with unifocal as well as multifocal lesions, with low- and high-grade histology, with and without comedonecrosis, and those with tumor size (either clinical or pathological) < 2 cm and 2–5 cm in diameter. However, more than one-fifth of DCIS patients treated with BCS and radiotherapy have some kind of breast event by 10 years, and radiotherapy has no effect on the frequency of contralateral breast events.

The use of a systemic therapy, such as tamoxifen, is the only way to reduce contralateral recurrence (CBCR). In two large randomized trials, tamoxifen, 20 mg daily for 5 years, was added either to BCS alone or BCS plus radiotherapy. A meta-analysis of

Table 3.4 Value of Adding Tamoxifen to BCS Alone or to BCS Plus Radiotherapy in Patients With DCIS: Results of a Meta-Analysis of Two Large International Trials

Patient Group Outcome	Number of Events	Risk Ratio	95% CI
All Patients			
Any breast event	740	0.73	0.64, 0.83
DCIS ipsilateral	302	0.75	0.61, 0.92
DCIS contralateral	54	0.50	0.28, 0.87
IBC ipsilateral	303	0.79	0.62, 1.01
IBC contralateral	115	0.57	0.39, 0.83
Mortality	276	1.11	0.89, 1.39
Radiated Patients			
Any breast event	452	0.74	0.63, 0.88
DCIS ipsilateral	153	0.84	0.62, 1.15
IBC ipsilateral	161	0.75	0.56, 1.02

DCIS = ductal carcinoma in situ; IBC = invasive breast cancer
95% CI = 95% confidence interval
NSABP B-24 with 1799 patients randomized to one of 2 arms (BCS + XRT or BCS + XRT + TAM) and UK/ANZ with 1576 patients randomized to 1 of 4 arms) BC alone, BCS + XRT, BCS + TAM, or BCS + XRT + TAM). Tamoxifen (TAM), 20 mg daily, was given for 5 years in both trials. Only 2382 received whole breast radiotherapy (XRT): 1799 in NSABP B-24 and 523 in UK/ANZ. BCS = breast-conserving surgery or wide excision.
Adapted from Staley H, McCallum I, Bruce J. Postoperative tamoxifen for ductal carcinoma in situ. *Cochrane Database Syst Rev.* 2012;10:CD007847.

these studies demonstrated that it reduced the chances of developing an IBE in both the ipsilateral and contralateral breast[21] (Table 3.4). However, the effect in the ipsilateral breast was smaller (~15%–25% reduction in risk of an IBE) and statistically not significant since the tamoxifen effect was additive to radiotherapy effect in most of the patients. The reduction in contralateral IBEs was ~50%. Although the direct evidence is limited to a small number of events in one trial, it appears that tamoxifen is less effective than radiotherapy in reducing IBEs in the ipsilateral breast. Tamoxifen added to BCS plus radiotherapy reduced IBEs by only 7% (p = NS) while radiotherapy added to BCS plus tamoxifen reduced IBEs by 73% (p < 0.0001).[22] Maximum reduction of IBEs will be achieved by use of BCS plus radiotherapy plus tamoxifen.

Exemestane has been shown in a prevention trial to reduce recurrences in a subset of patients with DCIS,[23] but no trial of any size or length of follow-up designed specifically to evaluate this treatment for DCIS has been completed.

Even though adding radiotherapy and tamoxifen to BCS reduces IBEs, these treatments have side effects and do not improve survival. For this reason, there is an ongoing effort to identify a subset of DCIS patients for whom BCS alone might be considered sufficient treatment. A number of uncontrolled trials, mostly retrospective but two prospective, have been conducted to evaluate BCS alone in highly selected populations.[24] The largest prospective study followed 565 patients with non-palpable, low- or intermediate-grade lesions ≤ 2.5 cm in diameter histologically (77% of those in the low- to intermediate-grade group had lesions < 1 cm), surgical margins > 3 mm (50% had margins ≥ 10 mm and 71% ≥ 5 mm), and no residual microcalcification on mammography for a median of 6.2 years; another 105 patients with similar treatment and follow-up had high-grade lesions ≤ 1 cm in size. For the low- to intermediate-grade lesions, the rate of ipsilateral recurrence at 7 years was 10.5% (95% CI; 7.5%–13.6%) and contralateral recurrence 4.8% (2.7%–6.9%). For the high-grade lesion the numbers, respectively, were 18.0% (10.2%–25.9%) and 7.4% (1.4%–13.3%). Invasive cancers constituted 53% and 35%, respectively, of the low/intermediate- and high-grade recurrences. There were no significant differences in recurrence rates among those with low/intermediate-grade tumor based on patient age (< 45 vs. ≥ 45 years), margin size (< 10 vs. ≥ 10 mm), or lesion size (< 10 vs. ≥ 10 mm). The results of other BCS alone studies are not more compelling, and none has succeeded in defining a group with a sufficiently low risk after at least a 15-year period of follow-up to conclude that this is equivalent to BCS with radiation therapy.

MANAGEMENT SUMMARY FOR DCIS

To minimize the likelihood that DCIS will recur in either breast, it should be fully excised. This can be done either by wide excision (BCS) or mastectomy, and the decision between them depends on what percentage of the breast must be removed to eliminate all DCIS and whether the patient feels the remaining breast is cosmetically acceptable. It is rare that DCIS will reach such a large size that BCS cannot be considered, but it is not uncommon for a patient to have multifocal tumor manifest by microcalcification in several or all four quadrants of the breast, or to have tumor at the

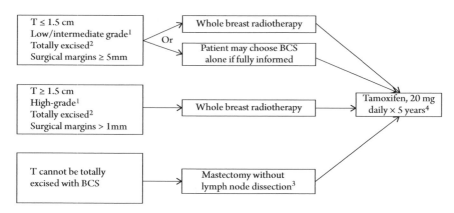

Figure 3.3 Guidelines for managing DCIS. [1] In addition to histology, newer predictive factors described in the text, such as ER and/or HER2 status or the DCIS Recurrence Score might be used to define tumors with how proliferative activity. [2] No evidence of tumor or suspicious microcalcification in other areas of breast on radiological studies after excision. [3] If there is a reason to suspect microscopic invasion (e.g., a very large, palpable tumor), sentinel node biopsy might be performed. [4] Tamoxifen is especially recommended for those with ER+ tumors. Exemestane might be considered for postmenopausal women.

excision margin even after several attempts at re-excision. The use of MRI identifies more of these multifocal tumors and leads to increased use of mastectomy, but there is no evidence yet that this improves outcomes, including survival. There is no indication for either a node biopsy or node dissection in any patient with a pure DCIS—that is, without evidence of at least microinvasion. However, initial biopsies may give a misleading result if the amount of tissue is very limited, and excision may provide evidence that the lesion is actually invasive. If there is reason to suspect this might be the case, a sentinel node biopsy might be performed at re-excision in order to avoid two surgical procedures. No survival benefit has been demonstrated for bilateral mastectomy.

If BCS is chosen, it should be followed by whole breast radiotherapy and 5 years of tamoxifen.

Since there is no evidence that any treatment improves survival, patients with small, low-grade tumors who wish to avoid the toxicity of radiation therapy and are willing to accept a 10%–20% chance of either an invasive or in situ recurrence at some point in the future might reasonably select wide excision alone or with tamoxifen. See Figure 3.3 for the schema for choosing among treatment options for patients with DCIS.

REFERENCES

1. Allred DC, Wu Y, Mao S, et al. Ductal carcinoma in situ and the emergence of diversity during breast cancer evolution. *Clin Cancer Res.* 2008;14:370–8.

2. Allred DC. Ductal carcinoma in situ: terminology, classification, and natural history. *J Natl Cancer Inst Monographs.* 2010;41:134–8.

3. Polyak K. Is breast tumor progression really linear? *Clin Cancer Res.* 2008;14:339–41.

4. Sontag L, Axelrod DE. Evaluation of pathways for progression of heterogeneous breast tumors. *J Theor Biol.* 2005;232:179–89.

5. Korkaya H, Liu S, Wicha MS. Breast cancer stem cells, cytokine networks, and the tumor microenvironment. *J Clin Invest.* 2011;121:3804–9.

6. Boecker W, ed. *Preneoplasia of the Breast: A New Conceptual Approach to Proliferative Breast Disease.* Munich: Elsevier GmbH; 2006.

7. Allred DC. Pathology and biological features of premalignant breast disease. In: Harris JR, Lippman ME, Morrow M, et al., eds. *Diseases of the Breast.* 4th ed. Philadelphia: Wolters Kluwer and Lippincott Williams & Wilkins; 2010:321–2.

8. Simpson PT, Reis-Filho JS, Lakhani SR. Lobular carcinoma in situ: biology and pathology. In: Harris JR, Lippman ME, Morrow M, et al., eds. *Diseases of the Breast.* 4th ed. Philadelphia: Wolters Kluwer and Lippincott Williams & Wilkins; 2010:333–40.

9. Wapnir IL, Dignam JJ, Fisher B, et al. Long-term outcomes of invasive ipsilateral breast tumor recurrences after lumpectomy in NSABP B-17 and B-24 randomized clinical trials for DCIS. *J Nat Cancer Inst.* 2011;103:478–88.

10. Gajdos C, Tartter PI, Bleiweiss IJ, et al. Mammographic appearance of nonpalpable breast cancer reflects pathologic characteristics. *Ann Surg.* 2002;235:246–51.

11. Coopey SB, Mazzola E, Buckley JM, et al. The role of chemoprevention in modifying the risk of breast cancer in women with atypical breast lesions. *Br Cancer Res Treat.* 2012;136:627–33.

12. Silverstein MJ, Lagios MD. Choosing treatment for patients with ductal carcinoma in situ: fine tuning the University of Southern California/Van Nuys Prognostic Index. *J Natl Cancer Inst Monogr.* 2010;2010:193–6.

13. Wang SY, Shamliyan T, Virnig BA, et al. Tumor characteristics as predictors of local recurrence after treatment of ductal carcinoma in situ: a meta-analysis. *Br Cancer Res Treat.* 2011;127:1–14.

14. Azu M, Abrahamse P, Katz SJ, et al. What is an adequate margin for breast-conserving surgery? Surgeon attitudes and correlates. *Ann Surg Oncol.* 2010;17:558–63.

15. Rudloff U, Jacks LM, Goldberg JI, et al. Nomogram for predicting the risk of local recurrence after breast-conserving surgery for ductal carcinoma in situ. *J Clin Oncol.* 2010;28:3762–9.

16. Yi M, Meric-Bernstam F, Kuerer HM, et al. Evaluation of a breast cancer nomogram for predicting risk of ipsilateral breast tumor recurrences in patients with ductal carcinoma in situ after local excision. *J Clin Oncol.* 2012;30:600–7.

17. Solin LJ, Gray R, Baehner FL, et al. A multigene expression assay to predict local recurrence risk for ductal carcinoma in situ of the breast. *J Natl Cancer Inst.* 2013;105:701–10.

18. Kumar AS, Bhatia V, Henderson IC. Overdiagnosis and overtreatment of breast cancer: rates of ductal carcinoma in situ: a US perspective. *Breast Cancer Res.* 2005;7:271–5.

19. Tuttle TM, Jarosek S, Habermann EB, et al. Increasing rates of contralateral prophylactic mastectomy among patients with ductal carcinoma in situ. *J Clin Oncol.* 2009;27:1362–7.

20. Early Breast Cancer Trialists' Collaborative Group, EBCTCG. Overview of the randomized trials of radiotherapy in ductal carcinoma in situ of the breast. *J Natl Cancer Inst Monographs.* 2010;41:162–77.

21. Staley H, McCallum I, Bruce J. Postoperative tamoxifen for ductal carcinoma in situ. *Cochrane Database Syst Rev.* 2012;10:CD007847.

22. Cuzick J, Sestak I, Pinder SE, et al. Effect of tamoxifen and radiotherapy in women with locally excised ductal carcinoma in situ: long-term results from the UK/ANZ DCIS trial. *Lancet Oncol.* 2011;12:21–9.

23. Goss PE, Ingle JN, Ales-Martinez JE, et al. Exemestane for breast-cancer prevention in postmenopausal women. *N Engl J Med.* 2011;364:2381–91.

24. White J. Do we need to irradiate all small invasive breast cancers and DCIS? *Am Soc Clin Oncol Educ Book.* 2013;2013:40–4.

4

NATURAL HISTORY OF INVASIVE
BREAST CANCER

CLINICAL BREAST CANCER: LONG COURSE
AND HETEROGENEITY AMONG PATIENTS

Two key characteristics of this disease are paramount in interpreting and understanding research results and in managing patients.

- Breast cancer has a long natural history. Even untreated, some patients will live for nearly 20 years[1] (see Figure 4.1). The survival curve for the Middlesex Hospital Series is consistent with other studies of untreated breast cancer patients,[2] but since these are patients who chose to have no treatment at a time when most patients had some form of surgery, there is always a question of whether they are truly representative. The treated patients at Johns Hopkins in the same era had a remarkably similar survival curve.[3] The median survival of the Middlesex and Hopkins groups were 2.7 and 3.0 years. More than 90% (but not all) of the patients in both series died as a result of breast cancer. In the Middlesex series the 5-, 10-, and 15-year survivals were 18%, 3.6%, and 0.8%, respectively.
- There is marked heterogeneity between patients in rate of growth and pattern of metastases. Long before it was possible to distinguish patient subsets on the basis of surface receptors or genetic profiles (see Chapter 7), physicians were struck with the fact that some patients died of breast cancer very rapidly and others only after many years, even though their presenting signs and symptoms were similar. There have been a number of attempts to identify and characterize patient subsets from large survival data sets. One of these is shown in Figure 4.2, which includes two groups, one with an annual mortality of 2.5% (60% of all the patients in the registry) and the other with an annual mortality of 20% (the remaining 40%).[4]

Patients in the US cancer registry (Figure 4.2) and in the Syracuse registry[5] (Figure 4.1) were mostly diagnosed 50–100 years after the patients in the untreated series from Middlesex Hospital. Clearly the overall survival curves are much better for the patients treated more recently. A logical supposition to explain this difference is better treatment in the more recent patient groups. However, it is also possible that the cohort with a 2.5% annual mortality was not represented at all in the patients of the earlier era. This might be the result of a change in the way the patients in the two eras were identified; patients in the nineteenth and early twentieth centuries were diagnosed on the basis of signs and symptoms, and in the Middlesex series all patients had autopsy-proven breast cancer. By the mid-twentieth century, breast cancer was defined primarily by histological findings in patients who had little more than a tiny

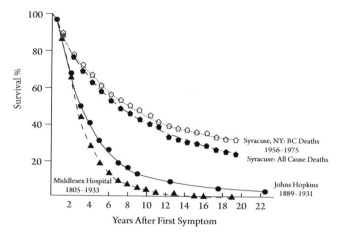

Figure 4.1 Long-term survival of breast cancer patients untreated or treated only with radical or modified radical mastectomy. Middlesex Hospital series: 250 patients self-selected to have no treatment of their breast cancer between 1805 and 1933 at the Middlesex Hospital in London, England [Bloom HJG, Richardson WW, Harries EJ. Natural history of untreated breast cancer (1805–1933). *Br Med J.* 1962;2:213–20]; Johns Hopkins series: 392 patients treated with a Halsted radical mastectomy between 1889 and 1933. (These include Halsted's patients reported in his seminal papers on this operation.) [Lewis D, Rienhoff WF. Results of operations at the Johns Hopkins Hospital for cancer of the breast: performed at the Johns Hopkins Hospital from 1889 to 1931. *Ann Surg.* 1932;95:336–400]; Syracuse series: 3,558 patients treated between 1956 and 1975, 90% with mastectomy (64% with a radical mastectomy) in the decades just before adjuvant systemic therapy was introduced for the treatment of early breast cancer [Mueller CB, Ames F, Anderson GD. Breast cancer in 3,558 women: age as a significant determinant in the rate of dying and causes of death. *Surgery.* 1978;83:123–32].

lump. It is likely that good prognosis cancers, such as tubular or even many lobular cancers, would not have been in that original series because they do not always form easily palpated masses.

We cannot rule out the possibility that many or most of the patients in the cohort with a 2.5% annual mortality would not be diagnosed with breast cancer and would die of other causes before a symptomatic mass appeared in the breast if we did not biopsy all asymptomatic lumps found on routine exams and microcalcifications seen on mammograms. These patients with "histologic breast cancer" that have little malignant potential might constitute as many as half of all breast cancers diagnosed today. This also means that when we evaluate treatments in randomized trials we cannot prevent or delay death in as many as half of the patients because they do not have a fatal disease.

IMPLICATIONS OF NATURAL HISTORY FOR INTERPRETING CLINICAL DATA AND TREATING PATIENTS

Because of the prolonged course, it is impossible to draw many conclusions about the effects of treatment on mortality without prolonged follow-up. It took more than two

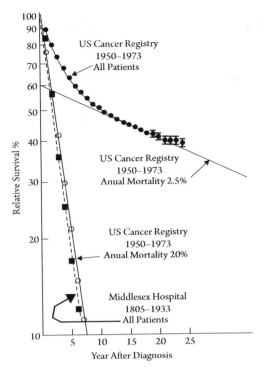

Figure 4.2 Heterogeneity in mortality rates in subsets of breast cancer patients. Mortality analysis of US breast cancer patients treated between 1950 and 1973 and compiled by the End Results Section, Biometry Branch, National Cancer Institute, compared with mortality of the Middlesex Hospital untreated patients from Figure 4.1, each plotted on a semi-logarithmic plot. The survival curve for all patients in the US registry suggests that there are at least two distinct patient groups, one with a high mortality rate (20% per year) with all patients dying within 10 years, and a second with a lower mortality rate (2.5% per year) with much longer survival. The Middlesex Hospital untreated patients appear to be more homogeneous, all of them having an annual mortality of 20% [Fox MS. On the diagnosis and treatment of breast cancer. *J Am Med Assoc.* 1979; 241:489–94].

decades of follow-up to demonstrate the survival advantage from more effective local therapy, and the earliest sign of reduced mortality from adjuvant systemic therapy did not appear until at least 5 years of follow-up (see Chapters 9 and 10). Because of the heterogeneity of the disease, groups of patients selected by any method other than randomization are likely to have different survivals independent of any treatment they are given. Many attempts have been made to match patients using staging systems (see Chapter 6) or, more recently, molecular markers (see Chapter 7), but in most cases these efforts have been unsuccessful because there are so many unknown variables that affect breast cancer patient survival. This is the reason that radical mastectomy seemed to be so effective in trials where these patients were matched to those given less extensive surgery, but was found to have no survival benefit at all when later evaluated in randomized trials.

A number of factors that contribute to disease heterogeneity have been identified and used to define patient subsets that are often managed differently. These factors

Table 4.1 Factors Used to Define Breast Cancer Patient Subsets and Whether They Are Prognostic or Predictive

	Has Prognostic Value?	Has Predictive Value?	Discussed in Chapter
Histology	Yes	No	5
Stage: TNM	Yes	No	6
Nodal status (pathological)	Yes	No	5, 6, 9, 10
Tumor grade	Yes	Yes	5, 7
Patient age	Yes	Yes	9, 10
Menopausal status	Yes	Yes	10, 11, 12
Disease-free Interval	Yes	Yes	12
Sites of metastases	Yes	No	12
Hormone receptor status	Yes	Yes	7, 10, 12
Ki-67, S-phase	Yes	No	7, 10
HER2/neu status	Yes	Yes	7, 10, 12
Triple negative: ER–/PR–/HER2–	Yes	?	7, 10,11,12
Microarrays	Yes	?	7, 10

may be prognostic in that they provide information about the pace of the patient's disease and the likelihood of metastases and duration of survival regardless of treatment, are predictive in providing information on how the tumor will respond to therapy, or both. (Prognostic factors may be used to select therapy even if there is no evidence of an interaction between the factor and response to treatment because it is thought that more toxic treatments can be justified only in those patients with the worst prognosis, and this sometimes leads to confusion between prognostic and predictive factors.) Some of the factors that have proven useful to define patient subsets are shown in Table 4.1. However, there is still considerable survival and therapeutic response heterogeneity within each of these patient subsets. For example, even some patients with very large tumors and lymph node metastases will survive for decades and die of other causes with minimal or no treatment (see the Middlesex Hospital survival curves in Figure 4.1). One reason for this may be that in a cohort of patients defined by a factor, such as a hormone receptor or HER2/neu, the actual number of tumor cells affected by this factor may vary from a few to almost all.

Preclinical Disease

The interval from the malignant transformation of a single breast cell to the point at which a tumor can be detected is also very prolonged. If breast cancer cells double at a constant rate every 100 days, this interval will be 6–10 years (Figure 4.3).[6] Observed or estimated doubling times for individual patients using clinically evident tumors and a variety of different techniques have ranged from a few days to several years. Estimates of average doubling times from serial mammograms prior to diagnosis in

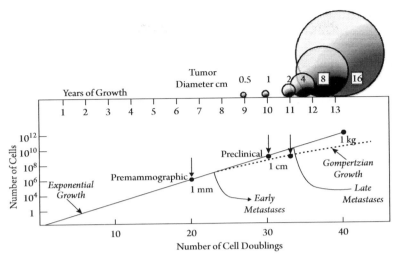

Figure 4.3 Hypothetical model of preclinical growth. It is assumed in this model that breast cancer cells double, on average, once every 100 days. A mass in the breast can be reliably detected by physical examination (or self-examination) when it is about 1 cm (assume 10^9 cells) in diameter and by mammogram at about 1 mm ($< 10^6$ cells). Under these assumption it would take 20–30 doublings, or 6.5–10 years, before a single cancer cell would grow into a detectable mass. This illustrates the long preclinical history of breast cancer, but the assumptions may seriously underestimate or overestimate the growth of any individual's cancer. Growth may, in fact, be intermittent in the earliest phases, and as tumors get larger they "outgrow" the blood supply, so that doubling times lengthen (Gompertzian growth). The likelihood of metastases increases as the tumor grows.
Source: Modified from Gullino PM. Natural history of breast cancer. *Cancer.* 1977;39:2697–703.

individual patents have ranged from 60 to 268 days.[7] Tumors in younger women may have a shorter tumor volume doubling time (mean 80 days for those < 50) than in older patients (157 for patients aged 50–70 and 188 days for those > 70 years.)[7] However, the preclinical biology of both primary cancers and metastatic cells is more complex than that suggested by the exponential growth curve in Figure 4.3. Tumor growth, even in the earliest phases, is unlikely continuous since cancer cells may remain dormant for long periods and then grow again as a result of facilitating factors, such as the growth of new blood vessels. As tumors reach clinical size and begin to outgrow their blood supply, growth slows and follows Gompertzian kinetics, so estimates of tumor growth rates from clinically detectable masses may overestimate the preclinical growth rate. Since a 1 cm mass is not necessarily composed entirely of tumor cells, it may be detected before there are 10^9 cancer cells, and cancers are often detected on mammogram before a mass is clearly identifiable.

THE METASTATIC PROCESS: CIRCULATING AND DISSEMINATED TUMOR CELLS

Metastases to regional lymph nodes and distant organs increase as the size of the tumor increases (see Chapter 6). This led to the hypothesis that breast cancer spread relatively late in the preclinical period and first traversed regional lymphatic channels.

It was assumed that removal of the tumor was urgent (thus the practice of biopsy under general anesthesia with immediate mastectomy if a frozen section showed tumor cells), and that removal of more tissue, including regional lymph nodes, skin, and fascia (radical mastectomy), and earlier diagnosis using tools such as mammography would decrease the frequency of distant metastases. The failure of such radical procedures to improve patient survival led to the "alternative hypothesis," which posited that the tumor is well established at distant sites before the tumor can be identified in the breast and that metastases leave the breast via both lymphatics and intramammary blood vessels.[8] (This is sometimes referred to as the Fisher hypothesis because Dr. Bernard Fisher popularized the idea and generated substantial evidence in support of the "alternative" hypothesis.) The fact that screening mammography and the early use of systemic therapy (Chapter 10) have both improved breast cancer survival suggests that both hypotheses have some validity.

Studies of circulating tumor cells (CTCs) in the blood and disseminated tumor cells (DTCs) in the bone marrow of patients without clinical evidence of metastases have provided additional support for the alternative hypothesis.[9] (There are a number of different ways to identify such cells, such as magnetic beads coated with an antibody to a cell adhesion molecule or RT-PCR, but it is not certain that all of the identified cells are important to the metastatic process, or that any assay has identified all potentially important cells.) CTCs and DTCs seem to occur with the same frequency in small (presumably early) and large tumor masses. They have even been found in patients who ostensibly have DCIS without evidence of invasion[10] and as long as 22 years after diagnosis in a patient who is metastases free.[11] From preclinical models it is estimated that < 1% of DTCs become overt tumors.[9] The presence of CTCs has prognostic value for patients with early, non-metastatic disease, after the diagnosis of distant metastases, and during or after systemic therapy of these metastases (see Chapter 12). In a meta-analysis of 49 studies with 6,825 patients, the presence of CTCs in patients with early disease was associated with an HR of 2.85 (95% CI, 2.19–3.75) for disease recurrence and an HR of 2.78 (95% CI, 2.22–3.48) for death. For those with metastases the presence of CTCs had an HR of 1.78 (95% CI, 1.52–2.09) for a short time to progression and an HR of 2.33 (95% CI, 2.09–2.50) for death.[12]

Showers of CTCs enter the circulation throughout most or all of the time the cancer is growing within the breast, but mutations are required to give some tumor cell clones the ability to adapt and survive in a new microenvironment outside the breast. It is not clear whether these critical mutations occur only in the intramammary tumor or in DTCs lodged in the bone marrow or other organs.[13] Differences in genetic aberrations in the primary and DTCs suggest that DTCs undergo evolution after leaving the breast, and this is one explanation for the apparent dormancy of many breast cancers after initial diagnosis and removal of the primary.[14] This suggests that many or most of the DTCs found in a routine bone marrow biopsy at the time the primary is diagnosed have limited or no malignant potential—that is, little potential for causing the patient's death. In a pooled analysis of nine studies with 4,703 patients, 31% were found to have bone marrow micrometastases at the time of diagnosis.[15] This included 25% of those with primary tumors < 2 cm in size and 26% of those without regional nodal involvement. (Nine percent of the patients had stage pT4 tumors, and 60% of them had micrometastases.) Although the patients with marrow micrometastases had a significantly higher probability of any recurrence, distance recurrence, or death from breast cancer, it is remarkable that ~ 60% of the patients with micrometastases had not recurred by 10 years of follow-up, and for the 299 patients with micrometastases who were otherwise considered at low risk of recurrence, the 10-year distant disease-free survival appeared to be closer to 90%. It is tempting to aggressively treat these DTCs with adjuvant systemic therapy (see Chapter 10) with the aim of eradicating all remaining occult breast cancer, but in animal models of DTCs these cells are generally relatively unresponsive to cytotoxic drugs.

CLINICAL BEHAVIOR OF METASTASES

The same heterogeneity and prolonged clinical course is seen after metastases are detected. The hazard of recurrence varies over time. Recurrences are most common in the first 5 years after primary diagnosis, with a peak occurring between years 2 and 3[16] (see Figure 4.4) Following year 5, the risk of recurrence steadily decreases, but the first evidence of recurrence may be several decades or more after complete removal of the primary tumor. There is no time when a patient may be assured that there is no chance of recurrence. In addition, the shape of the hazard curve may vary depending on tumor characteristics. For example, in Figure 4.4 the hazard of recurrence at 2 years is substantially and significantly higher for patients with hormone receptor negative (HR–) tumors (nearly 19%) compared to HR+ tumors (~11%).[16] By the year 5, the positions have reversed; those with HR+ tumors are at greater risk (5%) compared with HR– (3%). Similar non-proportional hazard rates have been reported for tumors differing in size, the number of involved axillary lymph nodes, tumor grade, intrinsic molecular subtypes, and the molecular prognostic signatures Oncotype DX and MammaPrint.[17] Patients might reasonably be followed more intensely during intervals of greatest risk, but the possibility of metastases should be considered whenever a

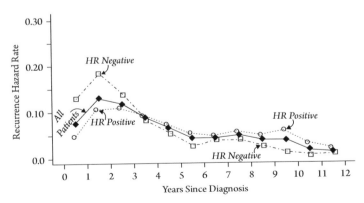

Figure 4.4 Annual hazard of recurrence of all, HR+ and HR– tumors. Recurrence rates for 3,585 pre- and postmenopausal patients enrolled in seven Eastern Cooperative Group Trials between 1978 and 1988, subdivided into HR+ ($n = 2,257$) and HR– ($n = 1,305$) tumors. All patients received treatment to the primary cancer; subsequently, 861 had no further therapy, 651 received adjuvant chemotherapy, and 1,986 received adjuvant chemotherapy plus tamoxifen.
Reprinted with permission from Saphner T, Tormey DC, Gray R. Annual hazard rates of recurrence for breast cancer after primary therapy. *J Clin Oncol.* 1996;14:2738–46.

patient presents with new symptoms of any type for the remainder of her or his life. It has been suggested that the biology and the response to therapy of early and late recurring tumors may be different (see Chapter 12). Most tests of statistical significance assume non-proportional hazard rates, which is clearly not the case for breast cancer recurrence. This needs to be taken into consideration (but usually is not) in statistical analyses of clinical breast cancer data.

Breast cancer most commonly metastasizes to bone, lung, liver, pleura, and brain, but it has been reported in many other sites—actually in almost every organ of the body—less frequently [18] (see Table 4.2).

Locoregional recurrences in the skin overlying the ipsilateral breast or chest wall and in axillary, supraclavicular, or internal mammary nodes occur in 15%–20% of all patients, with rates higher or lower than this depending on the number of positive axillary lymph nodes at presentation (see Chapter 9). More than half of these occur on the

Table 4.2 Most Common Sites for Breast Cancer to Metastasize

Metastatic Site	Cancer Registry 1986–1992 15-Year Cumulative Incidence[a]	Autopsy Studies 1943–1947 Median (Range) from 7 studies[a]	As the Only Site of Metastases
Number of patients with metastases	1,357	2,050	
	Frequency (%) Site Involved		**Frequency (%)**
Bone	62	71 (49–75)	3–5
Lung	32	71 (57–77)	2–12
Liver	32	62 (50–71)	4–6
Pleura	31	50 (36–65)	
Lymph nodes, distant[b]	24	67 (64–76)	
Brain	15	22 (10–36)	
Ovary	–	21 (15–23)	
Adrenal Gland		41 (34–54)	
Skin[c]		30 (19–36)	
Other sites[d]	18		

[a] Includes only patients with distant relapse.

[b] Exclusive of lymph nodes in the axilla, supraclavicular regions, and internal mammary chain

[c] Includes skin overlying the breast or chest wall following mastectomy

[d] "Other sites" include skin outside breast/chest wall, ovaries, spinal cord, eye, heart, and other organs not elsewhere classified

Cancer registry data are from British Columbia Cancer Agency in Kennecke H, Yerushalmi R, Woods R, et al. Metastatic behavior of breast cancer subtypes. *J Clin Oncol.* 2010;28:3271–7; autopsy data are averages take from 7 independent studies from Lee YT. Patterns of metastasis and natural courses of breast carcinoma. *Cancer Metast Rev.* 1985;4:153–72.

chest wall, about a quarter in the supraclavicular region, and somewhat less than 15% in the axilla. Skin lesions can be readily detected on a careful physical examination. They may manifest as diffuse erythema but more likely appear first as small nodules that eventually fungate and ulcerate without treatment or response to treatment. One manifestation of skin involvement is *en cuirasse*, a fibrous thickening of the chest wall that may progress to encasement of the entire chest wall. This may be due to plugging of skin lymphatics followed by lymphedema that eventually becomes fibrosed.[19] The presence of an in situ component of a biopsied chest wall or high axillary nodule suggests that this may be a new breast cancer that has developed from normal breast cells left behind after surgery. Invasive breast cancers may result from either cancer cells from the original primary that were not adequately treated or from hematogenous spread,[20] but in either case local recurrences are almost always the harbinger of distant metastases.

Metastases to the lung are usually asymptomatic or minimally symptomatic in their early stages. Lesions seen in lung parenchyma are either well-defined nodules, often asymptomatic, or streaky linear markings at the lung base, characteristic of lymphangetic carcinomatosis. Like en cuirasse of the skin, this is thought to result from plugged lymphatics and tumor emboli in arterioles with secondary fibrosis. It is more likely to cause dyspnea and non-productive cough, is often unresponsive to therapy (because even if the tumor emboli are destroyed the fibrosis persists), and is frequently a source of misery for patients with advanced disease. Pleural effusions are also an important cause of dyspnea and occur in breast cancer patients with and without other evidence of pulmonary metastases.

BONE METASTASES

Bone metastases are particularly important in the natural history and management of breast cancer. Between 70% and 80% of patients have bone metastases on autopsy, but given the difficulty of identifying small foci of metastases in an organ as large as bone in which complete evaluation requires demineralization, it is plausible that this number is really substantially higher (see earlier discussion of CTCs). Bone and/or bone marrow may be the first stop in the metastatic cascade for most or all patients with breast cancer, in which case targeting the metastatic process in bone as part of adjuvant systemic therapy or early after the first evidence of metastases at any site may prevent or delay the appearance of bone metastases (see Chapters 10 and 12).

It is not clear which breast cancer patients are most likely to develop metastases to the bone, but those with ER+ tumors who develop metastases are more likely to have predominantly or exclusively bone rather than visceral metastases. There are a number of genes that appear to promote metastases to bone, including parathyroid hormone-related protein (PTHrP), interleuken-8, integrin $\alpha_v\beta_3$, interleukin-11, and CTGF.[21] Gene expression profiles using microarray analyses have repeatedly demonstrated that patients with either basal-like or non-basal triple negative tumors are less likely to have metastases to bone[22,23] (see Chapter 7). In one of the largest of these studies (3,726 patients with a follow-up of 14.8 years), 66.6% and 71.4% of the luminal A and B patients, 65% and 59.6% of the HER2+, ER/PR positive or negative, and only 39% and 43.1% of the basal-like or non-basal triple negative tumors had bone metastases.[23]

Patients with high levels of bone turnover may also be more susceptible to developing bone metastases. Breast cancer micrometastases in bone secrete factors that activate osteoclasts, resulting in increased osteolysis (Figure 4.5). The osteoclasts and resorbing bone, in turn, release tumor growth factors, thus creating a vicious cycle in which the tumor cells and osteoclasts develop interdependence.[24–27] Breast cancer patients with high serum levels of bone sialoprotein, a non-collagenous bone matrix protein, are more likely to develop bone but not visceral metastases,[28] and breast cancer patients with high serum C-terminal or N-terminal propeptide of type I collagen

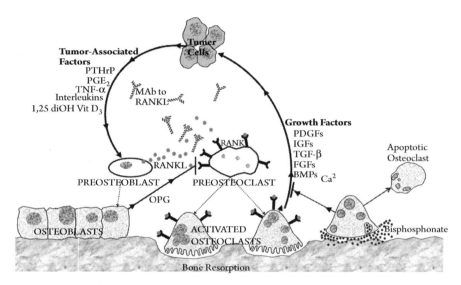

Figure 4.5 Molecular events involved in establishing breast cancer metastases in bone and their relationship to current treatments of bone metastases. Although the reasons why some, most, or all circulating breast cancer cells preferentially hone to the microenvironment of the bone is not entirely clear, once there these cells set up a "vicious cycle" in which they stimulate bone resorption by osteoclasts and are, in turn, stimulated to grow by growth factors released from osteoclasts and the resorbing bone. Tumor cells secrete factors, including PTHrP (parathyroid–hormone-related peptide), PGE_2 (prostaglandin E2), TNF-α (tumor necrosis factor), several different interleukins, and 1,25 diOH VitD$_3$ (1,25-dihydroxyvitamin D$_3$), that stimulate osteoblast precursor cells to produce RANKL (the ligand for RANK, the receptor activator of NF-κK) and/or reduce the production of OPG (osteoprotegerin). RANKL binds to RANK on the surface of the osteoclasts, causing osteoclastogenesis and activation. OPG, which is reduced by tumor-associated factors, would normally block the binding of RANKL to RANK. The osteoclasts thus activated cause bone resorption (osteolysis) and release tumor growth factors, including PDGF (platelet-derived growth factor), IGF (insulin-like growth factor), TGF-ß (transforming growth factor-ß), FGFs (fibroblast growth factor), BMPs (bone morphogenetic proteins), and extracellular Ca^{2+}. Relatively new therapies for managing and preventing bone metastases include monoclonal antibodies (MABs) to RANKL and bisphosphonates that affect the function and survival of osteoclasts.

Sources: Based on data from Roodman GD, Dougall WC. RANK ligand as a therapeutic target for bone metastases and multiple myeloma. *Cancer Treat Rev.* 2008;34:92–101; Fornier MN. Denosumab: second chapter in controlling bone metastases or a new book? *J Clin Oncol.* 2010;28:5127–31; Green J, Clezardin P. The molecular basis of bisphosphonate activity: a preclinical perspective. *Sem Oncol.* 2010;37 Suppl 1:S3–11.

are more likely to have relapse in bone and also to have metastases exclusively in bone.[29]

These observations on the "seed" (the tumor cell) and the "soil" (the microenvironment for metastases in the bone) provide the rationale for ongoing studies that may define the breast cancer patients most likely to benefit from treatments that target bone. At present, however, there is insufficient understanding of these mechanisms to use these observations in treatment guidelines.

Breast cancer metastases are mostly found in marrow-containing, axial skeleton, especially the spine, pelvis, skull, ribs, clavicle, proximal femurs, and humeri. Although it is common to find asymptomatic metastases (even a large number of them in a single patient) on routine radiological evaluations, about two-thirds of bone metastases are first identified because of pain.[30] Pain is usually confined to one or a few spots, and the patient may feel tenderness if pressure is applied or have pain on weight bearing. However, a patient may also present with diffuse "aches and pains" more suggestive of an arthritic process. The pain often disturbs the patient's sleep. Classically the pain is thought to persist and to increase steadily over time, but untreated bone pain may wax and wane over many months. Occasionally, relatively severe pain subsides after a week or 10 days, even without treatment. Some bone pain is related to fractures, microfractures, or tumor infiltration of nerves such as the dorsal nerve roots of vertebrae. However, bone pain occurs even without these complications, and the mechanism through which pain occurs is not entirely understood. It has been hypothesized that it may, in part at least, be related to increased osteoclast activity and bone resorption.[31]

On X-ray the lesions are predominately lytic with a substantial blastic component (in contrast to prostate bone lesions, which are predominately blastic, or multiple myeloma lesions, which may be purely lytic). This gives the lesions a moth-eaten appearance on plain films. There may be a lag time of some months between the patient's first symptoms and the appearance of lytic lesions because more than 30%–50% of bone must be destroyed and decalcified before the lesion can be seen on a plain film. Metastases can usually be identified on bone scan during this interval. Although routine bone scans for asymptomatic breast cancer patients have been shown to have little value in improving breast cancer outcomes, any patient with new onset of muscular-skeletal pain and a history of breast cancer should have a bone scan in the face of a negative plain film even though the abnormalities on scan are non-specific. Other modalities, especially PET-CT, are not much more sensitive than bone scans, but they are increasingly being used today in place of a bone scan because non-osseous sites can be evaluated with the same test.[32,33]

Between 25% and 35% of patients with bone metastases will have metastases only in bone. These patients have a better survival than those with both bone and visceral or only visceral metastases. Up to 20% of these patients may be alive 5 years after the appearance of the metastases.[34]

Patients with bone metastases will, on average, experience a skeletal-related event (SRE) every 3 to 6 months.[35] In addition to pain, about a third of these patients will experience pathological fractures, hypercalcemia that may be life threatening, spinal cord compression or cauda equina syndrome, spinal instability leading to kyphosis, and other nerve compression syndromes.[35,36] Bone metastases are the major source of pain for breast cancer patients and, along with resulting SREs, are the biggest threats to their quality of life, but newer bone modeling agents have substantially reduced morbidity from skeletal metastases (see Chapter 12).

CENTRAL NERVOUS SYSTEM METASTASES

About 15% of patients with advanced breast cancer will be diagnosed with central nervous system (CNS) metastases, but another 15% will have occult lesions found only at autopsy. One-year survival is about 20%, and in one series 2- and 5-year survival was 8% and 1.3%, respectively.[37] Median survival is generally better for brain metastases from breast cancer compared with other tumors types; in one series it was 13.8 months compared to < 7 months, respectively.[38] Age ≥ 60, a poor performance status, and a basal molecular subtype (see Chapter 7) are associated with a worse survival for breast cancer patients with brain metastases: 3.4 months versus 15–25 months for those < 60 with a good performance and luminal or HER2 subtype.

In autopsy studies, 13% of patients with CNS metastases have no distant metastases, and 42% of these are solitary lesions in the brain.[39] In one series, 40% of brain metastases identified on CT scan were solitary. It has been suggested that these patients should be treated with local therapies, such as surgery and radiation therapy, and might have prolonged survival as a result[39] (see Chapter 12).

Breast cancer more frequently metastasizes to the leptomeninges than other cancers. Though it is uncommon, it may account for up to 8% of CNS metastases in patients with HER2+ tumors, and it is more often seen in those with lobular or triple negative cancers.[40]

METASTASES AND MOLECULAR MARKERS

Patients with basal and HER2+ tumors have a higher incidence of brain metastases than other tumor subtypes defined by molecular markers (see Table 4.3). Various

Table 4.3 Sites of Metastases in 1,357 Patients With Advanced Breast Cancer, Subdivided by Molecular Subtype

Molecular Subtype	Percentage of Patients with Metastases at Each Site					
	Brain	Liver	Lung	Bone	Distant Nodes	Pleural or Peritoneal
Luminal A	7.6	28.6	23.8	66.6	15.9	28.2
Luminal B	10.8	32.0	30.4	71.4	23.3	35.2
HER2+ and ER/PR+	15.4	44.4	36.8	65.0	22.2	34.2
HER2+ and ER/PR–	28.7	45.6	47.1	59.6	25.0	31.6
Basal-like	25.2	21.4	42.8	39.0	39.6	29.6
Triple negative, non-basal	22.0	32.1	35.8	43.1	35.8	28.4

See Chapter 7 for discussion of molecular subtypes.
Adapted from Kennecke H, Yerushalmi R, Woods R, et al. Metastatic behavior of breast cancer subtypes. *J Clin Oncol.* 2010;28:3271–7.

studies indicate that between 30% and 50% of patients with HER2+ tumors develop brain metastases. The median time to the appearance of brain metastases is shorter (2.1 months) in patients with HER2+ tumors than those with HER2− (8.9 months), but the time to CNS metastases in patients under treatment with trastuzumab is significantly longer (13.1 months, $p = 0.0008$, compared to those not given trastuzumab).[37] However, brain metastases in HER2+ patients continue to appear up to 4 years after the appearance of the first metastasis.[40] The use of trastuzumab to treat other metastases does not increase the likelihood that the patient will develop CNS metastases.

Patients with triple negative (HER2−/ER−/PR−), particularly those in the basal molecular subset, have a similar frequency of CNS metastases and a poor prognosis from the brain metastases. Although chemotherapy benefits these patients, it appears to have less impact on their survival (median < 6 months) than the anti-HER2 drugs have on the HER2+ subset.[41] Table 4.3 shows the sites of metastases in 1,357 patients with advanced breast cancer, subdivided by molecular subtype.

REFERENCES

1. Bloom HJG, Richardson WW, Harries EJ. Natural history of untreated breast cancer (1805–1933). *Br Med J*. 1962;2:213–20.
2. Johnstone PA, Norton MS, Riffenburgh RH. Survival of patients with untreated breast cancer. *J Surg Oncol*. 2000;73:273–7.
3. Lewis D, Rienhoff WF. Results of operations at the Johns Hopkins Hospital for cancer of the breast: performed at the Johns Hopkins Hospital from 1889 to 1931. *Ann Surg*. 1932;95:336–400.
4. Fox MS. On the diagnosis and treatment of breast cancer. *JAMA*. 1979;241:489–94.
5. Mueller CB, Ames F, Anderson GD. Breast cancer in 3,558 women: age as a significant determinant in the rate of dying and causes of death. *Surgery*. 1978;83:123–32.
6. Gullino PM. Natural history of breast cancer. *Cancer*. 1977;39:2697–703.
7. Peer PG, van Dijck JA, Hendriks JH, et al. Age-dependent growth rate of primary breast cancer. *Cancer*. 1993;71:3547–51.
8. Fisher B, Anderson SJ. The breast cancer alternative hypothesis: is there evidence to justify replacing it? *J Clin Oncol*. 2010;28:366–74.
9. Redig AJ, McAllister SS. Breast cancer as a systemic disease: a view of metastasis. *J Intern Med*. 2013;274:113–26.
10. Husemann Y, Geigl JB, Schubert F, et al. Systemic spread is an early step in breast cancer. *Cancer Cell*. 2008;13:58–68.
11. Meng S, Tripathy D, Frenkel EP, et al. Circulating tumor cells in patients with breast cancer dormancy. *Clin Cancer Res*. 2004;10:8152–62.
12. Zhang L, Riethdorf S, Wu G, et al. Meta-analysis of the prognostic value of circulating tumor cells in breast cancer. *Clin Cancer Res*. 2012;18:5701–10.
13. Klein CA. Parallel progression of primary tumours and metastases. *Nat Rev Cancer*. 2009;9:302–12.
14. Goss PE, Chambers AF. Does tumour dormancy offer a therapeutic target? *Nat Rev Cancer*. 2010;10:871–7.
15. Braun S, Vogl FD, Naume B, et al. A pooled analysis of bone marrow micrometastasis in breast cancer. *N Engl J Med*. 2005;353:793–802.

16. Saphner T, Tormey DC, Gray R. Annual hazard rates of recurrence for breast cancer after primary therapy. *J Clin Oncol.* 1996;14:2738–46.

17. Jatoi I, Anderson WF, Jeong JH, et al. Breast cancer adjuvant therapy: time to consider its time-dependent effects. *J Clin Oncol.* 2011;29:2301–4.

18. Lee YT. Patterns of metastasis and natural courses of breast carcinoma. *Cancer Metast Rev.* 1985;4:153–72.

19. Haagensen CD. *Diseases of the Breast.* 3rd ed. Philadelphia: W. B. Saunders; 1986.

20. Bruce J, Carter DC, Fraser J. Patterns of recurrent disease in breast cancer. *Lancet.* 1970;1:433–5.

21. Kominsky SL, Davidson NE. A "bone" fide predictor of metastasis? Predicting breast cancer metastasis to bone. *J Clin Oncol.* 2006;24:2227–9.

22. Smid M, Wang Y, Zhang Y, et al. Subtypes of breast cancer show preferential site of relapse. *Cancer Res.* 2008;68:3108–14.

23. Kennecke H, Yerushalmi R, Woods R, et al. Metastatic behavior of breast cancer subtypes. *J Clin Oncol.* 2010;28:3271–7.

24. Roodman GD, Dougall WC. RANK ligand as a therapeutic target for bone metastases and multiple myeloma. *Cancer Treat Rev.* 2008;34:92–101.

25. Fornier MN. Denosumab: second chapter in controlling bone metastases or a new book? *J Clin Oncol.* 2010;28:5127–31.

26. Guise T. Examining the metastatic niche: targeting the microenvironment. *Semin Oncol.* 2010;37 Suppl 2:S2–14.

27. Green J, Clezardin P. The molecular basis of bisphosphonate activity: a preclinical perspective. *Sem Oncol.* 2010;37 Suppl 1:S3–11.

28. Diel IJ, Solomayer EF, Seibel MJ, et al. Serum bone sialoprotein in patients with primary breast cancer is a prognostic marker for subsequent bone metastasis. *Clin Cancer Res.* 1999;5:3914–9.

29. Lipton A, Chapman JA, Demers L, et al. Elevated bone turnover predicts for bone metastasis in postmenopausal breast cancer: results of NCIC CTG MA.14. *J Clin Oncol.* 2011;29:3605–10.

30. Front D, Schneck SO, Frankel A, et al. Bone metastases and bone pain in breast cancer: are they closely associated? *JAMA.* 1979;242:1747–8.

31. Smith HS. Painful osseous metastases. *Pain Physician.* 2011;14:E373–403.

32. Morris PG, Lynch C, Feeney JN, et al. Integrated positron emission tomography/computed tomography may render bone scintigraphy unnecessary to investigate suspected metastatic breast cancer. *J Clin Oncol.* 2010;28:3154–9.

33. Houssami N, Costelloe CM. Imaging bone metastases in breast cancer: evidence on comparative test accuracy. *Ann Oncol.* 2012;23:834–43.

34. Coleman RE, Smith P, Rubens RD. Clinical course and prognostic factors following bone recurrence from breast cancer. *Br J Cancer.* 1998;77:336–40.

35. Coleman RE. Clinical features of metastatic bone disease and risk of skeletal morbidity. *Clin Cancer Res.* 2006;12:6243s–9s.

36. Mercadante S. Malignant bone pain: pathophysiology and treatment. *Pain.* 1997;69:1–18.

37. Mehta AI, Brufsky AM, Sampson JH. Therapeutic approaches for HER2-positive brain metastases: circumventing the blood-brain barrier. *Cancer Treat Rev.* 2013;39:261–9.

38. Sperduto PW, Kased N, Roberge D, et al. Summary report on the graded prognostic assessment: an accurate and facile diagnosis-specific tool to estimate survival for patients with brain metastases. *J Clin Oncol.* 2012;30:419–25.

39. Tait CR, Waterworth A, Loncaster J, et al. The oligometastatic state in breast cancer: hypothesis or reality. *Breast.* 2005;14:87–93.
40. Brufsky AM, Mayer M, Rugo HS, et al. Central nervous system metastases in patients with HER2-positive metastatic breast cancer: incidence, treatment, and survival in patients from registHER. *Clin Cancer Res.* 2011;17:4834–43.
41. Lin NU, Amiri-Kordestani L, Palmieri D, et al. CNS metastases in breast cancer: old challenge, new frontiers. *Clin Cancer Res.* 2013;19:6404–18.

5

HISTOLOGY OF BREAST CANCER

Until the early part of the twentieth century, breast cancer was diagnosed because of signs and symptoms: usually a hard mass in the breast that adhered to the skin, enlarged lymph nodes that caused pain in the axilla, and cachexia. By 1920, the failure to cure these symptomatic patients with radical surgery led to increasing treatment of patients with only a small mass and evidence of cancerous cells on frozen section, even though it was recognized that some patients with "pathologically malignant" and "clinically benign" disease would be treated.[1] It was less than 60 years from the publication of Virchow's seminal work that led to widespread acceptance of an abnormal cell as the essential element of the development and spread of cancer, but even then it was clear that the cells in different tumors had different characteristics that correlated with different outcomes.

INFILTRATING DUCTAL CARCINOMA (IDC)

The most common breast cancer histology is infiltrating ductal carcinoma (IDC), or infiltrating breast cancer not otherwise specified (NOS), which accounts for 70%–80% of all breast cancers. Grossly this tumor may be rock-hard ("scirrhous") due to extensive desmoplastic tumor stroma, or softer if very cellular, and cytologically the field may be dominated by either stroma or cancer cells.[2] The cells may differ little from normal breast epithelium or may be very pleomorphic and may appear as glands, nests, trabeculae, or sheets of cells (Figure 5.1). There may be no, limited, or extensive DCIS accompanying the invasive cells, and there may be few or numerous mitoses. (For more on the significance of extensive DCIS, see Chapter 9, and on mitoses, see Chapter 7.) These differences occur both between and within tumors. Information on the behavior of breast cancer is based primarily on tumors with IDC.

BREAST CANCERS OF SPECIAL TYPE

Some tumors appear to have more homogeneous cellular characteristics associated with other distinctive qualities such as gross tumor appearance, findings on physical examination or mammogram, molecular markers, prognosis, or response to therapy[2-4] (see Table 5.1).

Invasive Lobular Carcinoma (ILC)

The most common of these special types is invasive lobular carcinoma, which accounts for 5%–15% of all breast cancers. The classic or pure form of ILC consists of sheets of small, uniform cells that invade the tumor in a single-file (Indian file) pattern that

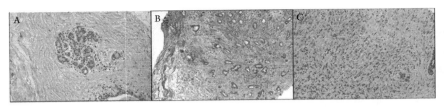

Figure 5.1 A: Normal lobule with an interlobular duct. B: Low-power view of invasive duct carcinoma. Glands are haphazardly arranged with variability in size and shape. C: Infiltrating lobular carcinoma with single cell invasion and cell filing (or "Indian filing"). The blue background is characteristic of ILC. These are typical histologic sections of IDC and ILC carcinoma, but there are many variations of each.
Source: Singh M, *Digital Atlas of Breast Pathology.* Department of Pathology, Stony Brook University Medical Center.

suggests strands with little desmoplastic reaction[2] (Figure 5.1C). IDC and ILC probably arise from the same cells: the terminal duct lobular unit. On physical examination or mammography there may no mass, only breast thickening, and it is not uncommon for this tumor to grow quite large before it can felt by either physician or patient. ILC (and LCIS) are unique in their lack of E-cadherin, an adhesion molecule, and this may account for some of the physical characteristics. These tumors are more often multifocal. It is generally thought that they have a greater propensity to be bilateral, and this is sometimes used as a rationale for performing bilateral mastectomy. However, not all studies demonstrate this increased tendency to bilaterality.[2] The incidence of ILC in the United States increased from 1987 to 1999 and then decreased from 1999 to 2004.[5] This correlated with increased use of postmenopausal hormone replacement therapy in the first period and decreased use in the second period, leading to a hypothesis that ILC may be more closely related to hormone usage than some other cancers. ILCs are less likely than IDCs to metastasize to lung, liver, and brain, and more likely to go to serosal surfaces of the abdomen, ovary, uterus, gastrointestinal tract, bone marrow, and leptomeninges. They have also been shown to be less responsive to chemotherapy.[4] In spite of these differences in the biological behavior of IDC and ILC, when matched for size and lymph node status they appear to have the same overall prognosis. Between 4% and 6% of tumors have mixed ductal and lobular features and cannot be placed in either class.

Other cancers of special type together constitute less than 10% of breast cancers, but some of the features of these special cancers may occur in a tumor that is predominantly IDC. Multiple variants have been identified that may not behave quite like the "pure" or "classic" type. There is often inconsistency in the assignment of type by different pathologists. If the assignment of type is not unequivocally IDC and this assignment is to be used in making treatment decisions, more than one pathologist, including one who is considered an expert, should review the histology.

As a rule of thumb, the pure form of cancers have a better prognosis than IDC (see Table 5.1). This is clearly true for tubular, mucinous, cribriform, adenoid cystic, and secretory carcinomas. This may be because they grow slowly and present with small size, or because they have a reduced tendency to metastasize, often manifest by few or no involved lymph nodes. Pure tubular cancers are often found on

Table 5.1 Breast Cancers of Special Type

Histological Type	%	Histology of the "Pure" Type	Predominant Molecular Characteristics of Pure Type	Prognosis Compared to IDC and Key Clinical Characteristics
Invasive lobular	5–15	Small, uniform cells invading in single-file strands; often multifocal	ER+ 92% HER2+ 5% • E-cadherin ➔ • Luminal subtype	• Survival similar • Often thickening with no mass on mammogram or examination • May have greater bilaterality • Unique patterns of metastases (see text)
Tubular	< 2–5	Multiple tubules formed by single layers of well-differentiated cells.	ER+ 95% HER2+ 0% • Luminal subtype	• Best prognostic type if "pure" • Often diagnosed as an incidental finding • May constitute up to 25% of mammogram detected cancers
Mucinous or colloid	1–2	Small clusters of cells in pools of extracellular mucin	ER+ 95% HER2+ 0% • Neuroendocrine features • Luminal subtype	• Prognosis almost equal to tubular • Often no mass on PE or mammogram • More often in older patients
Invasive cribriform	1–4	Nests of cells banded by dense connective tissue and lacunae give Swiss cheese appearance	ER+ 100% HER2+ 100%	• Better than average prognosis • Cribriform DCIS often present
Adenoid cystic	0.1	Similar to adenoid cystic cancer of salivary gland with small cells and variable architecture	ER+ 0% HER2+ 0% • Some are basal-like	• Better than average prognosis; metastases may exist for many years • Usually lymph node negative
Medullary	1–9	Syncytial with absent glandular features, marked lymphoplasmacytic infiltrate	ER+ 9% HER2+ 1% • BRCA1 associations • Some are basal-like	• Prognosis highly variable • Enlarged axillary nodes may be reactive rather than due to cancer metastases
Invasive papillary	1–2	Sheets of cells alternating with papillae consisting of a fibrovascular core covered by intermediate-grade cancer cells.	ER+ 100% HER2+ 0%	• Average prognosis • May have lobulated appearance on mammogram • Enlarged nodes may be reactive rather than a result of cancer metastases.

Type	%	Histology	Molecular	Clinical
Invasive micropapillary	1–2	Islands of intermediate grade cells in well-defined clear spaces within a mass of cancer cells NOS	ER+ 71% HER2+ 41% • Often p53+ • Distinct molecular subtype in luminal	• Worse than average prognosis • High frequency of metastases to multiple nodes, which may have micropapillary areas • Frequent lymphatic vessel invasion
Metaplastic	<5	Some cells transformed either to non-adenocarcinoma, epithelia cell (e.g., squamous), or mesenchymal cell (e.g., spindle cell, osseous. myoid)	ER+ 6% HER2+ 2% • Often p53+ • Basal-like	• Average prognosis • Tumors often grow to large size over short period of time
Neuroendocrine or cancers with endocrine differentiation	2–5	Parts of tumor have glandular appearance similar to carcinoid or oat cell cancers. May be argyrophilic.	ER+ 100% HER2+ 0% • Some have endocrine markers • Luminal subtype	• Average prognosis • Symptoms related to endocrine function of tumors, very rare
Invasive apocrine	<1–4	Cells with abundant cytoplasm that may have eosinophilic granulation	ER+ 17% HER2+ 33% • May have AR • Distinct molecular subtype	• Average prognosis
Secretory	<0.1	Well-differentiated cells form glands and spaces with vacuolated eosinophilic secretion	ER+ 24% HER2+ 4%	• Better than average prognosis, especially in young patients • Low rate of lymph node and distant metastases

IDC = invasive ductal carcinoma; PE = physical examination; NOS = not otherwise specified (such as IDC); AR = androgen receptor

Five less common types of the 17 identified in the WHO classification are not included in this list. For all tumor types, there is considerable variation in the histologic presentation and molecular or clinical characteristics of different tumors within the classification, but to be considered one of these special type 90% of the cells should be of the histologic type described. Since all but a few of these are very uncommon, the frequency that these are observed varies in various published series. The percentage of tumors that were scored as ER+ or HER2+ also varied among studies; this is the median value, but in most cases the range of observed values was narrow.

Sources: Histological descriptions, clinical outcomes, and molecular characteristics from Dillon DA, Guidi AJ, Schnitt SJ. Pathology of invasive breast cancer In: Harris JR, Lippman ME, Morrow M, et al., eds. *Diseases of the Breast.* 4th ed. Philadelphia: Lippincott Williams & Wilkins; 2010:374–407; Weigelt B, Horlings HM, Kreike B, et al. Refinement of breast cancer classification by molecular characterization of histological special types. *J Pathol.* 2008;216:141–50; and Weigelt B, Reis-Filho JS. Histological and molecular types of breast cancer: is there a unifying taxonomy? *Nature Rev Clin Oncol.* 2009;6:718–30.

screening mammograms and have the best prognosis of all breast cancers. The survival of patients with either tubular or adenoid cystic carcinoma is generally no worse than an age-matched population without cancer. Adenoid cystic tumors may metastasize and then grow very slowly for decades, regardless of treatment. Treating these tumors as garden-variety IDC may be over-treatment, but inappropriately assigning this diagnosis when, in fact, the patient has a mixed tumor or a different histological type may result in under-treatment. Between 15% and 20% of tumors are "mixed," defined as several different histologies in which each component comprises > 10% of the area on the slide.

Studies of molecular markers and gene expression (see Chapter 7) in these special histological types are still limited, but the evidence thus far indicates that each has a consistent molecular signature and clinical behavior that may or may not be consistent with the expected behavior for that signature.[3,4] For example, tubular and mucinous tumors are almost all luminal, ER+ and HER2–, and, not surprising, these tumors have a good prognosis. On the other hand, cribriform tumors are ER+ and HER2+, but they, too, have a better than average prognosis. Adenoid cystic tumors are ER– and basal like, but contrary to expectations from their markers, these tumors grow very slowly. High-grade medullary tumors, which are basal-like, ER+, and HER2–, have a good prognosis in spite of the histological grade and poor molecular profile. Invasive micropapillary tumors are luminal and mostly ER+ but have a very aggressive clinical behavior. Most of the tumors of special type are in the luminal or basal-like intrinsic (molecular) subtypes, but invasive micropapillary and invasive apocrine tumors form distinct molecular subtypes. In gene expression assays, all of the tumors of a histological type are within the same intrinsic breast cancer subtype, but they do not necessarily cluster together, suggesting core similarities with variability as well. It remains to be demonstrated that these additional gene mutations have clinical meaning.

Non-adenomatous Tumors Presenting in the Breast

Metaplastic tumors have adenomatous features, coupled with areas in which the tumors have the features of another epithelia type cancer, such as squamous cell, or a non-epithelial cancer such as spindle cell, osteocartilagenous, or sarcoma. These are treated as breast cancer.

Tumors also arise in the breast that are not considered breast cancers, such as lymphomas and sarcomas, and these are treated in the same way as if arising in a different part of the body. Cancers arising in other organs, including the opposite breast, may metastasize to the breast. The cancers most commonly found as metastases in the breast are melanoma, lung cancer, prostate cancer, and carcinoids.[2] These may be extremely difficult to distinguish from a primary breast cancer. The appearance of multiple lesions in both breasts and the absence of in situ elements in the histology are clues that a lesion might be metastatic from another organ.

Phyllodes Tumor or Cystosarcoma

Phyllodes is a fibroepithelial tumor of the breast with benign and malignant variants that are distinguished primarily by the number of mitoses per high-powered field, the degree of atypia, and whether there is evidence of infiltration. These may grow quite large. About 15% of these tumors recur locally, and an even smaller percentage recurs at distant sites. Treatment is wide local excision with clear margins exceeding 1–2 cm.[6] Often this is not achieved because the correct diagnosis is not made at the time of initial biopsy and re-excision is not performed. Node dissection and adjuvant therapies are not indicated for these tumors.

TUMOR GRADE

Tumor grade, when used with other clinical features, has proven to be one of easiest and the most reliable ways to define prognostic subgroups. Grade has been defined either entirely on nuclear features or, more commonly, on a combination of nuclear and cytoplasmic characteristics. The definitions of grade have evolved from the first description in 1925 through Scarff-Bloom-Richardson (often abbreviated as SBR on pathology reports) in the 1950s to the Nottingham Grading System (NGS) developed in the 1980s. All of the systems used for the last half-century have combined an assessment of nuclear and cytoplasmic characteristics with mitotic activity to segment the patients into three groups with increasing risk of recurrence or death from breast cancer. The Nottingham criteria and the microscopic appearance of the three histologic grades are shown in Figure 5.2. A major problem with using grading systems is their subjectivity and reproducibility, but the increasingly precise definitions of the elements and the assignment of numerical values seem to have improved reproducibility.

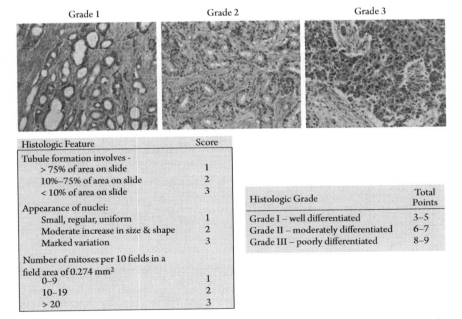

Histologic Feature	Score
Tubule formation involves -	
> 75% of area on slide	1
10%–75% of area on slide	2
< 10% of area on slide	3
Appearance of nuclei:	
Small, regular, uniform	1
Moderate increase in size & shape	2
Marked variation	3
Number of mitoses per 10 fields in a field area of 0.274 mm^2	
0–9	1
10–19	2
> 20	3

Histologic Grade	Total Points
Grade I – well differentiated	3–5
Grade II – moderately differentiated	6–7
Grade III – poorly differentiated	8–9

Figure 5.2 Nottingham tumor grading system with examples of the microscopic appearance of grade 1, grade 2, and grade 3 breast cancer.
Source: Rakha EA, Reis-Filho JS, Baehner F, et al. Breast cancer prognostic classification in the molecular era: the role of histological grade. *Breast Cancer Res.* 2010;12:207.

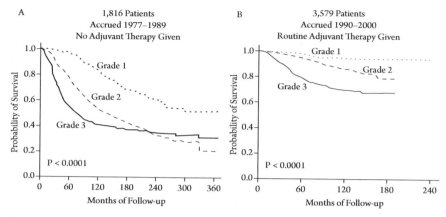

Figure 5.3 Nottingham histologic grade and breast cancer specific survival in two cohorts, the first accrued at an earlier date and not given adjuvant therapy (A) and the second accrued at a later date when adjuvant endocrine was given to receptor-positive patients and adjuvant chemotherapy to receptor-negative patients. Both sets of patients were consecutively seen at the Nottingham City Hospital, Nottingham, UK. In series A, 18% of patients had grade 1, 36% grade 2, and 46% grade 3 tumors. In B, 19% of the patients had grade 1, 39% grade 2, and 42% grade 3 tumors.

Source: Rakha EA, Reis-Filho JS, Baehner F, et al. Breast cancer prognostic classification in the molecular era: the role of histological grade. *Breast Cancer Res.* 2010;12:207.

In studies of inter-observer and intra-observer variability published since 1990, the kappa scores for the NGS have ranged from 0.54 to 0.83, with most of them in the mid-60s. [7] This suggests substantial but far from perfect reproducibility. The frequency of grade 1 tumors in various studies ranges from 17% to 28%, grade 2 from 36% to 49%, and grade 3 from 24% to 46%.[7] Grade 3 tumors recur earlier than those of other grades, but the recurrence rate after the first 5–10 years of follow-up is not substantially different from that of grade 2 patients not given adjuvant systemic therapy (see Figure 5.3).

Lymphatic vessel invasion (LVI) is not included in most combination scoring systems of grade, but its presence is associated with a higher frequency of lymph node involvement, shorter time to and higher likelihood of recurrence, and worse overall survival.[8] It retains its value in a multivariate model that includes tumor grade and size. Blood vessel invasion is also prognostic, but it occurs less frequently than LVI.

Tumor necrosis and perineural invasion are additional indicators of adverse outcomes.

TUMOR SIZE, MULTIFOCALITY AND MULTICENTRICITY

The size of the tumor on histological evaluation is now used preferentially in the TNM grading system (see Chapter 6). If there are multiple lesions, the AJCC recommends that the size of the largest invasive area of a single lesion be used as the "T"; the diameters of the various foci should *not* be added together.[9] Tumors are often categorized as multifocal (MF) when two or more lesions are identified in one quadrant, or multicentric

(MC) when two or more lesions are found in more than one quadrant. The incidence of MF/MC tumors will depend on the method of ascertainment and varies from 21% to 63% without the use of MRI and, on average, 16% more when MRI is used.[10] MC tumors are associated with a higher incidence of local failure and most often are treated with mastectomy, but many MF tumors are treated with breast-conserving surgery. The frequent use of MRI has led to the discovery of more MF/MC tumors and consequently an increased use of mastectomy over breast-conserving surgery, but it is not clear that MRI use improves outcomes. Two tumors are not necessarily associated with a worse survival than one, in spite of their association with other poor prognostic factors such as the number of involved lymph nodes, but there are inconsistencies in published data regarding the prognostic importance of MF/MC.[11,12] For this reason, this information is used in choosing local treatment, since it is axiomatic that all tumor tissue should be removed, but it is not used in decisions regarding adjuvant systemic therapy.

COMPLETE EXCISION, TUMOR MARGINS, AND EXTENSIVE DCIS

Ideally the surgeon will remove all tumor tissue, along with a rim of normal tissue around the tumor, since tumor remaining at the margin is associated with a higher rate of local recurrence, even when radiotherapy is administered after lumpectomy or mastectomy. To accurately ascertain the margins of excision, the removed specimen is routinely inked. However, there is no consensus regarding the optimal or minimal size of this normal tissue rim.

Biopsy specimens will usually have some foci of ductal carcinoma in situ (DCIS). However, when there is an extensive intraductal component (EIC), usually defined as $\geq 25\%$ of the invasive area of the tumor on a microscopic cross section as well as in grossly normal adjacent tissue, there is an increased probability of a local recurrence. When a lesion consists primarily of DCIS with one or more foci of invasive carcinoma, it may also be classified as EIC. In a study with relatively long follow-up by the investigators who originally defined this entity, the local and distant recurrence rates in 166 EIC+ tumors were 21% and 13%, respectively.[13] In 418 EIC– tumors these rates were 6% and 20% ($p < 0.05$). The absence of increased distant recurrences and nearly identical overall survival of EIC+ and EIC– patients suggests that this is a marker of multifocality within the breast, not a more aggressive form of the disease. When first described, EIC+ tumors were routinely treated with mastectomy rather than breast-conserving surgery (BCS) and radiotherapy, but more recent studies using newer mammographic and other radiological techniques have enabled more complete excision of the multiple tumor foci in these patients, thus enabling them to have BCS.

LYMPH NODES

The pathological lymph node status is generally considered the single most informative prognostic factor used either alone or as part of the TNM system (see Chapter 6). With increasing use of sentinel lymph nodes biopsies and limited node dissections (see Chapter 9), the total number of nodes available for examination is decreasing. The number of lymph nodes examined will vary with the procedures used and the diligence of the surgeon and pathologist, but if an inadequate number is removed there is a danger of under-staging and, as a consequence, under-treating the *node-positive* patient. If a treatment decision, such as the use of adjuvant radiotherapy or chemo-therapy, depends on knowing accurately the number of positive lymph nodes, a minimum of 6–10 should be removed.[14] Some would place this as high as 16[15] (see Chapters 9 and 10 on local and adjuvant therapy for further information on using the number of positive nodes in making treatment decisions.)

There is also a danger of over-staging the *node-negative* patient. Older studies used to establish the prognostic value of axillary nodes often did not consider microme-tastases or lymph nodes identified by any means other than H & E staining in the total count. More recently, micrometastatic lymph nodes have been defined as tumor deposits > 0.2 mm and < 2.0 mm, and the importance of these, especially when found in a sentinel lymph node (SLN) biopsy, is under intense study. Deposits < 0.2 mm are defined as isolated tumor cells (ITCs) and are even more controversial. Although the prognostic importance of micrometastases (MM) and nodes identified with immu-nohistochemical staining (e.g., cytokeratin stains) (IHC) is variable from one study to another, the most important point may be that outcome differences between those with only MM or ITC and those with no evidence of nodal involvement of any kind is very small. At present it is not recommended that this information be used to justify more extensive dissection of the axilla or the use of either radiotherapy or adjuvant systemic therapy.[16]

REFERENCES

1. Bloodgood JC. Diagnosis and treatment of border-line pathological lesions. In: Robbins GF, ed. *Silvergirl's Surgery: The Breast*. Austin, TX: Silvergirl; 1914:199–201.

2. Dillon DA, Guidi AJ, Schnitt SJ. Pathology of invasive breast cancer In: Harris JR, Lippman ME, Morrow M, et al., eds. *Diseases of the Breast*. 4th ed. Philadelphia: Lippincott Williams & Wilkins; 2010:374–407.

3. Weigelt B, Horlings HM, Kreike B, et al. Refinement of breast cancer classification by molecular characterization of histological special types. *J Pathol*. 2008;216:141–50.

4. Weigelt B, Reis-Filho JS. Histological and molecular types of breast cancer: is there a unify-ing taxonomy? *Nature Rev Clin Oncol*. 2009;6:718–30.

5. Eheman CR, Shaw KM, Ryerson AB, et al. The changing incidence of in situ and inva-sive ductal and lobular breast carcinomas: United States, 1999–2004. *Cancer Epidemiol Biomarkers Prev*. 2009;18:1763–9.

6. Guillot E, Couturaud B, Reyal F, et al. Management of phyllodes breast tumors. *Breast J*. 2011;17:129–37.

7. Rakha EA, Reis-Filho JS, Baehner F, et al. Breast cancer prognostic classification in the molecular era: the role of histological grade. *Breast Cancer Res*. 2010;12:207.

8. Mohammed RA, Martin SG, Mahmmod AM, et al. Objective assessment of lymphatic and blood vascular invasion in lymph node-negative breast carcinoma: findings from a large case series with long-term follow-up. *J Pathol*. 2011;223:358–65.

9. *AJCC Cancer Staging Manual*. 7th ed. New York: Springer; 2010.

10. Houssami N, Ciatto S, Macaskill P, et al. Accuracy and surgical impact of magnetic reso-nance imaging in breast cancer staging: systematic review and meta-analysis in detection of multifocal and multicentric cancer. *J Clin Oncol*. 2008;26:3248–58.

11. Lynch SP, Lei X, Chavez-MacGregor M, et al. Multifocality and multicentricity in breast cancer and survival outcomes. *Ann Oncol.* 2012;23:3063–9.

12. Weissenbacher TM, Zschage M, Janni W, et al. Multicentric and multifocal versus unifocal breast cancer: is the tumor-node-metastasis classification justified? *Breast Cancer Res Treat.* 2010;122:27–34.

13. Schnitt SJ, Harris JR. Evolution of breast-conserving therapy for localized breast cancer. *J Clin Oncol.* 2008;26:1395–6.

14. Weir L, Speers C, D'Yachkova Y, et al. Prognostic significance of the number of axillary lymph nodes removed in patients with node-negative breast cancer. *J Clin Oncol.* 2002;20:1793–9.

15. Somner JE, Dixon JM, Thomas JS. Node retrieval in axillary lymph node dissections: recommendations for minimum numbers to be confident about node negative status. *J Clin Pathol.* 2004;57:845–8.

16. Pesce C, Morrow M. The need for lymph node dissection in nonmetastatic breast cancer. *Annu Rev Med.* 2013;64:119–29.

6

CLINICAL AND PATHOLOGICAL STAGING

Clinical staging of cancer was initiated in the mid-twentieth century to identify those patients whose tumors had likely spread beyond the field of surgery and who would be unlikely to benefit from local therapy, even radical mastectomy with adjuvant radiotherapy. Although there were a number of proposed systems, the TNM (tumor, nodes, and distant metastases) system emerged as the standard, and the American Joint Committee on Cancer (AJCC), a group with representatives from multiple organizations involved with the study and care of cancer patients, was formed to define the key elements based on survival data.[1] In recent years the AJCC has collaborated closely with the Union for International Cancer Control (UICC; formerly the International Union Against Cancer) to create a system that is used worldwide.

Since the natural course of breast cancer varies enormously from one patient to another, it is difficult to know whether differences in outcomes from two series of patients treated differently is a result of the treatment or the intrinsic differences in the patients selected for each group (see Chapter 4). Early on it was hoped that staging would place patients in groups with nearly identical survival or recurrence rates prior to treatment and that outcomes for these groups could be compared after treatment to determine which therapy was more effective. Unfortunately, such comparisons led to the erroneous conclusion that radical surgery was superior to less extensive forms of treatment. Subsequent randomized trials demonstrated that these conclusions were erroneous and that this was an inappropriate use of staging (see Chapter 9).

Because it was routine practice to stage patients prior to the introduction of adjuvant systemic therapy for early breast cancer (see Chapter 10), the clinical and pathological staging system that was developed to address surgical questions was also adopted for defining which patients should receive adjuvant systemic therapy. In retrospect, this was probably inappropriate. Adjuvant systemic therapy is given because it is assumed that a patient has undetectable micrometastases in distant organs, and the important question is which will respond to a proposed drug. The classic staging system was developed to identify those patients who did *not* have distant metastases and thus would benefit from local treatment alone.

Originally, staging was based entirely on clinical findings prior to any treatment because it was meant to define the appropriate surgery. However, as it was used (inappropriately) to compare outcomes and make postsurgical treatment decisions, pathological findings were gradually introduced into the staging system, in part because they can be measured with greater precision. For example, in the original TNM, nodal status was determined entirely on physical examination. Later it was based on the results of axillary node dissection.

The TNM (Tumor, Nodes, and Distant Metastases) System Tumor (T)

For most tumors, the "T" is determined by the size of the tumor; T1 is < 2 cm, T2 is 2–4.9 cm, and T3 is ≥ 5 cm. Whenever possible, the size should be based on pathological findings (pT), preferably the longest dimension of *the invasive component only*, measured on a single histological slide of either a core or excisional biopsy. If the tumor is too large to do this, the measurement should be made on the gross specimen. Tumor size has been shown consistently to be of prognostic importance independent of other prognostic fractures, such as the number of involved nodes (see Figure 6.1).

Lesions are classified as T4 and generally are considered inoperable if the tumor is attached to either the chest wall (T4a, T4c) or the skin (T4b, T4c), or if there are satellite nodules, edema (sometime characterized as peau d'orange because of the similarity to the skin of an orange), or ulceration.

Inflammatory carcinoma, a particularly aggressive form of cancer, is also considered a T4 lesion (T4d) and on physical exam is characterized as having diffuse erythema and peau d'orange covering at least one-third of the breast. In the original descriptions of this tumor, no mass could be palpated. However, more recent studies have included patients with masses, leading to the possibility that these tumors are not the same, and possibly much less aggressive, than the tumors in older reports. The edema is the result of lymphatics plugged with cancer cells, and the diagnosis of inflammatory breast cancer requires a skin biopsy to demonstrate this phenomenon. Dermal lymphatic invasion (DLI) itself has a poor prognosis, but not as bad as that of inflammatory carcinoma with DLI.

T1 lesions include all tumors < 2 cm in size, but physicians often subdivide T1 into T1mi (≤ 1 mm, considered microinvasive), T1a (>1 to ≤ 5 mm), T1b (> 5 to ≤ 10 mm) and T1c (> 10 to ≤ 20 mm). In general, these subdivisions are more important for research than for clinical decision-making.

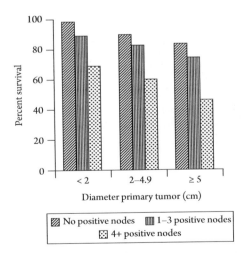

Figure 6.1 Relationship between tumor size and the percentage of patients alive at 5 years subdivided by the number of lymph nodes with tumor metastases: no positive nodes, 1–3 positive nodes, 4+ positive nodes.

Reprinted with permission from *AJCC Cancer Staging Manual*. 7th ed. New York: Springer; 2011:359.

Nodes (N)

When staging was primarily clinical, N1 designated palpable (firm or hard) but freely movable ipsilateral axillary lymph nodes (many of which proved to be tumor-free on pathological evaluation) at levels I and/or II of the axilla. (The axilla is conventionally divided into three regions defined by the pectoralis minor muscle. Level I is closest to the breast; level III is furthest away and includes infraclavicular and apical nodes.) N2 designated nodes that were fixed to each other (matted) or to other structures, such as the chest wall or skin, at levels I and/or II, and N3 indicated that infraclavicular or supraclavicular nodes, with or without nodes at levels I and II, were palpable. If ipsilateral internal mammary nodes are found *in addition to ipsilateral axillary nodes*, the nodal stage is also N3.

Full pathological staging is somewhat less precise today because the surgeon removes fewer nodes, and the pathologist invests less time trying to identify all negative nodes (see Chapter 9 on sentinel node biopsy). Today most patients have only level I or level I and II nodes removed because the incidence of lymphedema increases when nodes higher in the axilla are removed surgically, especially if they are both removed *and* treated with radiotherapy.

The odds of having distant metastases and the chance of eventually dying of breast cancer increases with each additional positive node.[2,3] In a recent study, the 15-year cause-specific survival of patients with one, two, or three positive lymph nodes was 77%, 70%, and 63%, respectively; these differences were statistically significant.[3] But by convention tumors have been grouped into those with no nodes (pN0), 1–3 nodes (pN1a), 4–9 nodes (pN2a), and ≥ 10 nodes (pN3). Survival outcomes related to these groupings from NSABP Trial B-04 with 15-year follow-up are shown in Figure 6.2.[4]

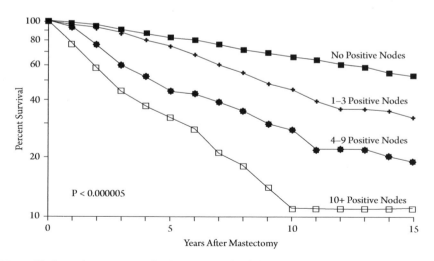

Figure 6.2 Survival over 15 years of 596 patients, subdivided by the number of positive axillary nodes, treated with radical mastectomy and no adjuvant systemic therapy on NSABP protocol B-04, which accrued patients between 1971 and 1974.

With permission from Fisher ER, Costantino J, Fisher B, et al. Pathologic findings from the National Surgical Adjuvant Breast Project (Protocol 4): discriminants for 15-year survival. National Surgical Adjuvant Breast and Bowel Project Investigators. *Cancer.* 1993;71:2141–50.

To be considered a "positive node," at least one area of metastases in the node must be larger than 0.2 mm in diameter and/or have > 200 cells. However, if no metastases are > 2.0 mm, the node is considered to have micrometastases and is classified as pN1mi. Patients who are pN1mi are generally treated much the same as any other pN1 patient. If there are isolated tumor cells (ITC's) in the nodes not meeting the criteria for pN1mi (size 0.2 – 2.0 mm), the patient is considered to have a pN0 tumor and "(i+)" is added after the designation (see Chapter 5 for further discussion on the importance of ITC's). This may change in the near future. If there are both ITCs and nodes with metastases > 0.2 mm, the ITCs are included in the total node count. Except for ITCs, only nodes with metastases that can be seen with an H & E stain are counted; ITCs include cells detected with immunohistochemical stains.Intramammary nodes are counted as axillary nodes and are considered to be level I.

Contralateral nodes in the axilla, internal mammary chain, or supraclavicular fossa would be counted as distant metastases and staged as M1.

Most breast cancers drain to axillary lymph nodes and only 8%–22% drain to internal mammary nodes.[5] However, internal mammary nodal metastases *without* involvement of axillary nodes occurs with a frequency of < 1%. For this reason, it is uncommon for information about internal mammary nodes to change the tumor stage. However, if nodes in the axilla are negative but internal mammary nodes are identified by CT, ultrasonography, or fine needle aspiration (but not by lymphoscintigraphy), the nodal stage is N2b or pN2b; if nodes are found in both regions the nodal stage is N3b or pN3b. Internal mammary nodes found to be positive on sentinel node biopsy without other evidence of involvement are classified as pN1b.

Metastases (M)

A classification of M1 is based entirely on the presence of unequivocal metastases outside the breast and *ipsilateral* regional (axillary, supraclavicular, and internal mammary) nodes using a combination of clinical findings, radiological studies, and histological evidence of cancer on H & E stained biopsy tissue. Beyond inquiring about symptoms that might be associated with breast cancer metastases and a complete physical examination, there are no required evaluations to rule out distant metastases for routine staging at the time the primary is diagnosed. A site need not be biopsied to confirm metastases if the clinical evidence is compelling. For example, a biopsy might be performed on a patient with a single suspicious lesion on a bone scan but not in a patient with multiple lytic lesions in the spine, ribs, pelvis, humeri, and/or femurs.

Circulating tumor cells (CTCs; see Chapters 4 and 12) and microscopic or molecularly positive deposits without either clinical or radiological evidence of metastases do not make a tumor M1. These may be designated as cM0(i+). There is good evidence that these findings have prognostic import, but insufficient follow-up and appropriate measures to reduce false positives are not yet in place to include them in the AJCC staging system.

CLINICAL AND PATHOLOGICAL STAGES USING TNM

Survival outcomes of various combinations of T, N, and M have been determined over the years, and those with similar outcomes have been grouped together to form

Table 6.1 Criteria for AJCC Stages Based on TNM Criteria

	T	*N*	*M*
Stage 0	Tis	N0	M0
Stage 1			
1A	T1	N0	M0
1B	T0 or T1	N1mi	M0
Stage 2			
IIA	T0 or T1	N1	M0
	T2	N0	M0
IIB	T2	N1	M0
	T3	N0	M0
Stage 3			
IIIA	T0, T1, or T2	N2	M0
	T3	N1 or N2	M0
IIIB	T4	N0, N1, or N2	M0
IIIC	Any T	N3	M0
Stage 4	Any T	Any N	M1

Tis = in situ tumor.

T and N status may be based on either pathological (preferred) or clinical findings, and a "p" (e.g., pT1) or "c" before the T or N indicates the basis of the classification. M is always based on clinical evidence of metastases.

Data adapted from *AJCC Cancer Staging Manual.* 7th ed. New York: Springer; 2011.

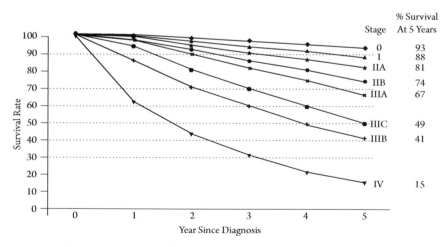

Figure 6.3 Observed overall survival (not breast cancer specific survival) for 211,645 breast cancer patients diagnosed in 2001–2002, subdivided by AJCC stage.

Taken from the National Cancer Data Base of the Commission on Cancer of the American College of Surgeon and American Cancer Society. Reprinted with permission from *AJCC Cancer Staging Manual.* 7th ed. New York: Springer; 2011:360.

four clinical/pathological stages. Although there are other subclassifications or divisions within stages (e.g., stage IA or IB), the stages used most frequently in clinical practice and for which robust survival data are available are summarized in Table 6.1. Additional detail about definitions of the groups shown here can be obtained from the AJCC Manual.[1] The 5-year survival for these groups are illustrated in Figure 6.3.

When a patient presents with simultaneous, bilateral primaries, each is staged separately. The prognosis is determined by and therapeutic decisions, such as the use of adjuvant systemic therapy, are made using information from the tumor with the highest stage.[6]

REFERENCES

1. *AJCC Cancer Staging Manual.* 7th ed. New York: Springer; 2010.

2. Nemoto T, Vana J, Bedwani RN, et al. Management and survival of female breast cancer: results of a national survey by the American College of Surgeons. *Cancer.* 1980;45:2917–24.

3. Dai Kubicky C, Mongoue-Tchokote S. Prognostic significance of the number of positive lymph nodes in women with T1-2N1 breast cancer treated with mastectomy: should patients with 1, 2, and 3 positive lymph nodes be grouped together? *Int J Radiat Oncol Biol Phys.* 2013;85:1200–5.

4. Fisher ER, Costantino J, Fisher B, et al. Pathologic findings from the National Surgical Adjuvant Breast Project (Protocol 4): discriminants for 15-year survival. National Surgical Adjuvant Breast and Bowel Project Investigators. *Cancer.* 1993;71:2141–50.

5. Pendas S, Giuliano R, Swor G, et al. Worldwide experience with lymphatic mapping for invasive breast cancer. *Sem Oncol.* 2004;31:318–23.

6. Robinson E, Rennert G, Rennert HS, et al. Survival of first and second primary breast cancer. *Cancer.* 1993;71:172–6.

7

MOLECULAR FACTORS AS
PROGNOSTIC/PREDICTIVE TOOLS
AND THERAPEUTIC TARGETS

During nearly a century of close observation, clinicians established that there were subsets of breast cancer patients with distinctly different likelihoods of dying from the disease, rates of growth, and response to treatment (see Chapters 4, 5, 12). Laboratory scientists are now identifying the molecules that define these patient subsets and that may serve as either biomarkers of prognosis and response or targets of future therapy. This process has required increased understanding of the biology of the disease at the cellular and molecular level. Central to this is an understanding of the role of hormones, especially estrogen and its receptor, in the pathophysiology of breast cancer.

ESTROGEN AND PROGESTERONE RECEPTORS

Varying levels of estrogen receptors (ER) and/or progesterone receptors (PR) are present on ~ 70% of breast cancers. There are two isoforms of ER: ERα and ERβ. Mice lacking ERα, which appears in only 10%–20% of normal human breast cells, are unable to develop ductal trees or to lactate, while those lacking ERβ develop normally.[1] The role of ERβ in normal and cancerous cells is less well understood than ERα, and there is no clinical role for its measurement at this time. When ER is used without further delineation, it refers to ERα. The best-understood functions of these receptors are as tissue-specific, ligand-specific transcription factors[1-3] (see Figure 7.1). In model systems, breast cancer cells exposed to estrogen may grow rapidly; removal of estrogen or the use of anti-estrogens may slow growth and in many situations results in apoptosis or autophagy.[4] However, there are also non-genomic and ligand-independent ER functions, as well. Interactions with various growth factors, tyrosine kinase receptors (especially those for EGF, HER2, and IGF1), and signal transduction pathways are important in understanding resistance to endocrine therapy. The interactions with PI3K/Akt are particularly important since this pathway, which blocks apoptosis and promotes tumor growth, is hyperactive as a result of mutations in 28% to 47% of breast cancers.[5] This is second only to PTEN mutations, which occur in 37% to 44% of breast cancers and also augment activity in the PI3K/Akt pathway. The interaction between PI3K and ER is bidirectional. PI3K signaling will increase ligand-dependent activation and cause ligand-independent activation of ER, and estrogen-activated ER in or near the plasma cell membrane, where PI3K resides, appears to rapidly initiate signaling in the PI3K, MAPK, and IGF1 pathways (see Figure 7.1).

In the first assays of ER and PR (ligand-binding assays, LBA, or dextran-coated charcoal assay, DCC), radiolabeled steroids were incubated with tumor cytosols,

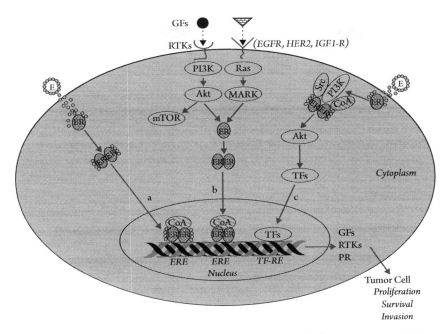

Figure 7.1 Some molecular effects of estrogen (E) and estrogen receptor (ER) in a breast cancer cell. In the classic genomic pathway (a), cytoplasmic estrogen receptor is activated by estrogen, forms a dimer and complexes with co-activators (CoA) and co-repressors while binding to estrogen response elements (ERE) in DNA. This results in transcription of mRNA for various growth factors (GFs) and receptor tyrosine kinases (RTKs), as well as more ER and progesterone receptors (PR), and ultimately leads to tumor cell proliferation, improved cell survival, and tumor invasiveness. ER can also be activated (i.e., phosphorylated) without estrogen (b, ligand-independent activation of ER), and the ER/coactivator complex then binds to DNA and EREs and facilitates transcription in the same way that the estrogen-activated complex does. ER located near or tethered to the plasma cell membrane may be activated by estrogen and then interacts directly with RTKs or RTK ligands on or near the membrane (c, non-genomic ER activity), causing activation of the signal transduction pathways associated with these RTKs and the formation of transcription factors (TF) that bind to TF response elements (TF-RE) on the DNA.

Adapted from Osborne CK. Receptors. In: Harris JR, Hellman S, Henderson IC, et al., eds. *Breast Diseases*. 2nd ed. Philadelphia: J. B. Lippincott; 1991:301–25; Musgrove EA, Sutherland RL. Biological determinants of endocrine resistance in breast cancer. *Nature Rev Cancer*. 2009;9:631–43; and Le Romancer M, Poulard C, Cohen P, et al. Cracking the estrogen receptor's posttranslational code in breast tumors. *Endocr Rev*. 2011;32:597–622.

and results were reported in femtomoles of receptor protein per mg of total cytosol protein (fmol/mg). This method was used to demonstrate the relationship between ER/PR levels and response to therapy, but it has been largely replaced by immunohistochemical assays (IHC) that use monoclonal antibodies to identify ER and PR on individual tumor cells from fresh, frozen, or paraffin-embedded tissue. IHC assays were developed through comparisons with LBA results. There is no standard IHC assay, and there have been problems in assuring high-quality, reproducible test results in many labs around the world. The most common problem is false negative reports due to poor technique (e.g., periods of > 4–6 hours from obtaining tissue to fixation or the lack of appropriate internal controls) and inexperience in interpreting the assay results.

All IHC reports should include the proportion of tumor cells that stained positive, the intensity of the staining, and an overall interpretation of the results as receptor positive (ER+ and/or PR+), receptor negative, or uninterpretable.[6] The consensus cut point for calling a tumor positive is ≥ 1% of stained cells because it has been shown that patients with < 1% do not benefit, and those with >1% do. There are a number of scoring systems (Allred, H-score, and quick score) that combine information on the proportion of positive cells and the intensity of staining that may be more sensitive and discriminatory than simply reporting whether there are more or less than 1% positive cells, but none of these is universally accepted as a standard. A third approach to measuring ER/PR is to use mRNA, and this is routinely done as part of the 21-gene recurrence assay (see further discussion later in this chapter). It appears to be as or more accurate than either LBA or IHC assays, but currently it is not available routinely outside a multigene assay.

About 75% of all breast cancers will be ER+, 45% PR+, 40% ER+PR+, and 1%–2% ER–PR+.[7] There is controversy about whether the ER–PR+ category is real since the cell needs ER to generate PR (see Figure 7.1).

A prognostic factor provides information on likely outcomes, such as recurrence or survival, independent of the effects of treatment, while a predictive factor provides information on likely response to treatment. ER and PR are both prognostic and predictive factors. Even ER+ tumors *not* treated with endocrine therapy are associated with a better overall and disease-free survival during the first 5 years of follow-up[8] (see Figure 7.2) In the study shown in the Figure 7.2, PR was also prognostic for time to first recurrence. As illustrated in Figure 4.4 in Chapter 4, these differences in outcomes

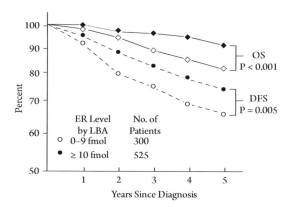

Figure 7.2 Prognostic value of ER for disease-free survival (DFS) and overall survival (OS) in 825 node-negative patients enrolled in NSABP Trial B-06 in which patients were randomized to one of three forms of local therapy. None of the patients received adjuvant endocrine therapy, but an unknown percent of the patients received endocrine therapy at the time of relapse. ER was measured using a ligand-binding assay (LBA).

Reprinted with permission from Fisher B, Redmond C, Fisher ER, et al. Relative worth of estrogen or progesterone receptor and pathologic characteristics of differentiation as indicators of prognosis in node negative breast cancer patients: findings from National Surgical Adjuvant Breast and Bowel Project Protocol B-06. *J Clin Oncol.* 1988;6:1076–87.

in untreated patients are seen primarily in the first 3–5 years after diagnosis. However, patients with ER positive tumors who are treated with endocrine therapy have better short-term and long-term survival as a result of the therapy, too.[9]

In general, ER+ tumors are relatively slower growing, which is reflected in their longer time to recurrence (or disease-free interval), and less aggressive, which is reflected in their greater likelihood of metastasizing to bone, skin, lymph nodes, and other soft tissues rather than to liver, lung, or brain. ER+ tumors occur at higher frequency in postmenopausal women, in older women regardless of menopause, in tumors with a low histological grade, in those with "good histologies" such as tubular, mucinous, and lobular (see Chapter 5), and those with a low proliferative thrust manifest as a low S-phase fraction or Ki-67 (see further discussion later in this chapter). Tumors that overexpress HER2/*neu* (HER2+) are less likely to be ER/PR+.

ER and PR also predict response to therapy. Patients whose tumors are ER+PR+ are more likely to respond, and the higher the ER, the more likely the response, measured either in tumor shrinkage for patients with metastases (see Table 7.1) or disease-free survival among those treated with adjuvant endocrine therapy.[10–12] In a meta-analysis of trials comparing 5 years of adjuvant tamoxifen with no endocrine therapy, the proportional reduction in breast cancer recurrence and mortality was 60% ± 6 and 36% ± 7, respectively, among those with ER ≥ 100 fmol/mg compared with 43% ± 5 and 23% ± 6 for those with ER levels of 10–99 fmol/mg.[12] There was no interaction with PR levels.

Table 7.1 Clinical Benefit Rate and Time to Treatment Failure in Patients with Different ER or PR levels

Receptor Level by IHC	ER		PR	
	Clinical Benefit Rate (%)	TTF (Months)	Clinical Benefit Rate (%)	TTF (Months)
All levels	60		61	
Low/Negative	25	5	46	5
Intermediate	46	4	55	2
High	66	10	70	10
p value	0.001	0.003	0.03	0.007
ER+PR+	62	9		
ER+PR–	55	8		

Clinical benefit rate is defined as a complete or partial response or stable disease for > 6 months, and time to treatment failure (TTF) is the interval from starting treatment to further tumor progression. ER or PR levels were measured by IHC in 205 patients with metastatic disease whose tumors were ER+ tumors by LBA and who were enrolled in a Southwest Oncology Group Trial evaluating tamoxifen therapy.

Data derived from Elledge RM, Green S, Pugh R, et al. Estrogen receptor (ER) and progesterone receptor (PgR), by ligand-binding assay compared with ER, PgR and pS2, by immuno-histochemistry in predicting response to tamoxifen in metastatic breast cancer: a Southwest Oncology Group Study. *Int J Cancer.* 2000;89:111–7.

Patients with ER+ tumors are also less likely to respond to chemotherapy. The pathological complete response (pCR) rate to neoadjuvant chemotherapy is 30%–40% in patients with ER–/PR– tumors, but only 2%–10% when tumors are ER+ and/or PR+[13] (see Chapter 11). A number of randomized trials have demonstrated that the effects of adjuvant chemotherapy on disease-free and overall survival are significantly less in ER+ than in ER– patients, especially those who are postmenopausal.[14] Patients with very high ER+ levels appear to derive no benefit at all (see Chapter 10).

ER and PR are routinely measured on all tumors at the time of initial diagnosis. However, some question the additive value of PR since all ER+ tumors should receive endocrine therapy at one or another time in their disease course, and patients with ER–PR+ may represent laboratory error (see earlier discussion). Although most decisions about therapy throughout a patient's course are based on the initial ER/PR measurements, there is evidence that as many as 25% of patients whose tumors are ER+ at diagnosis will be ER– at relapse.[15] The receptor value obtained closest in time to the treatment decisions appears to be the most predictive.

HER2/NEU (ERBB2)

HER2/neu, a tyrosine kinase receptor (RTK) that appears in small amounts on normal cells, including cardiac cells, is a phosphoprotein (p185^{ERBB2}) that is overexpressed on the surface of 20%–30% of breast cancers, almost always because of amplification of the gene on the short arm of chromosome 17q12. Like ER, it affects the cancer cell growth rate, and it is both a prognostic and a predictive factor.

The mechanisms through which HER2, dimerized with itself or other RTKs of the HER (ErbB) family, drives tumor cell growth by activating a number of signal transduction pathways in the cancer cell are illustrated in Figure 7.3.[16,17] The most important of these pathways is the PI3K/Akt pathway, which, among other things, suppresses apoptosis, thus giving the cancer cell a survival advantage. This pathway is often involved in resistance to chemotherapy. Another signal activated by HER2 is MAPK, and this leads to cell proliferation, migration, differentiation, and angiogenesis. Both of these pathways interact with ER, as well (Figure 7.1).

The most commonly used tests to evaluate for HER2 overexpression are immunohistochemical (IHC) assays using antibodies to p185^{ERBB2}.[18] These are ideally performed on fresh frozen tissue but, for practical reasons, are more often performed on paraffin-embedded tissue. Using guidelines developed by ASCO in cooperation with the American College of Pathology (ACP), a tumor is scored as 3+ and considered HER2 positive (HER2+) if there is uniform intense staining in > 30% of cells; a score of 2+, considered equivocal, is defined as non-uniform with weak intensity in > 10% of cells.[19,20] (see Figure 7.4). About 15% of tumors will stain 2+. The FDA has approved two IHC tests that use different antibodies: HercepTest by Dako and Pathway by Ventana. HER2 gene amplification can be evaluated using fluorescence in situ hybridization (FISH) in which a DNA probe that encodes HER2, labeled with a fluorescent tag, is bound to denatured DNA from the tumor (Figure 7.4). The results are usually reported as the ratio of HER2 gene copies to chromosome 17 centromeres or the number of HER2 gene copies per cell. The ASCO/ACP guidelines define a positive (FISH+) as a ratio > 2.2 or copy number great than 6.0, a negative as < 1.8 or < 4.0, and equivocal anything between these two. Three FISH tests have been approved by

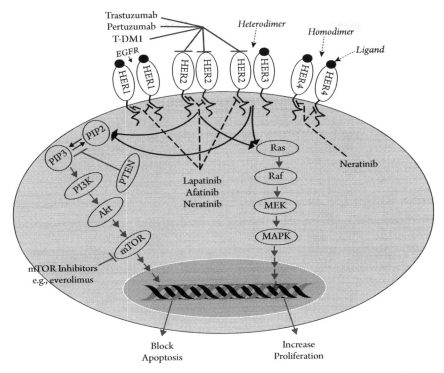

Figure 7.3 Four transmembrane tyrosine kinase receptors (RTKs) constitute the HER or ErbB family: HER1 (ErbB1 or EGFR), HER2 (ErbB2), HER3 (ErbB3), and HER4 (ErbB4). When activated either by ligands or spontaneously, RTKs form homodimers or heterodimers; only a few combinations are illustrated here. HER3 never exists as a homodimer and lacks kinase function, but the HER2:HER3 heterodimer is an especially powerful activator of signaling pathways. HER2 has no ligand but spontaneously forms homodimers that drive this pathway, as well. The PI3K/AKT and MAPK pathways are among the most important affected by these RTKs, and their activation leads to decreased apoptosis, increased cell survival, and increased proliferation. Monoclonal antibodies to the external domain of HER2 (trastuzumab, pertuzumab, and T-DM1) and small molecules that inhibit two to three of the internal domains (lapatinib, neratinib, and afatinib) have been used in the clinic to inhibit breast tumors with amplification of the HER2 gene.
Data from Yarden Y, Pines G. The ERBB network: at last, cancer therapy meets systems biology. *Nature Rev: Cancer.* 2012;12:553–63 and Baselga J, Swain SM. Novel anticancer targets: revisiting ERBB2 and discovering ERBB3. *Nature Rev: Cancer.* 2009;9:463–75.

the FDA: PathVysion by Abbott-Vysis, INFORM by Ventana, and PharmaDx FISH by Dako. There are two other modifications of FISH that have some technical advantages, perform as well but not necessarily better than FISH, and have been approved by the FDA: chromogenic in situ hybridization (CISH) and silver in vitro hybridization (SISH).

IHC is less expensive ($10 for reagents) than FISH ($140) and uses equipment and skills commonly available in most pathology laboratories, but results vary depending on which antibody is used, and there is considerable observer variability.[18] In several studies 94%–99% of patients with either IHC 0/1 or IHC 3+ tumors were

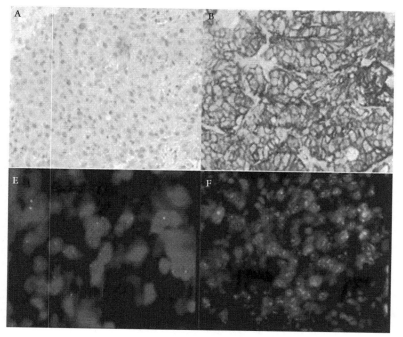

Figure 7.4 Images of paraffin embedded, invasive breast cancer with immunohistochemical (IHC) staining for erbB2 (P185) protein on the cytoplasmic membrane using the HercepTest™ (A and D) or fluorescence in situ hybridization (FISH) using the PathVysion™ probe targeting the chromosome 17 centromere (green dots) or the entire HER2 gene at 17q11.2-q12 (orange dots) (E and F). A is IHC negative and D ICH 3+. E has no amplification; only centromeres are readily seen. F is amplified with a HER2/centromere ratio > 2.2. Images obtained with a Micrometastasis Scoring System.
Reprinted with permission from Ellis CM, Dyson MJ, Stephenson TJ, et al. HER2 amplification status in breast cancer: a comparison between immunohistochemical staining and fluorescence in situ hybridisation using manual and automated quantitative image analysis scoring techniques. *J Clin Pathol*. 2005;58:710–4.

FISH– or FISH+, respectively. However, only 25%–48% of those with an IHC of 2+ were FISH+. For this reason, it is recommended that FISH be routinely performed on all IHC 2+ tumors. Tumors that are 2+ or 3+ by IHC but FISH– do not respond while those that are 0/1+ by IHC but FISH+ do respond to trastuzumab.

HER2 mRNA can also be used to determine HER2 status, but in practice this is only done as part of genomic tests (see discussion of Oncotype DX later in this chapter).

A tumor's HER2 status is less likely than ER status to change from primary diagnosis to relapse. In a longitudinal study, 8.7% of tumors HER2 positive at diagnosis were negative at relapse, and 5.8% of tumors negative at diagnosis were positive at relapse.[15]

Like ER, HER2 positivity is both prognostic[22] (Figure 7.5) and predictive. HER2- negative tumors rarely respond to therapies specifically targeting HER2, such as trastuzumab (see Chapter 12). The predictive value of HER2 in the selection of non-targeted therapies is less certain, but there are studies that suggest that paclitaxel and the anthracyclines have an advantage over regimens without these drugs only for

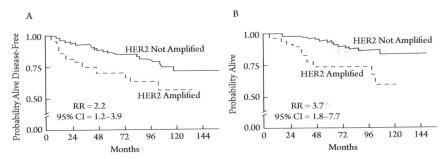

Figure 7.5 Disease-free (A) and overall survival (B) in 232 and 234 patient cohorts defined by HER2 gene amplification using FISH on archived tumors obtained from three universities. All cancers were diagnosed prior to 1990, had no axillary nodal metastases, and were surgically removed without radiation therapy or any form of adjuvant endocrine or chemotherapy. HER2 amplification was seen in 19% of the patients in each cohort. Minimal follow-up was 24 months.
Reprinted with permission from Press MF, Bernstein L, Thomas PA, et al. HER-2/neu gene amplification characterized by fluorescence in situ hybridization: poor prognosis in node-negative breast carcinomas. *J Clin Oncol.* 1997;15:2894–904.

tumors that are HER2+.[21] Some (but not other) trials have demonstrated a smaller benefit from a combination of cyclophosphamide, methotrexate, and 5-fluorouracil in patients whose tumors are HER2+ compared to those with HER– tumors. ER+/ HER2+ tumors are responsive to endocrine therapy, but generally less so than HER2– tumors.

The extracellular domain (ECD) of the HER2 RTK can be detected in the serum and/or pleural effusions of 25%–50% of patients with HER2+ disease. However, low levels can be detected in healthy women and those with HER– tumors, as well, and optimal cutoffs to define cancer are still uncertain. Correlations between either tumor load or clinical endpoints and circulating levels are inconsistent from one study to another.[23] The FDA has approved several types of ELISAs to measure ECD as a way of monitoring therapy, but only three of seven published studies demonstrated a correlation with response in HER2+ tumors to non-targeted therapy. ECD levels appeared to be no more predictive of benefit from anti-HER2 drugs. This test should not yet be generally used in making clinical decisions.

PROLIFERATION INDICES: KI-67 (MIB-1), S-PHASE FRACTION, MITOTIC SCORE

From the clinical observation that some breast cancers grow faster than others (Chapter 4) it is an easy step to hypothesize that tumors with a higher percentage of dividing cells (i.e., those with a high growth fraction) would have the worse prognosis. The earliest and still frequently used method for determining growth fraction is to simply count the number of mitotic figures in the tumor. Growth fraction can be determined by using flow cytometry to measure the fraction of cells in S-phase, but this has the disadvantage of requiring fresh tissue. Assays of cellular proteins present only during mitosis, such as Ki-67 or PCNA (proliferating cell nuclear antigen), are being developed. Most studies have demonstrated that all of these methods are prognostic and may also be predictive of response in at least some situations. All have been used as clinical decision-making tools and are usually part of any clinical algorithm that combines several prognostic markers.

Mitotic count (or mitotic index, MI) is an important component of histological grading (see Chapter 5). This is usually reported as the number of mitoses observed in 10 high-powered fields (hpf's) with empirically derived subdivisions such as low risk = ≤ 9 mitoses/10 hpf; moderate risk = 10–19 mitoses/10 hpf; and high risk ≥ 20 mitoses/10 hpf using a 0.59 mm diameter microscopic field.[24] There is more evidence for the prognostic power of mitotic count than any other way of measuring cellular proliferation.[25] In multivariate analyses combining multiple studies, the HR for high compared to low MI was 2.32 (95% CI, 1.76–3.06) for mortality and 2.39 (95% CI, 1.73–3.28) for recurrence.[26]

Ki-67 is a nuclear non-histone protein that is expressed only in G_1, G_2, and especially in S phases of the cell cycle. Its function is not certain. Another antibody targeting the same epitope, MIB-1, can be measured in paraffin-embedded tissue and is now used more frequently than Ki-67.[27] There is good correlation between Ki-67 level and mitotic counts. Patients with high ER generally have low Ki-67. The evidence that Ki-67/MIB-1 is a good prognostic factor is very strong but not entirely consistent from one study to the next. This seems to be in part due to the lack of either standard methodology for performing the assay or agreed-upon cut points. Two meta-analyses have been conducted, and both demonstrated a highly significant correlation between Ki-67 and outcomes.[28] In a multivariate analysis the HR for high compared to low Ki-67/MIB-1 levels was 1.73 (95% CI, 1.37–2.17) for mortality and 1.84 (95% CI, 1.62–2.10) for recurrence.

In preclinical systems, cells in S-phase respond better to chemotherapy than those primarily in G_0 even if the drug used is not considered to be cycle-dependent. Thus it is not surprising that there is considerable evidence from clinical studies that tumors with a high growth fraction are more responsive, too. A number of studies have demonstrated that patients with a high Ki-67 are more likely to have a pCR following neoadjuvant therapy, but Ki-67 is not predictive of response to endocrine therapy.[13] However, a fall in Ki-67 following neoadjuvant endocrine or chemotherapy is associated with a higher probability of a subsequent objective response and better overall outcome.

UPA (UROKINASE PLASMINOGEN ACTIVATOR) AND PAI-1 (PLASMINOGEN ACTIVATOR INHIBITOR)

uPA and PAI-1 are part of the plasminogen activating system, but they also appear to play a role in the migration, invasion, angiogenesis, and metastases of tumor cells by degrading extra-cellular matrix. Low levels of the two proteins have repeatedly been shown to be associated with a good prognosis, and they have been shown in a large prospective randomized trial to be predictive of benefit from chemotherapy in patients without lymph node involvement.[14] In this trial, patients with low levels received no adjuvant chemotherapy, while those with high levels of uPA and PAI-1 were randomized to receive adjuvant CMF (cyclophosphamide, methotrexate, and 5-fluorouracil) or no adjuvant treatment. At 10 years, 12.9% of low and 23.0% of the high uPA/PAI-1 tumors had recurred ($p = 0.011$). Adjuvant CMF reduced the risk of recurrence by

26% in the high uPA/PAI-1 tumors. The results of a second large trial utilizing other forms of chemotherapy are pending. No other marker has such robust evidence supporting its use, both as a prognostic and predictive factor. However, the test is not commonly used because the ELISA assay for uPA/PAI-1 requires fresh frozen tissue, and it has not been shown that its use adds to or is superior to established prognostic/predictive tools.

CA 15-3 OR CA 27.29 AND CEA

CA 15-3 and CA 27.29 are monoclonal antibodies to MUC-1, a glycoprotein secreted by breast cancer cells. These markers are elevated in 8%–20% of breast cancers around the time of diagnosis or the completion of local treatment; variations in results are likely related to the time when the sample was obtained relative to therapy and the mix of patient stages in the cohort studied. Elevated levels are associated with a poor prognosis, but these tests are not routinely obtained early on because of the likelihood of false positives.[21] It has been demonstrated in several studies that elevations of the markers occur, on average, 5–6 months before metastases can be detected, but because it has not been shown that this knowledge leads to improved outcomes, these tests are not routinely recommended prior to documentation of recurrence in more conventional ways. Between 75% and 90% of metastatic tumors will have an abnormal value, and the frequency increases each time the disease progresses further.[21,29] Those with visceral metastases, especially liver and bone, are most likely to have elevations. A fall in the level of the marker is associated with a longer time to disease progression, but a concordance between a change in the marker and progression or regression at other sites occurred only 50% of the time.[30] During the first 6–12 weeks following the initiation of therapy, there may be a sudden increase ("surge" or "spike") in the marker level in up to 20% of patients who eventually respond to treatment. This is thought to be related to tumor lysis and should not be used as a reason for discontinuing therapy. It is recommended that CA15-3 or CA 27.29 be used in conjunction with imaging studies and physical examination to monitor patients with metastatic breast cancer and that an increase in value after the first 3 months of therapy be accepted as evidence of disease progression in a patient with no other measurable sites of metastases.[21]

CEA (carcinoembryonic antigen) is elevated in only 50%–60% of patients with metastatic breast cancer, but the CEA is rarely abnormal in patients without elevated MUC-1 antigen levels.[21] It appears to have the same value and limitations as the CA 15-3 and CA 27.29, so it is recommended that it be obtained serially only if it is elevated and neither of the MUC-1 antigens is abnormal.

EMERGING BIOMARKERS WITH POTENTIAL VALUE

A number of molecular markers have been studied extensively and appear to have prognostic and/or predictive value but are not yet commonly used, usually because either data from studies are inconsistent, the quality of key studies is considered suboptimal, or no standard assay with widely agreed-upon cut points is yet available (see Table 7.2). Some of these markers are likely to be included in future multimarker arrays (see Table 7.2).

Table 7.2 Factors Found to Have Prognostic or Predictive Value for Patients With Breast Cancer but Not Yet Used Commonly for Management Decisions

Marker	Function/Role	Association with BC	Outcomes Related to OE or AMP
Cyclin D1	Cell cycle regulator (G1-S), especially of ER+ cells	OE in 50%, AMP in 15% of breast cancers	OE ProgF for better outcome in ER+ BC; AMP ProgF for early relapse; OE possibly PredF for poor response to anti-estrogens
Cyclin E	Cell cycle regulator (G1-S), possible role in breast tumorigenesis	Associated with BRCA1 mutations	OE of full protein or cleavage products; ProgF for poor DFS and OS, possible PredF for increased sensitivity to cisplatin & paclitaxel and resistance to anti-estrogens
Topoisomerase IIα	Repairs double-strand DNA breaks induced by cytotoxics, especially anthracyclines	Located on chromosome 17 near HER2 gene. AMP almost always in conjunction with HER2 AMP	AMP may be associated with increased sensitivity to the anthracyclines
p53	Tumor suppressor gene	Mutated in 20%–30% of all BC, more often in the more aggressive types, such as triple-negative and basal-like	Mutation/deletions ProgF in many studies, but results are inconsistent; use of IHC in paraffin-embedded tissues is unreliable. Possibly PredF for response to cytotoxic agents
Cathepsin D	Lysosomal protease OE & hyper-secreted in BC. It is mitogenic & degrades proteins in extracellular space, enables tumor cell invasion and angiogenesis		ProgF in many studies, but largest retrospective analyses suggest that the prognostic discrimination is relatively weak, especially in multivariate analyses

OE = overexpression or overexpressed; AMP = amplification or amplified; ProgF = prognostic factor; PredF = predictive factor; BC = breast cancer; DFS = disease-free survival; OS = overall survival.

From Harris L, Fritsche H, Mennel R, et al. American Society of Clinical Oncology 2007 update of recommendations for the use of tumor markers in breast cancer. *J Clin Oncol.* 2007;25:5287–312; and Weigel MT, Dowsett M. Current and emerging biomarkers in breast cancer: prognosis and prediction. *Endocr Relat Cancer.* 2010;17:R245–62.

GENOMIC PROFILE OF BREAST CANCERS: INTRINSIC MOLECULAR SUBTYPES

The biomarkers described earlier mostly represent the effect of one or a small number of genes, but it is unlikely that the abnormal behavior of a single gene accounts for all the pathological manifestations of most tumors, or that targeting a single gene will eliminate or suppress tumor growth. Recently attempts have been made to capture much more information about the relative expression of various genes in tumors compared to non-tumorous tissues. One measure of gene activity is its expression—or lack of expression—of mRNA, which can occur because a gene is either amplified or deleted, or because changes in its regulation (e.g., as a result of mutation) has caused it to produce abnormal amounts of mRNA. It seems plausible that some or many of the differences in gene expression between cancerous and non-cancerous tissues will explain the abnormal behavior of cancerous cells. Fortunately, the mRNA expression of multiple genes can be measured at one moment in time (a microarray). Analyses of microarrays demonstrate that there are not only numerous differences between cancerous and non-cancerous cells but also multiple differences in the relative expression of various genes in cancers ostensibly of the same histological type. Gene expression changes seen frequently have been grouped together, and the behavior of tumors within these groups seems to be more like that of other tumors in the group than that of tumors in other groups.

The relative activity (or "expression") of 496 genes (the "intrinsic genes") in 42 individual tumors is illustrated in Figure 7.6.[31] This is a common way of illustrating gene expression patterns. The clusters found in this study have subsequently been found in multiple other studies using different tumors and different methods of measuring gene expression. They have also been shown to correlate with more traditional classifications of breast cancers[32] (see Figure 7.7). At present, breast cancers are usually grouped into four molecular classes: basal-like, luminal A, luminal B, and HER2-like. The majority (50%–60%) of breast cancers are luminal, and most of these are ER+ and HER2–. Luminal As are histologically better differentiated or low grade, more universally responsive to endocrine therapy, and slower growing (thus smaller in size with fewer lymph nodes and a lower Ki-67 at diagnosis) than luminal Bs. By definition, HER2-like tumors are all HER2+, but they can be either ER+ or ER–. They tend to be high grade and advanced at diagnosis.

BASAL-LIKE AND TRIPLE NEGATIVE (TN) BREAST CANCER

Basal-like cancers, a category that became important clinically only after the introduction of gene expression profiles, include but are not synonymous with "triple-negative (TN) cancers," that is, tumors that are ER–, PR– and HER2–. About 80% of TN tumors are basal-like.[33] More than 75% of BRCA1 tumors are basal-like or TN. Although often discussed as a homogenous group, there are clearly distinct subsets with different clinical phenotypes; disparities in the mix of these subtypes from one study to another may affect outcome measures.[33] The presence or absence of cytokeratin 5 and EGFR may distinguish two of these subsets. Basal-like and TN tumors generally have the worst prognosis of all tumor types, at least in the first years after

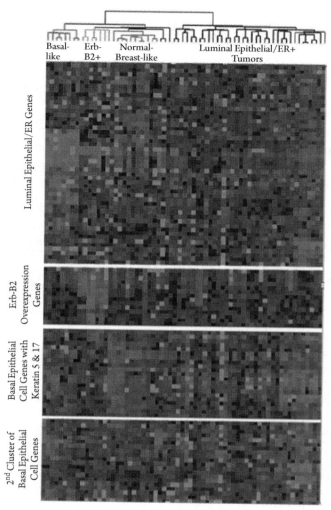

Figure 7.6 Intrinsic breast cancer subtypes defined from a cluster analysis of gene expression arrays (complementary DNA of tumor mRNA) in 65 tumor specimens from 42 patients using 496 genes (the "intrinsic gene set"); for these 496 genes there was greater variation in gene expression in tumor-to-tumor comparisons than in repeated measurements of a single tumor. In the figure, each column represents one tumor specimen; each row represents one gene. A red square represents increased expression of the gene represented by that row and the tumor represented by that column, relative to the expression of that gene in all other tumors in the study. Green represents decreased expression, and black average expression. Tumors with similar gene expression profiles are grouped together; the classifications of the tumors are shown in the dendrogram at the top. The classification of genes that clustered together is shown at the left edge of the figure.

Reprinted with permission from Perou CM, Sorlie T, Eisen MB, et al. Molecular portraits of human breast tumours. *Nature.* 2000;406:747–52.

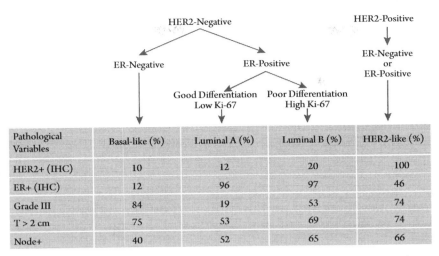

Pathological Variables	Basal-like (%)	Luminal A (%)	Luminal B (%)	HER2-like (%)
HER2+ (IHC)	10	12	20	100
ER+ (IHC)	12	96	97	46
Grade III	84	19	53	74
T > 2 cm	75	53	69	74
Node+	40	52	65	66

Figure 7.7 Relationship between molecular classification (basal-like, luminal A, luminal B, and HER2-like) and more traditional clinicopathological features of breast cancer.
Adapted from Sotiriou C, Pusztai L. Gene-expression signatures in breast cancer. *N Engl J Med.* 2009;360:790–800.

diagnosis (Figures 7.7 and 7.8), constitute ~ 15% of all breast cancers, and occur more frequently in black and Hispanic women. Risk factors for developing these cancers differ, as well.[33] In spite of speculation to the contrary, there is insufficient evidence to conclude that these tumors arise from different breast cells than other breast cancer subtypes. These tumors are more likely to metastasize to viscera than bone and seem to recur locally more often than other subtypes. Placing a patient in this subgroup has important therapeutic implications (see Chapter 12).

TN or basal-like tumors tend to recur at a much higher rate than other subtypes during the first 3–4 years following diagnosis, but after that there is no difference in the hazard of recurrence[34] (see Figure 7.8A). Once metastases are diagnosed, the median duration of survival (6–9 months) is also shorter than that of other tumor types. However, by 10 years of follow-up, the overall survival of HER2+ tumors (luminal B and HER2-like) diagnosed in the era prior to trastuzumab availability was worse[35] (see Figure 7.8B).

USE OF GENOMIC ASSAYS TO PREDICT CLINICAL OUTCOMES

A large number of tests of multi-gene function are under development, and two, OncotypeDX and MammaPrint, are commercially available and widely used (see Table 7.3). Each genomics (or "omics") test measures the expression of several to nearly 100 genes in the tumor cell, using either qRT-PCR or a microarray. These data are then correlated with clinical outcomes, such as time to recurrence, and the information from individual genes is weighted using complex algorithms to provide a test output. This may be a continuous variable defining risk, a risk category, or the molecular subtype of the tumor. Tests that use formalin-fixed paraffin-embedded tissue are

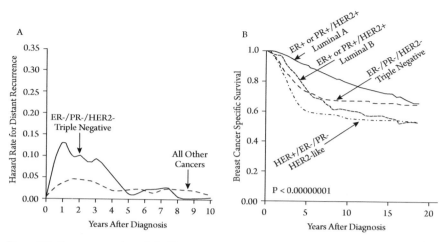

Figure 7.8 Recurrence and survival of breast cancer groups in molecular subtypes determined using immunohistochemical methods. A: The hazard rate for distant recurrence was determined for 61 triple negative patients and compared to 290 patients with non-triple negative cancer from a hospital database of 1,601 patients diagnosed between 1987 and 1997. About half of all the patients had received chemotherapy, half tamoxifen, and none trastuzumab prior to recurrence [Dent R, Trudeau M, Pritchard KI, et al. Triple-negative breast cancer: clinical features and patterns of recurrence. Clin Cancer Res 2007;13:4429–34]. B: 4040 patients entered into a regional database between 1986 and 1992 were retrospectively divided into four groups (2,620 luminal A, 221 luminal B, 258 HER-like, and 639 triple negative) to compare breast cancer–specific survival. Patients were treated with endocrine and chemotherapy but no trastuzumab.

Reprinted with permission from Cheang MC, Voduc D, Bajdik C, et al. Basal-like breast cancer defined by five biomarkers has superior prognostic value than triple-negative phenotype. *Clin Cancer Res.* 2008;14:1368–76.

more practical; this is true for all of the tests shown in Table 7.3, but some, such as MammaPrint and GGI, can use both. Most of the commercially available tests are performed in a central, CLIA approved laboratory, but Nanostring Technologies plans to market kits and equipment that will enable local laboratories to perform the MAP50.

The process of developing these tests is long and arduous. Some tests have gained considerable popularity and have even been used in clinical decision-making before reported tests outputs were shown to be misleading.[36] Before acceptance into routine clinical practice, the test should be shown to have clinical utility, which means that its use should be shown to improve patient outcomes at least as well or better than other approaches, ideally in a prospective randomized trial. Demonstrations of clinical utility are either missing or suboptimal for all the tests listed in Table 7.3, but OncotypeDX and MammaPrint are currently being evaluated in a several large, randomized trials.

Two different approaches to the initial creation of the tests have been employed. In a "bottom-up" approach, genes known to have clinical importance are combined in the assay. OncotypeDX is an example of this approach.[37] Initially, 250 candidate genes previously demonstrated to have some importance in the clinical behavior of breast cancer were selected; then an algorithm was developed to identify the minimal gene

Table 7.3. Multi-Gene Tests in the Clinic or Under Development in North America

Test (Alternative Names)	Company	Genes in Signature	Technique	No. of Patients/No. of Evaluable Studies*	Test Output
OncotypeDX	Genomic Health	21	qRT-PCR	4,219/21	Risk Score (RS) as Continuous Variable 1–100
MammaPrint	Agendia	70	Microarray	1,465/15	Risk Groups: "good" or "poor"
PAM50 (Prosigna)	Nanostring Technologies	50	qRT-PCR & Nanostring	1,496/2	Molecular Profile Subtype AND Risk of Relapse (ROR) Score as Continuous Variable 1–100
Breast Cancer Index (BCI, Theros)	bioTheranostics	7	qRT-PCR	539/2	Risk Score Indexed as Continuous Variable 1–10
Genomic Grade Index (GGI, MapQuant DX)	Ipsogen	97	Microarray	1,284/5	Genomic Grade "low" or "high"

qT-PCR = quantitative reverse-transcriptase–polymerase-chain-reaction.

*From systematic search of literature for evaluable patients in evaluable models designed to assess the clinical validity and utility of the test. From Azim HA, et al. Utility of prognostic genomic tests in breast cancer practice: The IMPAKT 2012 Working Group Consensus Statement. *Annals Oncol.* 2013;24(3):647–654.

set required to provide the best association with breast cancer recurrence. This proved to be 16 cancer-related and 5 reference genes (see Table 7.4).

In a "top-down" approach, genes found to be associated with clinical outcomes are selected without regard to or knowledge of their function. MammaPrint is an example of this approach. The genomes of 78 tumors were evaluated for 25,000 genes to identify genes significantly increased or decreased in at least three tumors; 231 of these genes were associated with disease recurrence, and eventually 70 genes were found to constitute an optimal gene set for the test.

There is considerable concordance in the classification of patients using these different methods in spite of the fact that each is measuring different genes. For example, MammaPrint and OncotypeDX have only one gene in common: SCUBE2.

Table 7.4 Genes Included in the OncotypeDX Test

Gene Group Function	Number of Genes in Group	Specific Genes
Proliferation and anti-apoptosis	5	Ki-67
		STK15 (seronine/threonine kinase 15)
		Survivin
		CCNB1 (cyclin B1)
		MYBL2
Estrogen sensitivity	4	ER
		PR
		BCL2
		SCUBE2
Invasiveness	2	MMP11 (Stromolysin 3)
		CTSL2 (Cathepsin L2)
HER2	2	GRB7
		HER2
Estrogen-related	2	GSTM1
		BAG1
Macrophage marker	1	CD68
Housekeeper or reference genes	5	ACTB (b-actin)
		GAPDH
		RPLPO
		GUS
		TRFC

Algorithm for Oncotype Recurrence Score (RS) = + 0.47 × HER-2 group score − 0.34 × estrogen group score + 1.04 × proliferation group score + 0.10 × invasion group score + 0.05 × CD-68 − 0.08 × GSTM-1 − 0.07 × BAG-1. Although the risk increases continuous with RS, patients with ER+ tumors and no lymph node involved are usually classified as having a low (RS < 18), intermediate RS (18–31) or high (RS > 31) risk of distant recurrence.

Adapted from Paik S, Shak S, Tang G, et al. A multigene assay to predict recurrence of tamoxifen-treated, node-negative breast cancer. *N Engl J Med.* 2004;351:2817–26.

All of the tests in Table 7.3 provide information on prognosis, and none has been specifically approved for selecting among treatment options. (Only MammaPrint has FDA approval, and CLIA laboratory certification does not address the indications for a test.) However, Oncotype and MammaPrint are both used frequently to decide whether to use adjuvant chemotherapy for node-negative patients (see Chapter 10), and as many as 25%–30% of treatment recommendations may be changed as a result of the test results. It is likely that the patient groups for whom these tests may be beneficial and their predictive value for specific types of therapy will expand rapidly in the next few years.

ALTERNATIVES TO CURRENTLY AVAILABLE GENOMICS TESTS

Comparative trials have not yet established that the genomics tests are superior to combinations of individual biomarkers measured with immunohistochemistry. Such IHC tests include Mammastrat, which has five markers (p53, NDRG1, SLC7A5, CEACAM5, HTP9C) and IHC4 (ER, PR, HER2 and Ki-67). At the same time, new technologies that allow efficient and relatively less expensive studies of the genome, such as next-generation sequencing, permit evaluation of mutations, intratumoral genomic heterogeneity, DNA methylation, the effect of single nucleotide polymorphisms (SNPs), and the effect of microenvironment. The process of defining breast cancer subtypes is likely to expand increasingly more rapidly. The era of using these technologies to personalize treatment has only just started.

REFERENCES

1. Musgrove EA, Sutherland RL. Biological determinants of endocrine resistance in breast cancer. *Nature Rev Cancer.* 2009;9:631–43.
2. Osborne CK, Schiff R. Mechanisms of endocrine resistance in breast cancer. *Annu Rev Med.* 2011;62:233–47.
3. Le Romancer M, Poulard C, Cohen P, et al. Cracking the estrogen receptor's posttranslational code in breast tumors. *Endocr Rev.* 2011;32:597–622.
4. Clarke R, Cook KL, Hu R, et al. Endoplasmic reticulum stress, the unfolded protein response, autophagy, and the integrated regulation of breast cancer cell fate. *Cancer Res.* 2012;72:1321–31.
5. Miller TW, Balko JM, Arteaga CL. Phosphatidylinositol 3-kinase and antiestrogen resistance in breast cancer. *J Clin Oncol.* 2011;29:4452–61.
6. Hammond ME, Hayes DF, Dowsett M, et al. American Society of Clinical Oncology/College of American Pathologists guideline recommendations for immunohistochemical testing of estrogen and progesterone receptors in breast cancer. *J Clin Oncol.* 2010;28:2784–95.
7. Osborne CK. Receptors. In: Harris JR, Hellman S, Henderson IC, et al., eds. *Breast Diseases.* 2nd ed. Philadelphia: J. B. Lippincott; 1991:301–25.
8. Fisher B, Redmond C, Fisher ER, et al. Relative worth of estrogen or progesterone receptor and pathologic characteristics of differentiation as indicators of prognosis in node negative breast cancer patients: findings from National Surgical Adjuvant Breast and Bowel Project Protocol B-06. *J Clin Oncol.* 1988;6:1076–87.

9. Jatoi I, Anderson WF, Jeong JH, et al. Breast cancer adjuvant therapy: time to consider its time-dependent effects. *J Clin Oncol.* 2011;29:2301–4.

10. Elledge RM, Green S, Pugh R, et al. Estrogen receptor (ER) and progesterone receptor (PgR), by ligand-binding assay compared with ER, PgR and pS2, by immuno-histochemistry in predicting response to tamoxifen in metastatic breast cancer: a Southwest Oncology Group Study. *Int J Cancer.* 2000;89:111–7.

11. Dowsett M, Allred C, Knox J, et al. Relationship between quantitative estrogen and progesterone receptor expression and human epidermal growth factor receptor 2 (HER-2) status with recurrence in the Arimidex, Tamoxifen, Alone or in Combination trial. *J Clin Oncol.* 2008;26:1059–65.

12. Early Breast Cancer Trialists Collaborative Group. Tamoxifen for early breast cancer: an overview of the randomised trials. Early Breast Cancer Trialists' Collaborative Group. *Lancet.* 1998;351:1451–67.

13. Colleoni M, Viale G, Goldhirsch A. Lessons on responsiveness to adjuvant systemic therapies learned from the neoadjuvant setting. *Breast.* 2009;18 Suppl 3:S137–40.

14. Bedard PL, Cardoso F. Can some patients avoid adjuvant chemotherapy for early-stage breast cancer? *Nature Rev Clin Oncol.* 2011;8:272–9.

15. Lindstrom LS, Karlsson E, Wilking UM, et al. Clinically used breast cancer markers such as estrogen receptor, progesterone receptor, and human epidermal growth factor receptor 2 are unstable throughout tumor progression. *J Clin Oncol.* 2012;30:2601–8.

16. Yarden Y, Pines G. The ERBB network: at last, cancer therapy meets systems biology. *Nature Rev: Cancer.* 2012;12:553–63.

17. Baselga J, Swain SM. Novel anticancer targets: revisiting ERBB2 and discovering ERBB3. *Nature Rev: Cancer.* 2009;9:463–75.

18. Shah S, Chen B. Testing for HER2 in breast cancer: a continuing evolution. *Pathol Res Int.* 2011;2011:903202.

19. Wolff AC, Hammond ME, Schwartz JN, et al. American Society of Clinical Oncology/ College of American Pathologists guideline recommendations for human epidermal growth factor receptor 2 testing in breast cancer. *J Clin Oncol.* 2007;25:118–45.

20. Ellis CM, Dyson MJ, Stephenson TJ, et al. HER2 amplification status in breast cancer: a comparison between immunohistochemical staining and fluorescence in situ hybridisation using manual and automated quantitative image analysis scoring techniques. *J Clin Pathol.* 2005;58:710–4.

21. Harris L, Fritsche H, Mennel R, et al. American Society of Clinical Oncology 2007 update of recommendations for the use of tumor markers in breast cancer. *J Clin Oncol.* 2007;25:5287–312.

22. Press MF, Bernstein L, Thomas PA, et al. HER-2/neu gene amplification characterized by fluorescence in situ hybridization: poor prognosis in node-negative breast carcinomas. *J Clin Oncol.* 1997;15:2894–904.

23. Leyland-Jones B, Smith BR. Serum HER2 testing in patients with HER2-positive breast cancer: the death knell tolls. *Lancet Oncol.* 2011;12:286–95.

24. Aleskandarany MA, Green AR, Benhasouna AA, et al. Prognostic value of proliferation assay in the luminal, HER2-positive, and triple-negative biologic classes of breast cancer. *Breast Cancer Res.* 2012;14:R3.

25. van Diest PJ, van der Wall E, Baak JP. Prognostic value of proliferation in invasive breast cancer: a review. *J Clin Pathol.* 2004;57:675–81.

26. Stuart-Harris R, Caldas C, Pinder SE, et al. Proliferation markers and survival in early breast cancer: a systematic review and meta-analysis of 85 studies in 32,825 patients. *Breast*. 2008;17:323–34.

27. Weigel MT, Dowsett M. Current and emerging biomarkers in breast cancer: prognosis and prediction. *Endocr Relat Cancer*. 2010;17:R245–62.

28. Luporsi E, Andre F, Spyratos F, et al. Ki-67: level of evidence and methodological considerations for its role in the clinical management of breast cancer: analytical and critical review. *Br Cancer Res Treat*. 2012;132:895–915.

29. Laessig D, Nagel D, Heinemann V, et al. Importance of CEA and CA 15-3 during disease progression in metastatic breast cancer patients. *Anticancer Res*. 2007;27:1963–8.

30. Duffy MJ, Evoy D, McDermott EW. CA 15-3: uses and limitation as a biomarker for breast cancer. *Clin Chim Acta*. 2010;411:1869–74.

31. Perou CM, Sorlie T, Eisen MB, et al. Molecular portraits of human breast tumours. *Nature*. 2000;406:747–52.

32. Sotiriou C, Pusztai L. Gene-expression signatures in breast cancer. *N Engl J Med*. 2009;360:790–800.

33. Foulkes WD, Smith IE, Reis-Filho JS. Triple-negative breast cancer. *N Engl J Med*. 2010;363:1938–48.

34. Dent R, Trudeau M, Pritchard KI, et al. Triple-negative breast cancer: clinical features and patterns of recurrence. *Clin Cancer Res*. 2007;13:4429–34.

35. Cheang MC, Voduc D, Bajdik C, et al. Basal-like breast cancer defined by five biomarkers has superior prognostic value than triple-negative phenotype. *Clin Cancer Res*. 2008;14:1368–76.

36. *Evolution of Translational Omics: Lessons Learned and the Path Forward*. Washington, DC: The National Academies Press; 2012.

37. Paik S, Shak S, Tang G, et al. A multigene assay to predict recurrence of tamoxifen-treated, node-negative breast cancer. *N Engl J Med*. 2004;351:2817–26.

8

DIAGNOSIS, WORKUP, AND FOLLOW-UP
OF BREAST CANCER PATIENTS

Most patients with breast cancer are diagnosed because of self-discovered masses (25% from self-examination and 18% accidentally) or symptoms; 43% are found on screening mammography.[1] More recently, the frequency of mammogram-detected cancers has increased to 56% in women aged 50–59, the group where mammography is known to be most effective and where it is most consistently recommended. Other key symptoms of breast cancer that lead patients to seek evaluation include the following:

- Changes in the size of one breast
- Nipple inversion or dimpling of skin away from the nipple
- Skin changes, such as redness, increased warmth in one part or over an entire breast, pitting of the skin giving the texture of an orange (peau d'orange), or skin puckering
- Nipple discharge other than milk, sometimes bloody, especially if in only one breast
- Thickening or hardening of part of the breast
- Breast pain (more often associated with benign breast conditions, especially if there is no mass, but 5% of breast cancer lesions are painful; it should not be assumed that pain means "benign")
- Enlarged lymph nodes in the axilla
- Symptoms of distant disease such as bone pain, respiratory symptoms, jaundice, cognitive dysfunction, or headache that could result from hypercalcemia or CNS metastases, or localized neurologic signs.

HISTORY AND ASCERTAINMENT OF RISK

In obtaining an initial history, information should be obtained on changes and the time course of change in the breast, as opposed to differences between the two breasts. Differences in the size of the breasts is normal, while a change in the size of one breast should be carefully evaluated. Thickening, especially in the inframammary fold, is common, and when present for a long time should not elicit concern. The waxing and waning of breast pain relative to the menstrual cycle is common and often associated with breast cysts.

A patient's risk of developing breast cancer is usually determined. If so, greater diligence may be given to evaluating a sign or symptom that might otherwise be just watched in a low-risk patient. However, 80% of women with breast cancer have no identifiable risk factors, and too much emphasis on risk may lead a clinician to devalue borderline findings or to be too casual in examining a patient at low risk. The most important risk factors are the following:

- Patient age: While risk does increase with age, breast cancers may rarely occur in teenagers, and 2.4% of all breast cancers occur among women aged < 35 and 6.6% in those < 40 (see Chapter 1).
- Prior breast cancer, such as an in situ cancer, or a biopsy proven premalignant lesion (see Chapter 3)
- Inherited genetic disorders: 3%–5% of breast cancers occur in women with BRCA1 or BRCA2 mutations. Other syndromes with increased risk include Li Fraumeni, Cowden's, and Peutz-Jeghers (see Chapter 1).
- Family history of breast cancer, especially in a first-degree relative: mother, sister, daughter, father, brother, son (see Chapter 1)
- Early menarche with early onset of regular menses and late first pregnancy (see Chapter 1)
- Increased breast density on mammograms (see Chapter 1)
- Radiation to the chest with inclusion of the breast prior to age 40.

CLINICAL BREAST EXAMINATION (CBE)

Many breast cancers cannot be detected on physical examination, but no method of cancer detection is more specific. In pooled results from six formal studies, the sensitivity of CBE was 54.1% and specificity 94.0%.[2] The duration of the CBE is the most important factor affecting the likelihood of finding a cancer. It has been calculated that the optimal duration is between 6 and 8 minutes.

CBE consists of careful inspection and palpation of the breast with the patient both sitting and supine.

Specific abnormalities to look for on inspection while the patient is sitting include the following:

- Any asymmetry in the size or shape of the breasts
- Inversion of the nipple
- Dimpling of the skin: This abnormality can usually be best seen if the patient is asked to contract her pectoralis muscles by first pressing her hands against her waist and then pressing her hands against her forehead so dimpling in the lower quadrants can be easily seen. The pectoralis muscles attach to Cooper's ligaments, which course through the breast and attach to the skin. Lesions growing in the breast, especially slow-growing lesions, often entangle these ligaments, causing them to shorten and in turn to tug on the skin.
- Localized swelling in one area of the breast: This may reflect an underlying mass, especially for a lobular cancer.

Look for changes in the skin overlying the breast while the patient is sitting and supine. Specifically identify the following:

- Areas of erythema with or without increased warmth of the skin: These areas may be very small or may encompass a substantial portion of the entire breast. Inflammatory breast cancer is a particularly aggressive form of the disease that classically was described as skin changes suggesting an infection, including erythema and warmth, without an underlying mass (see Chapter 6). It is often misdiagnosed as an infection and treated with antibiotics, thus delaying diagnosis (see Chapter 11).
- Patchy or extensive skin edema: This occurs when underlying lymphatics are plugged with tumor in patients with locally advanced or inflammatory breast cancer. These changes, along with erythema, may make the skin look like that of an orange—thus its designation as "peau d'orange."
- Flaking, nodularity, or small ulceration on or at the edge of the nipple: These may be the only signs of Paget's disease, another form of breast cancer that is characterized by tumor cells populating the undersurface of the nipple, either as the only manifestation of the cancer or accompanying a deeper mass that may or may not be readily felt during the CBE.

While the patient is sitting, compress the breast between both hands to detect masses. While this form of palpation is not as sensitive as examination while the patient is supine, there are some lesions, especially those immediately below the nipple, that can be appreciated more readily while the patient is sitting.

Look for lymphadenopathy in the supraclavicular, infraclavicular, and axillary areas. These examinations are usually performed best with the patient sitting.

The most demanding and time-consuming part of the CBE is palpation in the supine position. Although there has been considerable work in recent years to identify the most effective ways of performing this part of the CBE, there is no universally accepted approach (see Figure 8.1).[2-4] Breast tissues is not evenly distributed; 41% is in the upper outer quadrant, 34% behind the nipple, 14% in the upper inner quadrant, and 5% and 6%, respectively, in the inner and outer lower quadrants. Breast cancers have a similar distribution in the breast.

Cancerous lesions are classically hard, single, well defined, and have either regular or irregular edges. They may take almost any shape. Most cancers, especially early ones, are freely movable, but more advanced cancers may be fixed either to the fascia of underlying muscle or to overlying skin. When a well-defined lesion that is different from anything else in the breast and highly suspicious for cancer is found on the CBE, label it as a "dominant mass," since it cannot be called a cancer prior to histological evaluation but should be treated as such until proven otherwise by biopsy. Invasive lobular cancers are often difficult to define on CBE since they may be very large and may appear more as a thickening than a discrete mass. All mass lesions and areas of thickening should be measured with calipers.

Benign lesions, such as fibroadenomas or cysts, are more often very regular, round, slightly softer, and freely moveable. Breast "lumpiness" is common, especially in premenopausal women. It is often reassuring to patients to understand that this is normal and that lumpiness per se is not a risk factor for disease. Since it is not pathological, avoid describing it to the patient or in the record as "fibrocystic disease."

Prior to further evaluation of any suspicious findings, the results of the CBE should be carefully recorded. No other area of medicine is subject to more litigation than "failure to diagnose" breast cancer, but good record-keeping will reduce this risk

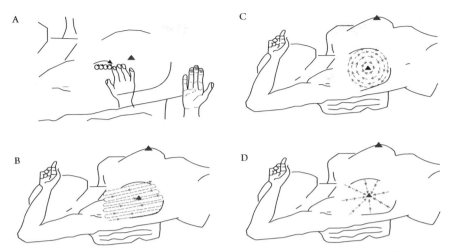

Figure 8.1 Clinical breast examination (CBE): Palpation of the breast. The patient should be on a flat surface but slightly turned with her hand resting on her head. This positions the breast so that it is not continuously shifting during the exam. The patient is usually more comfortable and able to maintain this position throughout the examination if a pillow or towel is placed under the ipsilateral shoulder. All breast tissue is then examined with several levels of pressure using the surface of the 2nd, 3rd, and 4th fingers of the examining hand, which moves in small circles about the size of a dime (A). Alternatively, breast tissue may be rolled between two fingers while they are alternating pressure, such as typing two keys on a typewriter or playing two keys on the piano (not shown). Three different patterns of palpation commonly used are (B) the vertical strip (MammaCare®), (C) concentric circles, and (D) radial spokes. In studies of breast self-examination, the vertical strip appears to encompass more breast tissue, but there are no direct comparisons of the three patterns of CBE by clinicians.
Modified from Barton MB, Harris R, Fletcher SW. The rational clinical examination. Does this patient have breast cancer? The screening clinical breast examination: should it be done? How? *J Am Med Assoc.* 1999;282:1270–80; McDonald S, Saslow D, Alciati MH. Performance and reporting of clinical breast examination: a review of the literature. *CA Cancer J Clin.* 2004;54:345–61; and Goodson WH, 3rd. Clinical breast examination. *West J Med.* 1996;164:355–8.

substantially while indicating appropriate follow-through after completion of the CBE. Describe the elements of the examination (e.g., palpation using vertical strip) and list pertinent negatives such as the lack of asymmetry, architectural distortion, nipple inversion, or skin dimpling. All lesions should be recorded on a diagram of the breasts; this includes non-suspicious lumps since this is helpful in evaluating change or the lack of change during future examinations. The information recorded on suspicious lesions should be sufficient to assign a clinical stage (see Chapter 6).

The discovery of a "dominant lesion" on CBE mandates either a biopsy or *very* close follow-up at short intervals, regardless of findings from other tests (see Figure 8.2) If a lesion is felt by the patient but not by the clinician, a repeat CBE should be performed within 2–3 months, or a second clinician should be asked to perform a CBE. When close follow-up is recommended, send the patient a written reminder of the follow-up visit. Call the patient if she misses an appointment after worrisome findings on a CBE. Note these actions in the patient's record.

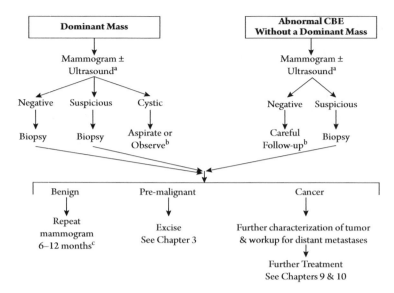

Figure 8.2 Algorithm for further evaluation after an abnormal CBE (clinical breast exam).
[a] Mammograms are often insufficiently sensitive in younger women, especially those aged < 30, because of breast density, in which case ultrasound is preferred. Both tests may be used together, especially when there is a concern about whether a mass is solid or fluid-filled.
[b] Follow-up CBE should be 6–12 weeks; a cyst that recurs within this time will need to be biopsied or excised. Follow-up mammograms for other abnormalities are usually repeated within 3 to 6 months.
[c] Interval depends on certainty of diagnosis.

FURTHER EVALUATION OF CBE FINDINGS

All abnormalities on CBE require some form of further evaluation (see Figure 8.2). If the patient has not already had a mammogram, one should be obtained to define better the extent of disease and the ideal location for biopsy. The breasts of younger women, especially those aged < 30, may be so dense that a mammogram is not helpful, in which case an ultrasound is preferred. For older women an ultrasound will help distinguish a solid from a cystic lesion. It is also helpful in distinguishing benign from malignant masses, but should generally not be used as the basis for *not* biopsying a dominant solid mass found on CBE.

Mammography

Today a suspicious lesion is as likely to be found initially on a screening mammogram prior to its discovery on breast self-exam or CBE. A diagnostic mammogram that includes magnification or other specialized views with proper breast compression is often required after an abnormality is found on a screening mammogram, especially if there are no abnormalities on CBE. The most common findings associated with malignancy are a mass or clustered microcalcifications (see Figure 8.3). Lesions that are irregular in shape (spiculated or lobulated rather than round or oval) and dense with poorly defined margins are more likely to be cancer. Calcifications that

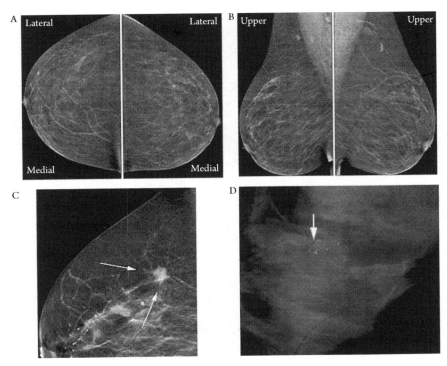

Figure 8.3 Mammograms. A: Craniocaudal views of normal breasts with the outer or lateral quadrants at the top. B: Lateral views of normal breasts with the upper portions of the breast at the top. The views of the two breasts are usually hung on the viewer as mirror images to facilitate comparison. C: A spiculated mass, the most common mammographic manifestation of cancer. D: Clustered microcalcifications, the second most common manifestation. The higher the density of a spiculated mass, the more likely it represents cancer. Microcalcifications may be clustered, as illustrated here, or linear. They represent involuted intraductal carcinomas that have calcified. They must be distinguished from larger calcifications that more often reflect benign changes in the breast.

are pleomorphic with a fine linear or branching linear pattern suggesting the outline of the duct are more likely to be cancerous. Usually at least five microcalcifications are required, but larger numbers are more often associated with malignancy. Breast asymmetry and changes in skin thickness may raise suspicion and lead to further investigation, but the risk of malignancy associated with these changes is much smaller. Breast density is now widely accepted as a risk factor for breast cancer (see Chapter 1) and is routinely reported, usually placing the patient in one of four categories: predominantly fatty (0%–25% dense), scattered fibroglandular densities (25%–50% dense), heterogeneously dense (51%–75% dense) and dense (> 75%). Some states require that the patient always be informed of their density classification, even though it is still uncertain how this information should be used in patient management.

Digital mammography, which replaces the conventional X-ray film with an electronic digital image, is rapidly replacing conventional mammography in the United States. These images can be more easily stored and transferred electronically. It is possible to modify contrast and brightness after the image has been obtained, and this may allow increased ability to detect certain abnormalities. It has not been possible to show that this methodology increases breast cancer detection, sensitivity, or specificity overall, but sensitivity is increased in patients with dense breast and those with ER– tumors.[5] A very recent modification of digital mammography is tomosynthesis, which generates a 3D image; its added value, if any, and role in patient management are still being assessed.

Mammographers differ in their skill at detecting and interpreting mammographic abnormalities. Very experienced mammographers will often carefully watch lesions that less experienced radiologists immediately biopsy. To increase consistency in the interpretation of mammograms, the American College of Radiologists has developed the BI-RADS classification, which is useful in determining whether a patient should have suspicious abnormalities biopsied and the interval for subsequent examinations if immediate biopsy is not indicated (see Table 8.1).[6]

Between 10% and 15% of mammograms are negative in patients with an abnormal CBE and histologically proven breast cancer. For this reason, biopsy of a dominant mass found on CBE should be performed, even if the mammogram is negative (see Figure 8.2).

Contrast-Enhanced Breast Magnetic Resonance Imaging (MRI)

MRI using a dedicated breast coil has greater sensitivity but less specificity than mammography. Today it is frequently used to define the extent of disease when choosing the type and planning the extent of local therapy. It is particularly useful for breast cancers not easily defined by mammograms, such as lobular, DCIS, or lesions in dense breasts. However, it has proven difficult to use MRI to ensure adequate surgical margins during breast-conserving surgery (BCS), and there are no trials demonstrating that its routine use will decrease local recurrences or improve survival.[7,8] Nonetheless, it is common practice to use MRI in this way, and this may be one reason that the percentage of patients receiving BCS is falling.[9] At this point, MRI should be reserved for the patients for whom it is known to have unique value, such as young women with dense breasts. In addition, it is a useful tool in evaluating and assessing response in patients undergoing neoadjuvant therapy (see Chapter 11).

Biopsy

Biopsy is indicated in almost all patients with a dominant solid mass and in patients with a CBE abnormality along with abnormalities on mammogram and/or ultrasound. Breast biopsy is performed with local anesthesia; hospitalization is not required. The lesion must be localized, and, depending on its characteristics, this is done with palpation, mammography (stereotactic or wire localization), ultrasound, or MRI. There are a number of different ways to biopsy the breast:

- Fine needle aspiration (FNA): The advantage of FNA is its ease of use, minimal patient discomfort, and rapidity of diagnosis. It is useful primarily for palpable lesions, but it can be used with ultrasound guidance. The cytologist *must* be very experienced. The frequency of inadequate specimens may exceed 25%. It is not possible to distinguish invasive and in situ lesions, and there is insufficient tissue for evaluation of ER or HER2. If the biopsy is not performed in centers with extensive experience, core needle biopsy is preferred, but FNA is very useful in evaluating palpable lymph nodes, skin nodules that may represent metastases, and sites of distant metastases. It is also used to aspirate simple cysts. It is safer than more extensive procedures in patients with coagulation disorders.

Table 8.1 American College of Radiology BI-RADS (Breast Imaging Reporting and Data System) Categories for Reporting Mammography Results

Category	Abnormalities Found on Mammogram	Probability of Malignancy	Recommendations
0: Incomplete	May need more views or prior mammograms for comparison	Unknown	Further evaluation
1: Normal	No abnormalities of any type seen	0%	Normal interval follow-up, usually annual
2: Benign	Benign nodules such as fibroadenomas, cysts, benign calcification	0%	Normal interval follow-up, usually annual
3: Probably benign	Does not fully fit benign or malignant category; might be asymmetry, nodules not clearly benign, or calcifications not fulfilling "micro" definition	< 2%	Shorter follow-up interval, possible every 6 months for 1–2 years
4: Suspicious abnormality	At least one lesion with some characteristics of cancer		
4a:	Radiologist has low level of concern	2%–9%	Consider biopsy
4b:	Radiologist has moderate level of concern	10%–49%	Consider biopsy
4c:	Radiologist has high level of concern	50%–94%	Consider biopsy
5: Highly suggestive	Spiculated masses and/or pleomorphic microcalcifications and/or skin retraction	≥ 95%	Biopsy recommended
6: Biopsy proven cancer		100%	Appropriate treatment

From D'Orsi CJ, Sickles EA, Mendelson EB, et al., eds. *American College of Radiology Breast Imaging Reporting and Data System BI-RADS.* 5th ed. Reston, VA: American College of Radiology; 2013.

- Core needle biopsy (CNB): Guided by palpation, mammography, ultrasound, or MRI, this is the procedure of choice in most centers because more tissue is removed than with FNA, resulting in greater accuracy; it allows the clinician to distinguish between in vitro and invasive cancer, and it provides sufficient tissue to measure ER and HER2. Stereotactic guidance is required when using CNB to evaluate microcalcifications.
- Vacuum-assisted CNB (VAB): This technique obtains larger samples, even with smaller gauge needles than required for ordinary CNB. It is particularly useful for microcalcifications and asymmetric densities that do not form a well-defined mass.[10] Compared to CNB, there are fewer sampling errors and false-negative findings.
- Excisional biopsy: Complete removal of the tumor, with or without wire localization prebiopsy, is less commonly done today as an initial procedure because of the ease of percutaneous needle biopsies, but full excision is eventually performed for all invasive tumors, usually as part of breast-conserving therapy and limited node sampling (see Chapter 9). It is performed initially for larger areas of microcalcifications, for lesions that cannot be well localized (including very deep lesions near the chest wall or superficial lesions near the nipple), after a negative FNA or CNB of abnormalities that on CBE or imaging appear to have a very high likelihood of being malignant, and after a CNB that has not adequately removed benign lesions. These include atypical ductal hyperplasia and LCIS (see Chapter 3), phyllodes tumors, and the first occurrence of fibroadenomas or papillomas. The complete removal of suspicious microcalcifications should be documented with specimen mammography at the time of biopsy and with a follow-up mammogram a month after biopsy. If there are remaining microcalcifications, an excisional biopsy is indicated, even if the first biopsy showed only benign changes. When malignant tissue is re-excised, evaluations of hormone receptors and HER2 should be repeated since some studies have shown discordance between values obtained with a CNB and excisional biopsy.

OTHER ABNORMALITIES ON CBE

Lesions other than a simple dominant mass may require additional procedures.

- Cysts: Suspected cysts are best evaluated by an ultrasound that will confirm the presence of fluid in the cyst and whether it is simple or complex. A simple cyst, especially one that is causing the patient pain, may be aspirated, guided by palpation or ultrasound. If the fluid is not bloody, it should be discarded; cytology is more often misleading than helpful. The mass should disappear following aspiration. This can be demonstrated by palpation or ultrasound, and it should be documented in the patient record. A CBE should be repeated approximately 6 weeks later to ensure that it has not rapidly recurred. Cancers may, on rare occasion, grow in the lining of a fluid-filled cyst. These cysts are more likely to be irregular in shape (rather than round or oval) with sharp margins, have bloody aspirates, and do not disappear with aspiration and/or recur rapidly after aspiration. Complex cysts need to be biopsied or excised, usually with localization techniques. An asymptomatic cyst that can be fully collapsed with aspiration and does not rapidly recur after aspiration does not need treatment or further evaluation.

- Nipple discharge: A spontaneous (i.e., not obtained by squeezing or pressing on the nipple) bloody (or guaiac positive) discharge from one breast and especially from one duct is worrisome in a women aged > 40. These patients should have an ultrasound and mammogram to rule out the possibility that the discharge is a manifestation of a deep-seated tumor or an intraductal papilloma. A ductogram, ductal lavage, or an MRI may be helpful, but cytology is not.
- Nipple ulceration: This is the classic sign of Paget's disease of the breast (also called Paget's disease of the nipple or mammary Paget's disease). It is scaly or raw with a yellow exudate that begins on the nipple and spreads to the areola. There may be a bloody discharge. It may cause pain or itching; patients with these symptoms and no physical findings should be carefully followed for the development of the nipple signs. There is usually a mass, either near the nipple or deep in the breast, which may or may not be felt on a CBE or found on mammogram. The diagnosis is best made with a full thickness biopsy of the nipple, but a punch biopsy will also provide evidence of disease that will need further surgical evaluation. Cytokeratin 7 should be measured, along with tests usually obtained for other forms of breast cancer (see further discussion later in this chapter). Management will depend on whether a mass is found. In all cases, the nipple and areolar complex are excised, but treatment may be either breast-conserving surgery or mastectomy.[11]
- Breast pain: Even though it is rarely associated with cancer, pain should never be used to eliminate the diagnosis. A history of a recurrent pattern of waxing and waning with menses and the existence of the pain over a long duration decreases the probability that it is associated with a malignancy. Biopsy should be avoided if there is no evidence of other abnormalities on examination or imaging studies. Close follow-up is recommended.
- Inflammatory skin changes: If there is a suspicion of inflammatory breast cancer, a separate skin biopsy should be obtained to determine if skin lymphatics are plugged with tumor, the hallmark of this diagnosis (see Chapter 11).
- Clinically apparent bilateral breast cancer occurs synchronously in 1%–2% of patients with early stage breast cancer. The use of MRI in patients without abnormalities on CBE or mammography may identify another 3%–4% of patients with a contralateral breast cancer.[12] However, nearly half of these could be in situ cancers, and the incidence of false positive MRIs exceeds 10%. The widespread use of MRI appears to have substantially increased the use of contralateral prophylactic mastectomy, even though there is no evidence that this improves overall survival.[13] MRI should be used judiciously, then, in patients who clearly have an increased risk of contralateral breast cancer, such as those with BRCA mutations or a history of mantle irradiation during childhood. The risk of bilateral breast cancer is also somewhat greater in younger women and those with first-degree relatives who had breast cancers diagnosed at a young age and/or in both breasts. Contralateral MRI may be appropriate for these patients, too, especially if the patient has dense breasts for which mammography has more limited value.

CHARACTERIZING AND STAGING A NEWLY DIAGNOSED CANCER

Once it is clear that the patient has breast cancer, information needed for selecting local and systemic therapies (see Chapters 9, 10, 11) should be obtained. These should be obtained on every patient:

- Clinical and pathological stage (T and N, see Chapter 6)
- Tumor grade (see Chapter 5)
- Hormone receptor status (ER and PR) (Chapters 7, 10, 11, 12)
- HER2 status (Chapters 7, 10, 11, 12)
- Some measure of the tumor's proliferative activity: A mitotic count will be available when the tumor is given a grade, but many centers routinely obtain a Ki-67 (or MIB-1) even though there are controversies regarding the assays (see Chapter 7).
- An assessment of distant metastases: Start with a careful history of possible signs and symptoms associated with dysfunction in the organ systems to which breast cancer most frequently metastasizes: bone, skin, lung, liver, and brain (see Chapter 4). For patients with stage I or II breast cancers, the likelihood of distant metastases is very low and further workup is *not* indicated if these patients are asymptomatic[14] (see Table 8.2). The frequency of false positive rates are 10%–22% for bone scans, 33%–66% for liver ultrasonography, and 0%–23% for chest radiography.[14] False negative rates for bone scans are about 10%. This means that patients at low risk of recurrence may often undergo extra (and sometimes painful and always anxiety-producing) biopsies to evaluate these false positive results. The probability

Table 8.2 Prevalence of Distant Metastases in Newly Diagnosed, Asymptomatic Breast Cancer Patients by Stage From Two Separate Analyses That Pooled Results

Evaluation	*Prevalence of Distant Metastases (% with 95% CI in parentheses)*		
	Stage I	*Stage II*	*Stage III*
Bone Scan[a]	0.5 (0.1–0.9)	2.4 (1.8–3.0)	8.3 (6.7–9.9)
Liver ultrasound[a]	0 (0)	0.4 (0.0–0.8)	2.0 (0.4–3.6)
Chest X-ray[a]	0.1 (0–0.3)	0.2 (0.0–0.4)	1.7 (0.8–2.6)
All Conventional Studies[b]	0.2	1.1	8
PET/CT[2]	NA	3.3*	26**

NA = not available; CI = confidence interval.

* based on one study, underscoring the paucity of data on the use of PET/CT in this setting

** based on four studies

[a] From Myers RE, Johnston M, Pritchard K, et al. Baseline staging tests in primary breast cancer: a practice guideline. *Can Med Assoc J.* 2001;164:1439–44; based on nine studies with 5,407 women diagnosed between 1985 and 1995.

[b] From Brennan ME, Houssami N. Evaluation of the evidence on staging imaging for detection of asymptomatic distant metastases in newly diagnosed breast cancer. *Breast.* 2012;21:112–23; based on 22 studies with 14,824 women.

of finding distant metastases increases for stage III patients. The chance of finding metastases in a workup that includes a CBC, liver function studies, a chest X-ray, a bone scan, and possibly some form of liver imaging (ultrasound, CT scan, or MRI) is sufficiently high to justify their use in patients with higher risk lesions. This evaluation should be done before making final decisions on local therapy since the results are likely to affect whether local therapy is appropriate and in which order local and systemic therapies are given when both are used (see Chapter 11). Tumor size and T stage (Chapter 6) may be a better predictor of distant metastases than the number or location of involved lymph nodes.[15] PET/CT scanning has greater sensitivity and specificity for distant metastases than more conventional studies and has the advantage of using only one test initially.[16] However, this does *not* justify its routine use to evaluate asymptomatic patients with stage I/II breast cancer. The American Society of Clinical Oncology (ASCO), as part of the American Board of Internal Medicine Foundation's "Choosing Wisely" initiative, has selected PET/CT scanning of asymptomatic breast cancers at low risk of recurrence as one of its five tests to avoid.[17,18]

Genetic profiling is of proven value in deciding whether chemotherapy will be effective in patients with early breast cancer (see Chapters 7 and 10). However, it is not indicated as part of the primary workup of a newly diagnosed breast cancer and, for now, should be restricted to patients for whom there is question about the potential value of adding chemotherapy to adjuvant endocrine therapy.

COUNSELING THE NEWLY DIAGNOSED PATIENT

Helping a new patient understand her risk of recurrence and treatment options may require several hours of physician time. This process requires the clinician to understand a patient's values and should be individualized to match the unique characteristics of each patient's tumor and personality.

- Accurately estimating the patient's likelihood of recurring or dying of breast cancer at specific time intervals (5, 10, and 20 years) is critically important (see Chapter 4). A patient may inappropriately choose toxic treatments of limited or unproven benefit if the clinician overestimates the risk of dying (and especially if toxicity is underplayed, as often happens when clinicians are discussing therapies they personally administer). On the other hand, a patient may decline treatments that are highly effective if the clinician underestimates risk (and especially if toxicity is overemphasized, as often happens when clinicians are discussing therapies administered by another specialty).
- A useful tool for estimating an individual patient's risk and likelihood of benefiting from one or another treatment strategy is Adjuvant! Online[19] (http://www.adjuvantonline.com/index.jsp). However, this information may be confusing to patients, underscoring the importance of providing sufficient interaction between clinician and patient to fully explain the predicted risk.[20] When multiple risk factors are considered together, both clinician and physician tend to focus on the bad ones, even if a bad factor is only one among many good factors.

- Learning to live with risk requires time and habituation, just as people get used to living with other risks, such as flying in a plane or driving a car. Reassuring patients that this will happen over time is often helpful in their early adjustment to the fact of having a cancer diagnosis.
- Since breast cancer patients have a lifelong chance, albeit small, of recurring, and the exact nature of the benefit from therapy is not clear (see Chapter 10), the word "cure" should be avoided. We do not know if we can cure any patient and, more important, any particular patient.
- The knowledge that most patients diagnosed with cancer do not die of it, regardless of the therapy given, may empower a patient to make therapeutic decisions primarily on the evidence of benefit (or lack thereof), rather than her fear of death from the disease.
- An overemphasis on recurrence and death may lead a patient to sublimate issues of body image and sense of self. Provide the patient with an opportunity to discuss issues of cosmesis and reassure her that these are common concerns of most patients with breast cancer.
- Encouraging the patient to pursue treatments other than surgery, radiation, endocrine and chemotherapy allow her to reassert her sense of self-control, something that is usually lost in the pressurized atmosphere of modern medicine. These include support groups, exercise programs, acupuncture, and Chinese herbs (to name just a few).

FOLLOW-UP AFTER COMPLETION OF PRIMARY THERAPY

Randomized trials have failed to demonstrate that more intensive follow-up with extensive laboratory or radiologic testing leads to better disease-free or overall survival than a periodic follow-up visit with a physician experienced in monitoring cancer patients.[21] It is not clear that this person needs to be a cancer specialist, but there are many examples of patients suffering needless anxiety and pain because of a delay in the diagnosis of metastases by a generalist who fails to think of cancer. Breast cancer has a long natural history, and metastases may first occur 20 and 30 years after completion of the initial therapy. Clinicians without this knowledge sometimes discount the possibility of breast cancer as the cause of new symptoms, even in the face of a patient's query.

Many organizations have suggested a follow-up routine.[21] Most include the same elements and about the same frequency. The one promulgated by ASCO is shown in Table 8.3. The examination most supported by evidence is regular mammography since patients with one breast cancer remain at higher than average risk of another throughout their lifetime. The risk of a second breast cancer is usually stated to be 0.5%–1% per year, but this varies from one to another series and probably overestimates the risk, especially in populations treated with adjuvant endocrine therapy (see Chapter 10). ASCO has included the use of surveillance markers and imaging modalities in the follow-up of asymptomatic breast cancers as another of its five practices to avoid.[17]

Table 8.3 Recommended Follow-up After Completion of Primary Therapy

Evaluation/Patient Characteristics	Timing and Frequency
History and physical examination with a careful CBE that includes all breast tissue, the skin overlying the breast and chest wall, and regional lymph nodes	
Year 1–3	Every 3–6 months
Year 4–5	Every 6–12 months
Year 6+	Annually
Mammograms	
Patients stable after primary treatment	Annually
After breast-conserving surgery	No earlier than 6 months after completion of radiation therapy, then annually
Patients with residual abnormalities of uncertain stability	Every 6–12 months
Genetic counseling for those with bilateral breast cancer in patient or relative; two or more first- or second-degree relatives diagnosed with breast cancer; first-degree relative with breast cancer diagnosed age < 50; a first- or second-degree relative with ovarian cancer; a male relative with breast cancer; Ashkenazi Jewish heritage.	Any time after diagnosis
Breast self-examination	Monthly
Pelvic examination	Regularly
Patients who have received tamoxifen should be instructed to seek immediate evaluation for vaginal bleeding.	When symptomatic
Routine blood tests: CBCs, liver function studies	Not recommended
Imaging studies in asymptomatic patients: chest X-rays, bone scans, live ultrasound, CT scans, PET scans, breast MRI	Not recommended
Tumor marker studies: CEA, CA 15-3, CA 27.29	Not recommended

Khatcheressian JL, Hurley P, Bantug E, et al. Breast cancer follow-up and management after primary treatment: American Society of Clinical Oncology clinical practice guideline update. *J Clin Oncol*. 2013;31:961–5.

REFERENCES

1. Roth MY, Elmore JG, Yi-Frazier JP, et al. Self-detection remains a key method of breast cancer detection for U.S. women. *J Womens Health (Larchmt)*. 2011;20:1135–9.
2. McDonald S, Saslow D, Alciati MH. Performance and reporting of clinical breast examination: a review of the literature. *CA Cancer J Clin*. 2004;54:345–61.

3. Barton MB, Harris R, Fletcher SW. The rational clinical examination. Does this patient have breast cancer? The screening clinical breast examination: should it be done? How? *JAMA*. 1999;282:1270–80.

4. Goodson WH, 3rd. Clinical breast examination. *West J Med*. 1996;164:355–8.

5. Kerlikowske K, Hubbard RA, Miglioretti DL, et al. Comparative effectiveness of digital versus film-screen mammography in community practice in the United States: a cohort study. *Ann Intern Med*. 2011;155:493–502.

6. D'Orsi CJ, Sickles EA, Mendelson EB, et al., eds. *American College of Radiology Breast Imaging Reporting and Data System BI-RADS*. 5th ed. Reston, VA: American College of Radiology; 2013.

7. Hylton N. Magnetic resonance imaging of the breast: opportunities to improve breast cancer management. *J Clin Oncol*. 2005;23:1678–84.

8. Houssami N, Turner R, Macaskill P, et al. An individual person data meta-analysis of preoperative magnetic resonance imaging and breast cancer recurrence. *J Clin Oncol*. 2014;32:392–401.

9. Katipamula R, Degnim AC, Hoskin T, et al. Trends in mastectomy rates at the Mayo Clinic Rochester: effect of surgical year and preoperative magnetic resonance imaging. *J Clin Oncol*. 2009;27:4082–8.

10. O'Flynn EA, Wilson AR, Michell MJ. Image-guided breast biopsy: state-of-the-art. *Clin Radiol*. 2010;65:259–70.

11. Sandoval-Leon AC, Drews-Elger K, Gomez-Fernandez CR, et al. Paget's disease of the nipple. *Br Cancer Res Treat*. 2013;141:1–12.

12. Lehman CD, Gatsonis C, Kuhl CK, et al. MRI evaluation of the contralateral breast in women with recently diagnosed breast cancer. *N Engl J Med*. 2007;356:1295–303.

13. Morrow M. Prophylactic mastectomy of the contralateral breast. *Breast*. 2011;20 Suppl 3:S108–10.

14. Myers RE, Johnston M, Pritchard K, et al. Baseline staging tests in primary breast cancer: a practice guideline. *Can Med Assoc J*. 2001;164:1439–44.

15. Chu QD, Henderson A, Kim RH, et al. Should a routine metastatic workup be performed for all patients with pathologic N2/N3 breast cancer? *J Am Coll Surg*. 2012;214:456–61; discussion 61–2.

16. Niikura N, Costelloe CM, Madewell JE, et al. FDG-PET/CT compared with conventional imaging in the detection of distant metastases of primary breast cancer. *Oncologist*. 2011;16:1111–9.

17. Schnipper LE, Smith TJ, Raghavan D, et al. American Society of Clinical Oncology identifies five key opportunities to improve care and reduce costs: the top five list for oncology. *J Clin Oncol*. 2012;30:1715–24.

18. Brennan ME, Houssami N. Evaluation of the evidence on staging imaging for detection of asymptomatic distant metastases in newly diagnosed breast cancer. *Breast*. 2012;21:112–23.

19. Ravdin PM, Siminoff LA, Davis GJ, et al. Computer program to assist in making decisions about adjuvant therapy for women with early breast cancer. *J Clin Oncol*. 2001;19:980–91.

20. Engelhardt EG, Garvelink MM, de Haes JH, et al. Predicting and communicating the risk of recurrence and death in women with early-stage breast cancer: a systematic review of risk prediction models. *J Clin Oncol*. 2014;32:238–50.

21. Khatcheressian JL, Hurley P, Bantug E, et al. Breast cancer follow-up and management after primary treatment: American Society of Clinical Oncology clinical practice guideline update. *J Clin Oncol*. 2013;31:961–5.

9

TREATMENT OF THE BREAST AND REGIONAL LYMPH NODES
SURGERY AND RADIATION THERAPY

Traditionally the primary aim of surgery has been to remove all tumor and, as a result, to give the patient the same life expectancy she would have had if the cancer had never developed—that is, to "cure" the patient. Radiation therapy was first used to treat breast cancer in the late nineteenth century, and the radiotherapist's goal has always been the same as that of the surgeon. However, local eradication of tumor is a worthwhile end in itself. Untreated or uncontrolled disease in the breast may eventually cause pain, ulcerate, weep, and become malodorous. Tumor-laden regional lymph nodes may cause arm swelling, pain, and loss of upper extremity function because they obstruct lymph flow and compress nerves in the brachial plexus.

In the 1880s, surgeons led by William Halsted and Willy Meyer hypothesized that the spread of breast cancer was an orderly process initially limited to the lymphatics and subcutaneous tissues and that removing more tissue substantially reduced the likelihood of tumor recurrence. When they compared the frequency of local recurrence from their procedures with that reported in earlier decades using less extensive (or less "radical") surgery, they appeared to have improved local control. However, they were unable to demonstrate that this more radical procedure improved survival, and an "alternate" but less intuitive hypothesis that breast cancer spreads to distant organs via the bloodstream long before the cancer could be detected in the breast began to take hold. This hypothesis is often attributed to Bernard Fisher and is used to argue that improved local control will not necessarily improve survival.

DOES IMPROVED LOCAL CONTROL OF BREAST CANCER RESULT IN IMPROVED SURVIVAL?

Since some type of surgery has been the primary breast cancer treatment for more than 3,500 years, one might assume this question was settled quite some time ago. However, proof to meet today's standards would require a randomized trial in which half the patients received no surgical treatment at all. No such trial has ever been conducted.

An alternative approach is to compare limited with more extensive local treatment, much as we sometimes demonstrate the value of a drug by comparing a low dose with higher doses. Most trials of this type have failed to demonstrate a statistically significant advantage for the more extensive treatment. In a pivotal trial addressing this issue, 1,850 patients were randomized to treatment with total mastectomy, lumpectomy, or lumpectomy plus breast irradiation.[1] After 20 years of follow-up, nearly 40% of the women treated with lumpectomy had an ipsilateral breast cancer recurrence, compared to only 14% of those who had both lumpectomy and radiotherapy ($p < 0.001$) (Figure 9.1). Similar differences existed whether the patients had involved lymph nodes or not. However, no differences in disease-free, distant-disease free, or overall survival have emerged yet.

A meta-analysis of 78 trials enrolling over 42,000 women found a somewhat different result. In studies where the use of more extensive therapy reduced the local recurrence rate by < 10%, no survival advantage ensued, but in those where the reduction in local recurrence was > 10%, there was a significant improvement in overall survival for those with more extensive treatment. The first inkling of this survival benefit became apparent 5 to 10 years following diagnosis[2] (Figure 9.2).

Taken together, these observations provide solid evidence that the extent of local treatment does make a difference in the survival of some patients, but this effect is

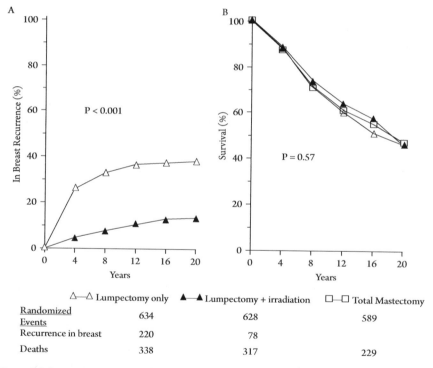

Figure 9.1 Recurrences in the ipsilateral breast (A) and overall survival (B) 20 years after 1,851 women in NSABP Trial B-06 were randomized to lumpectomy alone, lumpectomy plus irradiation of the breast but not the axilla, or total mastectomy. All patients had removal of levels I–II axillary lymph nodes. Patients with positive lymph nodes received adjuvant chemotherapy. There was a highly significant reduction in the frequency of recurrence (or new cancers) in the breasts of patients who received breast irradiation compared to those treated only with lumpectomy (A), but no evidence of a survival difference (B).

Reprinted with permission from Fisher B, Anderson S, Bryant J, et al. Twenty-year follow-up of a randomized trial comparing total mastectomy, lumpectomy, and lumpectomy plus irradiation for the treatment of invasive breast cancer. N Engl J Med. 2002;347:1233–41.

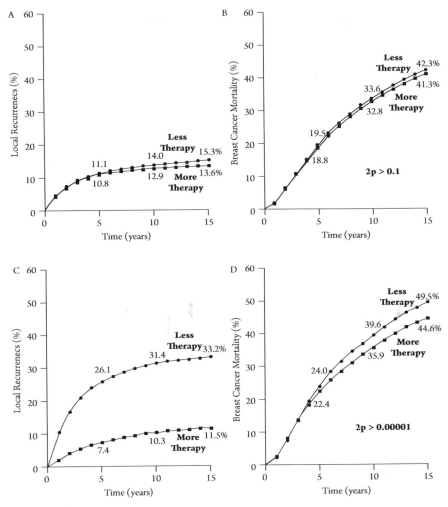

Figure 9.2 Relationship between effectiveness of therapy in improving local control and the effect of that therapy on patient survival. Data taken from a meta-analysis of 78 randomized trials (42,080 patients, 21,531 deaths) comparing the same surgery with or without radiotherapy (23,488 patients), more versus less surgery (with the same radiotherapy in both arms, 9,287 patients), or more surgery versus less surgery plus radiotherapy (9,305 patients). The first of each of these comparisons was designated as "more therapy." The trials were divided into those in which the difference in local recurrence rate between the two study arms at 5 years was < 10% (A and B: 12 trials, 16,804 patients, 43% node positive) or > 10% (C and D: 12 trials, 25, 276 patients, 51% node positive). From Early Breast Cancer Trialists Collaborative Group. Effects of radiotherapy and of differences in the extent of surgery for early breast cancer on local recurrence and 15-year survival: an overview of the randomised trials. *Lancet*. 2005;366:2087–106.

small enough that it can be demonstrated only in very large trials (or meta-analyses of multiple studies) with long follow-up. Key principles for the use of local treatment in the management of early breast cancer are outlined in Box 9.1. One of the challenges in using these observations on the relationship between local recurrence risk and survival is defining patients with a risk in excess of 10%–15%. The same treatment in patients with ostensibly the same characteristics yields very different local recurrence rates in the hands of different groups.[3] (For more on calculating risk of local recurrence, see later in this chapter on the use of radiation therapy.)

BREAST-CONSERVING SURGERY

Breast-conserving surgery (BCS) in which the tumor is excised with a > 2 mm tumor-free margin of breast tissue is a reasonable treatment for the vast majority of breast cancer patients with stage I–II breast cancer. Surgeons may differ on what they consider an optimal margin in any given patient, but most prefer that, at a minimum, there be no tumor cells at the inked margin of the tissue removed, and most attempt to have a margin > 2 mm. However, removal of excessive amounts of normal tissue can seriously compromise the final cosmetic result, especially if the breast is not large. Radiation therapy is routinely administered to remaining breast tissue (see section on Radiation Therapy).

The survival of patients treated with BCS and radiation has been shown to be equivalent to mastectomy in seven randomized trials and in a meta-analysis of these trials[2] (see Table 9.1).

It has not been possible to identify a group of patients whose survival will be predictably compromised by BCS. However, a higher local recurrence rate is associated with a number of factors, especially inadequate surgical margins, which may be difficult to obtain when there is multi-focal disease or an extensive intraductal component (Table 9.2). All of these factors may be considered relative contraindications for BCS, and oncologists will frequently differ in their recommendations to a patient.

Tumor size has become less of a barrier to BCS because of the use of neoadjuvant therapy to shrink tumor size before surgery and radiation therapy (see Chapter 11). Sometimes breast MRI is performed prior to surgery to assess multifocality, but it has not been demonstrated that this results in decreased frequency of local recurrence, and it may unnecessarily eliminate some patients who could be treated with BCS without problems. Molecular markers may identify less suitable candidates for BCS, but there are as yet insufficient data to recommend any of these tests for this purpose, including HER2 status or multi-gene profiles.

Patients for whom BCS is contraindicated or who choose mastectomy should be treated with a total mastectomy (Table 9.3). Some patients prefer mastectomy because they feel that this is the only way to ensure that "all disease has been removed" or because they cannot easily access radiotherapy facilities for the time required to complete radiation therapy. Although larger operations may improve locoregional control of the cancer, this can be achieved as effectively and with less toxicity by adding postmastectomy radiation therapy (see section on Radiation Therapy).

Important shortcomings from surgery to the breast are cosmetic, either because of the painful psychological adjustments from the loss of the breast after mastectomy or distortions in the breast contour, loss of sensation, and the buildup of scar tissue within the breast after lumpectomy.

Box 9.1 Key Principles in the Use of Local Therapy That Have Evolved From Randomized Clinical Trials and Meta-Analyses of These Trials

More extensive local treatment reduces the likelihood of a local recurrence.

- *More extensive local treatment includes either a larger operation, the addition of radiotherapy to any form of surgery, or a combination of both.*

Improved local control results in better survival.

- *The effects on local control are apparent within the first 5 years following treatment, but the survival benefits aren't apparent for at least 5 years and continue to increase for at least 15 years.*
  - *A local treatment difference that reduces the 5-year local recurrence risk by 20% would reduce the 15-year breast cancer mortality by 5.2% (SE 0.8, 2p_0.00001).[a]*

But—if the risk of local failure is small, the size of any survival benefit will be small.

- *The chances of a local failure in patients with small tumors, good prognostic factors, and no lymph node involvement is small enough that a survival benefit from adding radiotherapy to regional lymph nodes is likely to be clinically unimportant or impossible to demonstrate in clinical trials.*
  - *A local treatment difference that reduces the 5-year local recurrence risk by < 10% would reduce the 15-year breast cancer mortality by 1.0% (SE 0.9, 2p > 0.1).[1]*

Improved local control improves overall quality of life.

- *The psychological effect of a local recurrence is devastating.*
- *Infrequently, local recurrences cannot be eradicated, in which case they can be a source of pain, a constant reminder of the presence of disease, and a cause of lymphedema or neuritis.*

But—adverse effects must be weighed against the benefits.

- *More extensive removal of breast tissue results in poorer cosmetic outcomes or total loss of the breast.*
- *More extensive surgery, radiation therapy, or combinations of both increase the likelihood of lymphedema with concomitant disfigurement and loss of sensation and/or function, brachial plexopathy, rib fractures, and cardiac toxicity.*

The net benefit from adding radiation generally exceeds the adverse effects from more extensive local treatment.

[a] *Early Breast Cancer Trialists Collaborative Group. Effects of radiotherapy and of differences in the extent of surgery for early breast cancer on local recurrence and 15-year survival: an overview of the randomised trials. Lancet. 2005;366:2087–106.*

Table 9.1 A Meta-Analysis of Seven Randomized Trials in Which Mastectomy Was Compared With Breast Conserving Surgery (BCS) Plus Radiotherapy

	Mastectomy	BCS + Radiotherapy	p Value
Number randomized			
Total	2,042	2,083	
Node negative	1,432	1,438	
Node positive	610	645	
All cause mortality			
All patients	40%	41%	0.6
Breast cancer mortality			
All patients	32%	34%	0.3
Node negative	26%	27%	0.8
Node positive	47%	49%	0.9
Local recurrence risk at 5 years			
Node negative	5.3%	8.6%	< 0.00001
Node positive	7.9%	4.7%	0.7

Axillary lymph node dissection was performed in patients on both arms of each trial.

Data from Early Breast Cancer Trialists Collaborative Group. Effects of radiotherapy and of differences in the extent of surgery for early breast cancer on local recurrence and 15-year survival: an overview of the randomised trials. *Lancet.* 2005;366:2087–106.

BREAST RECONSTRUCTION

Following mastectomy, the breast can be reconstructed with excellent cosmetic results using implants or autologous tissue transferred from other parts of the body (Table 9.3). The reconstruction can be done at the same time as the mastectomy or delayed until some time later. Several surgical procedures over the course of a year are required for most patients to achieve an optimal cosmetic result. Patient priorities and practical considerations determine which of the reconstruction options best serves the patient's needs. The breast feels more natural (but does not have normal skin sensation) with the autologous procedures, but implants require less operative time and may look better, especially in a woman with small breasts. Implants may contract or rupture. There may be flap failure, and there will usually be some or extensive loss of muscle strength at the donor site following autologous procedures. The nipple-areolar complex is reconstructed late in the process using grafts, often from the contralateral nipple, and tattooing. Immediate reconstruction is thought to produce superior aesthetic results and greater patient satisfaction because the patient does not experience a time without a breast. However, the reconstructed breast does not look and feel like the breast that was removed, and some patients appreciate the reconstruction more if they have first had a period with no breast.

Table 9.2 Factors That Might Lead to the Use of Mastectomy Rather Than Breast Conserving Surgery and Radiation in Patients With Newly Diagnosed Breast Cancer

Factor	Comment
Large tumor relative to breast size, often defined as tumor > 5 cm	*Relative contraindication since the outcome affected is strictly cosmetic if tumor margins are clear*
Multi-focal tumor in the breast	*Usually based on mammogram (multiple foci of suspicious microcalcifications) or MRI and depends in part on whether all of the tumor can be removed surgically*
Extensive intraductal component	*>25% of the tumor around the invasive focus is DCIS; this is associated with higher frequency of residual disease on rebiopsy or mastectomy*
Positive margins	*Usually at least one attempt at re-excision will be made, but if all of the tumor cannot be removed the chances of local recurrence are increased substantially.*
Pregnancy	*Depending on the gestational age of the fetus, patient may be given neoadjuvant therapy with administration of radiation after delivery.*
Collagen vascular disease	*Likelihood of excessive reactivity of normal breast tissue in patients with lupus, scleroderma, and similar diseases leads to increased complications and a suboptimal cosmetic result.*
Young age, often defined as <35	*In randomized trials these patients have a higher local recurrence rate.*
BRCA1/2 mutations in tumor	*Associated with a higher local recurrence rate*

Note: Regarding an individual patient, experts often disagree.

The use of radiation therapy with reconstruction increases the frequency of complications and the risk of failure, often compromises cosmesis, and is difficult to sequence with surgery. There is no consensus regarding the optimal timing, but usually reconstruction is delayed in patients who need postmastectomy radiotherapy (see discussion later in this chapter).

There is no evidence that reconstruction compromises early detection of local recurrences.

RADIATION THERAPY TO THE BREAST AND/OR CHEST WALL AFTER SURGERY

As radiation therapy techniques have improved, resulting in both increased efficacy and substantially less toxicity, the amount of ostensibly normal breast and lymphatic tissue that is surgically removed has decreased. However, radiation therapy is *not* used

Table 9.3 Local Treatments of the Breast and Regional Lymph Nodes in Current Use or of Historical Importance

Form of Local Therapy	Definition
Radical mastectomy (Halsted radical mastectomy)	*Remove entire breast, major and minor pectoral muscles, all axillary lymph nodes at levels 1, II and III, and all fat, fascia, and adjacent tissues en bloc with minimal disruption of any tissue that might contain breast cancer or metastases from breast cancer.[a]*
Modified radical mastectomy	*Remove breast, nipple-areolar complex, enough skin to be able to cover the wound without tension, pectoralis fascia, and axillary lymph nodes*
Total mastectomy with sentinel lymph node biopsy	*Same as a modified radical mastectomy without removal of lymph nodes; the most common form of mastectomy in use today*
Skin-sparing mastectomy	*Same as total mastectomy except the maximal amount of skin overlying the chest wall is left for breast reconstruction*
Axillary lymph node dissection (ALND) accompanying breast conserving surgery	*Remove axillary lymph nodes at anatomical levels I and II, usually with the goal of removing at least 10 nodes.[b]*
Sentinel lymph node (SLN) biopsy	*Excision of the lymph node that first receives lymphatic drainage from the breast cancer. This node is identified using tracers—either technetium-99m and/or isosulfan blue dye—that are injected either around or near the areola or near the tumor. The dye can be identified visually and the radioactivity with a handheld device in the operating room.*
Breast-conserving surgery (BCS) (lumpectomy, partial mastectomy, quadrantectomy)	*Removal of the breast cancer with a rim of normal tissue, defined minimally as "tumor-free" at the inked margin or > 2 mm at all margins, depending on the clinical situation. When a larger amount of breast tissue is removed it is more often referred to as a partial mastectomy or quadrantectomy, but there is no agreed-upon definition for these terms.*
Prosthetic or implant-based reconstruction after mastectomy	*An implant containing either saline or silicone gel placed under the pectoralis muscle some months after mastectomy and temporary placement of a tissue expander.*
Autologous tissue reconstruction with a pedicled flap after mastectomy	*Transfer of either a transverse rectus abdominus myocutaneous (TRAM) or latissimus dorsi flap to the chest wall with the original vasculature intact in a pedicle.*
Autologous tissue reconstruction with a free flap after mastectomy	*Transfer of tissue from the rectus abdominus (TRAM), deep inferior epigastric perforator (DIEP), superficial epigastric artery (SIEA), superior or inferior gluteal artery perforator (SGAP or IGAP) muscle along with vasculature, which is reconnected, to thoracodorsal or internal mammary artery and vein in the thorax.*

(continued)

Table 9.3 Continued

Form of Local Therapy	Definition
Partial breast reconstruction after BCS	*Correction of defects, such as volume loss, skin retraction or nipple deviation, using autologous tissue reconstruction techniques, local rearrangement of tissue, augmentation with tissue from the contralateral breast, and transfer of fat tissue from other parts of the body.*
Whole breast irradiation (WBI)	*Typically 45–50 Gy (~ 2 Gy/day) delivered over 5–6 weeks in two opposing tangents that cover the anterior chest and lower axillary lymph nodes, followed by a 10–16 Gy boost with electron beam over another 1–1.5 weeks to an area encompassing and extending 1.5–2.0 cm beyond the surgical cavity. Contours to minimize dose to intrathoracic organs are determined by CT scan prior to starting treatment.*
Accelerated whole breast irradiation (AWBI) (hypofractionated whole breast irradiation, h-WBI)	*Radiation delivered to the whole breast at a dose-rate > 2 Gy/day for a smaller number of fractions than WBI, with or without a boost to the tumor bed. An AWBI schedule might consist of 42.5 Gy in 16 fractions, compared with a conventional dose-rate of 50 Gy in 25 fractions. See text regarding limitations.*
Accelerated partial breast irradiation (APBI)	*Delivery of a conventional dose of radiation to the tumor bed and a limited volume of surrounding tissue over a few days to 2 weeks using either multicatheter interstitial brachytherapy, balloon catheter brachytherapy, external 3D conformal external beam radiotherapy, or intraoperative external beam radiotherapy. Not yet an established therapy; see text regarding limitations.*
Postmastectomy radiation therapy	*Usually doses of about 50 Gy are delivered to the chest wall and to node-bearing areas in the axilla and above/below the clavicle that have not been surgically dissected, followed by a boost to the chest wall to bring the total dose there to about 60 Gy.*

[a] It is technically impossible to remove all breast tissue because it is attached closely to both skin and underlying structures.

[b] While there are considerable data relating the number of lymph nodes removed to interpretations of outcomes, this number is not universally accepted. The "number of nodes" listed on a pathology report is a function of both the number the surgeon has removed and the number the pathologist has counted. Positive nodes are usually easier to find.

in place of surgical excision of known cancerous tissue that can be readily removed from the breast and easily accessible regional lymph nodes.

Whole breast irradiation (WBI) is routinely administered after lumpectomy to most patients with stage I–II breast cancer. It has been demonstrated in randomized trials and in meta-analyses of these trials that this reduces the risk of locoregional recurrence by 50%–75% and significantly improves survival after 10–15 years of follow-up[4] (Figures 9.1 and 9.2). Nonetheless, radiation following BCS is sometimes omitted in patients with a low risk of recurrence and a shortened life expectancy because of age or comorbid conditions. Six hundred thirty-six women aged > 70 with clinical stage I, ER+ tumors were randomized to either tamoxifen alone or tamoxifen plus radiation therapy after BCS.[5] With a follow-up of 12 years the recurrence rate within the breast was 2% versus 9% ($p = 0.0001$), respectively, for those who did and did not receive radiation therapy. There were no differences in other endpoints, including breast-cancer specific and overall mortality. It is plausible that other groups of patients with very low risk of local recurrence might reasonably omit radiation therapy (e.g., those with luminal A tumors), but this cannot be recommended until more evidence with prolonged follow-up is available from randomized studies.

Radiation therapy is usually administered daily for about 6 weeks. This is a barrier to its use by patients who live some distance from centers with state-of-the-art equipment. In general, there are steep dose-response and dose-toxicity curves to radiation, and fractionation schedules (amount per day) have been developed by finding the daily dose that will maximize tumor control and minimize damage to either normal breast tissues or organs that are more sensitive to radiation, especially heart, lung, and nerves (see Table 9.4 for guidelines for using radiotherapy).

As improved radiation techniques have enabled a higher daily dose with fewer fractions (hypofractionation or h-WBI, Table 9.3), the possibility of shorter durations of treatment can be considered. A number of different fractionation schedules have been evaluated in randomized trials. A task force of the American Society of Radiation Oncology (ASTRO) concluded that trial data have demonstrated that h-WBI has equivalent efficacy and no more toxicity than WBI in patients who are 50+ years old, have pathologic stage T1-2, N0 breast cancer, have not had systemic chemotherapy, meet all other criteria for WBI (Table 9.2), and can receive a dose along the central axis that is within ± 7% of the prescription dose.[6] The use of h-WBI might reduce the duration of treatment by half, especially if no boost is administered to the tumor bed. This shorter course of treatment may enable more patients to have BCS and radiation instead of mastectomy.

When BCS with radiation was first evaluated, a boost was not always included as part of the therapy (Figure 9.1). However, it has been demonstrated in a randomized trial with 5,318 women that a 16Gy boost using electron beam or iridium implant reduced the local recurrence rate at 10+ years from 10.2% to 6.2% ($p < 0.0001$).[7] In women ≤ 40 years of age, the rates were 23.9% and 13.5% ($p = 0.0014$) for no boost versus boost. This is consistent with other studies that have demonstrated a higher risk of local recurrence after BCS in younger women, and it is plausible that this large reduction in local recurrence rate in younger women will translate into a survival advantage with longer follow-up (see earlier discussion). The use of a boost decreased the number of mastectomies performed because of local recurrence after BCS by 41%.

However, women receiving a boost had a 4.4% incidence of severe fibrosis compared to only 1.6% ($p < 0.0001$) in those without a boost.

In some of the h-WBI studies, a boost to the tumor bed was omitted, and in the patients selected for these trials this did not seem to have an adverse effect. For example, in a study of 1,234 women with tumors < 5 cm in size in breasts <25 cm wide who had pathologically negative lymph nodes and clear surgical margins, the 10-year local recurrence rate was 6.7% and 6.2% ($p = NS$) after conventional (50 Gy over 35 days) and hypofractionated (42.5 Gy over 16 days) irradiation, both without a boost.[8] There were no differences in cosmesis. (In this study, 25% of the patients were < 50 years of age, 71% had ER positive tumors, and 20% had tumors > 2 cm in size, but data from these subsets have not been presented separately.) Taken together, these data establish the importance of using a boost in patients with high-risk features for local recurrence and, at the same time, suggest that at least some patients—especially older patients with small, low-grade tumors, clear surgical margins, and no evidence of multifocality or DCIS adjacent to the tumor—might be safely treated without a boost.[9]

The goal of accelerated partial breast irradiation (APBI) is both to reduce the duration of radiation treatment to less than a week and to improve local control by increasing the dose to the tumor bed. Somewhere between 75% and 90% of local recurrences are in the quadrant of the original tumor,[7,10] and therefore it is anticipated that important residual cancer will be within the APBI fields. A number of different techniques involving brachytherapy and external beam irradiation have been used as APBI (Table 9.3), and at least four randomized trials, together enrolling > 3,300 women, have been undertaken. The results of these studies are very provocative, but the techniques in each of the four trials are quite different and the reported follow-up is generally short.[11]

In the largest of these studies women were randomized to whole breast radiotherapy (40–56 Gy, using a conventional dose schedule) or to TARGIT, which consists of a single dose of low energy X-ray therapy delivered into the tumor bed over 20–35 minutes immediately following the surgical removal of the tumor.[10,12] This delivers about 20 Gy to the surface of the tumor bed and 5–7 Gy at a depth of 1 cm. Most of the patients included in this trial had small, low-grade tumors that were estrogen receptor positive (ER+) and few or no lymph node metastases. The median follow-up is only 2.5 years. The ipsilateral breast recurrence is low in both arms (3.3 for TARGIT, 1.3% for whole breast, $p = 0.042$), but the difference in the arms is still below the non-inferiority lower bound set for the study. It is too early to embrace this treatment as a standard, but if these results hold up over time they will have a major impact on the local treatment of breast cancer.

Other large trials of APBI are accruing patients, and it is difficult to know how to use the data from the TARGIT trial in the routine management of patients with early breast cancer. Ideally, patients interested in this approach should be enrolled in a clinical trial, and treatment should be given only in centers with experience and a formal program evaluating the results. If not on a trial, APBI might be considered for those patients ≥ 60 years of age with tumors ≤ 2 cm in size, no pathologically involved lymph nodes, no evidence of multicentricity, no lymphovascular invasion, and whose tumors are also estrogen receptor positive.[11]

Postmastectomy radiation (Table 9.3) will inevitably decrease the likelihood of a recurrence on the chest wall, but it was not possible to demonstrate a net survival advantage (reduction in breast cancer mortality minus increase in non-breast cancer

Table 9.4 Guidelines for Using Radiotherapy in the Management of Early, Invasive Breast Cancer

Area to Be Irradiated	Indication, Exceptions, and Conditions
Breast tissue remaining after surgical excision of all tumor tissue	• *Whenever surgery is less than total mastectomy* • *Possible exceptions: age > 70, negative nodes, ER positive, comorbid disease (see text)* • *Hypofractionation and the omission of a boost after either conventional or hypofractionated irradiation may be appropriate in selected patients (see text).* • *The use of accelerated partial breast irradiation may be a reasonable alternative in the future (see text).*
Chest wall (after mastectomy)	• *Whenever risk of locoregional recurrence exceeds 10%–15%* • *When 4+ positive lymph nodes are found on ALND* • *When at least 1 node is positive and tumor size exceeds 4 or 5 cm (see text)* • *When there are < 4 positive nodes on ALND but one or more risk factors, such as large tumor, LVI, and/or young age (see text)*
Lymph nodes (along with radiation of breast or chest wall)	
Axillary lymph nodes	• *When ALND is not performed and an SLN biopsy is positive. This may be changing (see text).* • *A clinically detectable node is positive on biopsy.*
Supraclavicular nodes	• *Whenever the risk of locoregional recurrence exceeds 10%–15%*
Internal mammary nodes	• *Only when nodes are clinically or pathologically positive*

ALND = axillary lymph node dissection; SLN = sentinel lymph node.

mortality from toxicity of radiation therapy) in trials reported before the late 1990s. At that time, results from trials using modern radiotherapy techniques and meta-analyses with 15 years of follow-up were first published[2] (see analysis presented earlier).

Based on the observation that a 10% reduction in local recurrence rate during the first 5 years after treatment (Figure 9.2) would result in a significant improvement in survival 10 to 15 years after diagnosis, postmastectomy radiation therapy is generally added when the number of positive lymph nodes and the size of the lesion result in a local recurrence risk > 15%. This includes all patients with 4 or more positive lymph nodes and those with 1–3 positive lymph nodes who have larger tumors, usually defined as > 5 cm and categorized as T3 tumors[13] (Table 9.5).

Tumor size alone may not be associated with a sufficiently large risk to justify post-mastectomy radiotherapy. For example, in a group of 70 patients with tumors ranging from 5 cm (30% of the group) to > 11 cm but without lymph node involvement, the 5-year local failure rate after mastectomy and adjuvant systemic therapy was only 7.6%.[14] In a multivariate analysis using a Cox model that included patient age, menopausal status, number of lymph nodes sampled, hormone receptor status, and lymphatic vessel invasion (LVI), only the latter was associated with a higher local failure rate. When fewer than four nodes are involved, there is often a difference of opinion among oncologists as to whether postmastectomy radiation should be given, but usually a combination of several high-risk factors, such as size, patient age, surgical margins, and LVI are used to determine if the patient is at sufficiently high risk to justify the treatment.

Table 9.5 Locoregional Failure Rate 10 Years Following Mastectomy Without Any Additional Radiotherapy Related to the Number of Involved Lymph Nodes and Tumor Size in 2,098 Women Enrolled in Randomized Trials Evaluating Different Forms of Adjuvant Chemotherapy

Number of Involved Nodes and Tumor Size	Failure Rate (%)			
	Loco-regional*	Local *	Infra- Supra-Clavicular*	Axillary
1–3 Nodes				
T1	12.4	8.5	3.9	2.0
T2	12.1	7.5	4.1	1.1
T3	31.4	25.7	2.9	2.9
4–7 Nodes				
T1	19.9	12.3	7.7	2.4
T2	26.7	15.0	9.5	6.8
T3	44.8	25.7	15.9	6.2
≥ 8 Nodes				
T1	32.7	15.9	14.9	11.3
T2	32.7	15.9	15.7	6.8
T3	33.2	18.5	18.2	4.0

Note: 141 of these patients were randomized to an observation arm.

* All sites, including chest wall (local), infraclavicular or supraclavicular nodes, and axillary nodes, with or without distant failure as well.

T1, T2 and T3 = tumor sizes using AJCC staging definitions

Data from Recht A, Gray R, Davidson NE, et al. Locoregional failure 10 years after mastectomy and adjuvant chemotherapy with or without tamoxifen without irradiation: experience of the Eastern Cooperative Oncology Group. *J Clin Oncol.* 1999;17:1689–700.

While patients are receiving radiation, the most common adverse events are fatigue (usually mild) and skin changes in the radiation fields, including transient dry desquamation and an inflammatory response manifest as erythema and edema that is only rarely painful. With longer follow-up, there are varying degrees of telangiectasia and hyperpigmentation that may be permanent. After BCS and radiation there may be subcutaneous fibrosis leading to contraction of the breast around the scar, volume loss, and some architectural distortion of the breast, but this, too, is highly variable. Most patients are pleased with the cosmetic result, and 90% of the outcomes are scored by the patient as excellent or good. A radiation pneumonitis characterized by a dry cough, shortness of breath, and sometimes fever may appear 6–18 months after treatment, but this is almost always self-limited and requires no treatment. Radiographic changes in areas of irradiated lung are usually permanent but asymptomatic. Cardiac complications are uncommon with newer methods of radiation therapy and the use of CT-guided contours. However, caution is needed when cardiotoxic drugs, especially the anthracyclines, are administered concomitantly, before or after radiation therapy. Pathological rib fractures, often asymptomatic, may occur in 2%–3% of patients.

Although radiation therapy does cause myelosuppression and (uncommonly) suppression of other bone marrow elements, these are rarely a problem when radiation is used without cytotoxic systemic therapies.

However, when chemotherapy is given concomitantly or following radiotherapy, the two modalities are synergistic and may result in either increased morbidity or a reduction in chemotherapy dose sufficient to compromise its value. This is illustrated by a comparison of myelosuppression in patients randomized to receive adjuvant chemotherapy either before or after BCS and radiation therapy[15] (Table 9.6).

In this and two other randomized trials in which radiation therapy was delayed until the completion of adjuvant chemotherapy, there did not seem to be any compromise in local control or other endpoints as a result.[16] However, only 1,097 patients were enrolled in these three trials together. A population-based study using SEER and Medicare data concluded that a delay in the initiation of radiation therapy in patients *who are not receiving adjuvant chemotherapy* might be disadvantageous.[17] Because of the myelosuppression from using radiation with or before chemotherapy, it is now common practice to delay radiation until all adjuvant chemotherapy has been given, but the optimal way to integrate these two treatment modalities cannot yet be considered a completely settled issue.

MANAGING LYMPH NODES

From the late nineteenth century (when Halsted and Meyer reported that removing the breast and regional lymph nodes *en bloc* improved local control) until the 1990s, treatment of regional lymph nodes with surgery and/or radiation therapy was routine. When questions were raised about the contribution of nodal treatment to improved patient survival, the desire to obtain the prognostic information provided by the number of positive lymph nodes help to perpetuate the practice. This has changed in recent years with the introduction of the sentinel lymph node biopsy and the use of predictive and newer prognostic factors (see Chapters 4–7).

The adverse effects from treating regional lymph nodes are substantially greater than from treating the breast or chest wall. This is true for both surgery and radiation.

Table 9.6 Effect on Bone Marrow of Combining Radiotherapy of the Breast and Adjuvant Chemotherapy

Effect on Bone Marrow Elements	Radiotherapy Given Before Chemotherapy	Chemotherapy Given Before Radiotherapy	p value
	Percent of Patients Affected		
Nadir granulocyte count < 500/mm³			
In any cycle	80	68	0.05
On day 15 of			
Cycle 1*	76	53	< 0.001
Cycle 2*	13	16	0.70
Cycle 3*	53	31	0.002
Cycle 4*	19	16	0.59
Nadir platelet count < 50,000/mm³ in any cycle	0	2	0.25
Hemoglobin ≥ 6.5 g/dL in any cycle	3	3	1.00
Fever or neutropenia requiring hospitalization	17	7	0.02

In a randomized trial, 244 patients with stage I–II breast cancer treated with breast-conserving surgery received radiotherapy to the whole breast with a boost and radiation to regional nodes either before or after adjuvant chemotherapy consisting of cyclophosphamide, methotrexate, doxorubicin, 5-flurouracil, and prednisone.

*The authors attributed differences in the frequency of serious neutropenia between cycles to the fact that when a patient experienced neutropenia the drug dose was reduced or delayed per protocol in the next cycle. Thus all patients received full dose therapy on cycle 1, reduced doses in cycle 2, full doses again in cycle 3 because neutropenia was not observed in cycle 2, and reduced doses again in cycle 4.

Data from Recht A, Come SE, Henderson IC, et al. The sequencing of chemotherapy and radiation therapy after conservative surgery for early-stage breast cancer. *N Engl J Med.* 1996;334:1356–61.

The greater the extent of surgery and/or the higher the dose of radiation, the greater the risk of serious damage to lymphatics and nervous tissue. The two modalities are synergistic. Scarring of axillary tissue obstructs lymphatic flow, leading to lymphedema of the ipsilateral arm. The incidence in various reports has ranged from 6% to 70%, depending on the extent of the treatment used, the definition of lymphedema, the method of ascertaining cases, and the means of measuring it. In the days of the radical mastectomy, serious lymphedema or elephantiasis occurred in up to 10% of patients. It may occur months or years after the treatment and is often precipitated by a low-grade infection somewhere on the extremity. Brachial plexopathy occurs uncommonly after radiation but may lead to loss of upper or total arm function and/ or chronic pain. Both of these conditions occur with locoregional cancer recurrences, as well, and determining the cause of either lymphedema or brachial plexopathy can occasionally be a challenging clinical problem. These adverse events associated with treatment of lymph nodes have been an important incentive for decreasing the extent of nodal treatment or its elimination altogether.

In general, randomized trials specifically designed to evaluate nodal treatment in patients with no clinical evidence of lymph node involvement have failed to show any survival advantage for treating the nodes. The largest of these, NSABP B-04, randomized patients to treatment with a radical mastectomy, total mastectomy, or total mastectomy with radiation therapy to regional nodes[18] (see Figure 9.3). (All patients with clinically positive nodes received nodal treatment.) Although there was a significantly higher incidence of local recurrence on the chest wall for patients whose lymph nodes were untreated (i.e., the total mastectomy group), the differences in regional recurrence were very small. Differences in distant recurrence were not significant, and no differences in overall survival could be detected after 25 years of follow-up. About 40% of the women with clinically negative nodes were found to have pathologic node involvement in the radical mastectomy group. It might reasonably be assumed that among women randomized to total mastectomy without nodal treatment the percentage with positive nodes would be the same and that these untreated nodes would eventually be manifest as regional recurrences. On this basis, the expected number of patients with positive axillary nodes in the total mastectomy arm was ~ 146, but the observed number was only 68. This provides substantial evidence that most untreated histologically positive lymph nodes will not cause problems for the patient. This has been called the "recurrence gap" and has been reported in a number of other studies, as well.[19]

Involvement of the internal mammary nodes is common in patients with axillary nodal metastases, but randomized trials evaluating either surgical or radiation treatment of these have demonstrated no survival benefit and only a small local recurrence benefit.[19] The data from randomized trials evaluating local treatment of supraclavicular nodes is even more limited, but many studies evaluating postmastectomy and BCS radiation have included the supraclavicular fields. For this reason, the indication for treating this region after either of these surgical procedures is the same as for treating the chest wall postmastectomy (see Table 9.4).

Further insight into the value of radiotherapy for regional lymph nodes is likely to emerge from Canadian trial NCIC-CTG MA-20 in which 1,832 women were randomized after BCS and WBI to receive no additional radiation or radiotherapy to the supra/infraclavicular region, upper internal mammary nodes, and level III axillary nodes.[20] Eighty-five percent of these patients had 1–3 positive lymph nodes. After 5 years of follow-up there was a 2% reduction in regional recurrences (HR 0.59, $p = 0.02$), an improvement in disease-free survival ($p = 0.003$), and a trend toward improved overall survival ($p = -.07$) from the addition of radiation. Longer follow-up and better insight into the contribution of subgroups to these findings will be required before they are incorporated into standard practice.

SENTINEL LYMPH NODE BIOPSY AND AXILLARY LYMPH NODE DISSECTION

Sentinel lymph node biopsy (SLNB) (Table 9.3) is based on observations in several tumor types that an afferent lymphatic channel drains the area of the tumor to a first node in a nodal chain, and that this node reflects the status of other nodes in the chain.

Table 9.7 Evaluations of Axillary Lymph Node Dissection After a Sentinel Lymph Node Biopsy

	NSABP B32[a]			ACSOG Z0011[b,c]		
	SLNB + ALND	SLNB alone		SLNB + ALND	SLNB alone	
Number randomized	2,807	2,804		445	446	
Negative nodes in SLNB	1,975	2,011		0	0	
Length of follow-up	Mean 8 years			Median 6.3 years		
Tumor characteristics	*Percent of Patients*			*Percent of Patients*		
Tumor size ≤ 2 cm	84	84		68	71	
ER+	NA	NA		82	82	
Histology = grade 3	NA	NA		29	28	
Positive lymph nodes = 3	NA	NA		7	3	
≥ 4	NA	NA		14	1	
Micrometastases only				38	45	0.05
Treatment	*Percent of Patients*			*Percent of Patients*		
Mastectomy	12	13		0	0	
Lumpectomy	84	84		100	100	
Radiotherapy	82	82		89	90	
Adjuvant systemic therapy	85	84		96	97	
Adverse Events (AE)	*Percent of Patients*		*p value*	*Percent of Patients*		*p value*
Any surgical AE				70	25	≤ 0.001
Grade III AE	0.5	0.4		NA	NA	
Lymphedema at 1 year						
Subjective	NA	NA		13	2	≤ 0.0001
Measured	NA	NA		11	6	0.0786
Wound infections	NA	NA		8	3	0.0016
Seromas	NA	NA		14	6	0.0001
Outcomes	*Percent of Patients*		*p value*	*Percent of Patients*		*p value*
Local RR	2.7	2.4		3.1*	1.6*	0.11
Regional RR	0.4	0.7		0.5	0.9	0.45
Disease-free DF at 5 years	89.0	88.6		82.2	83.9	0.14
HR (95% CI)	1.05 (0.9–1.22)		0.54	0.82 (0.58–1.17)		

(continued)

Table 9.7 Continued

	NSABP B32[a]			ACSOG Z0011[b,c]		
	SLNB + ALND	SLNB alone		SLNB + ALND	SLNB alone	
Survival at 5 years	96.4	95.0		91.8	92.5	0.25
HR (95% CI)	1.20 (0.96–1.50)		0.13	0.79 (0.56–1.10)**		

In NSABP B-32 women with clinically negative lymph nodes were randomized before sentinel lymph node biopsy (SNLB) to have either no additional surgical axillary lymph node treatment or axillary lymph node dissection (ALND) if no nodes were positive on SNLB. Patients were stratified on the basis of the planned surgery (mastectomy or BCS). Mastectomy patients with a negative SNLB had no additional treatment to the nodes while BCS patients had tangential field radiation therapy that involved the lower axillary nodes. In ACSOG Z0011 women with positive nodes on SNLB were randomized to no additional surgical axillary lymph node treatment or ALND. All patients had BCS and tangential field whole breast irradiation that included the lower axillary node region, but no patient had radiation to a third field. Adjuvant systemic therapy was administered at the discretion of the physician but was not reported.

NA = not reported RR = recurrence rate HR = hazard ratio DF = disease-free.

* Recurrences at 5 years. ** Unadjusted HR for non-inferiority, $p = 0.008$

[a] Krag DN, Anderson SJ, Julian TB, et al. Sentinel-lymph-node resection compared with conventional axillary-lymph-node dissection in clinically node-negative patients with breast cancer: overall survival findings from the NSABP B-32 randomised phase 3 trial. Lancet Oncol. 2010;11:927–33.

[b] Giuliano AE, Hunt KK, Ballman KV, et al. Axillary dissection vs no axillary dissection in women with invasive breast cancer and sentinel node metastasis: a randomized clinical trial. *JAMA*. 2011;305:569–75.

[c] Lucci A, McCall LM, Beitsch PD, et al. Surgical complications associated with sentinel lymph node dissection (SLND) plus axillary lymph node dissection compared with SLND alone in the American College of Surgeons Oncology Group Trial Z0011. *J Clin Oncol*. 2007;25:3657–63.

In the largest study evaluating SLNB, NSABP B-32, sentinel nodes were identified using technetium-99m and isosulfan blue dye in 97.2% of all patients and in 98.9% of those with a hot spot.[21] Among those whose SLNB was negative, 9.8% were found to have a positive node at subsequent axillary dissection (ALND), but the overall accuracy of SLNB was 97.1%. As a result of this and other studies, SLNB is now routinely used in the management of axillary lymph nodes.

Until recently, patients with a positive SLN biopsy went on to have an immediate axillary lymph node dissection, and those with a negative biopsy received no further axillary treatment. However, two studies suggest that ALND provides no added benefit compared to SLNB alone. In one of these (NSABP B-32), patients with a negative SLNB were randomized to have ALND as well or SLNB alone.[22] In the other (ACSOG Z0011), patients with a positive SLNB were randomized to ALND or SLNB alone.[23] There were no significant differences in local or regional recurrences, disease-free survival, and overall survival (Table 9.7). However, there were highly significant differences in adverse effects. The majority of patients in both studies had T1 tumors. Other tumor characteristics are available only for the ACSOG study, but in that trial 82% of tumors were ER+. Patients treated with BCS had radiation to the lower axillary

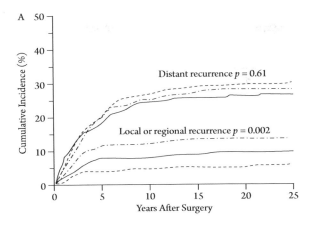

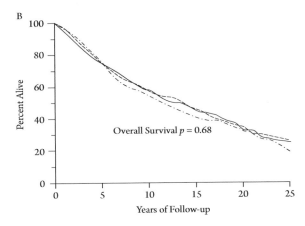

C	Radical Mastectomy	Total Mastectomy	Total Mastectomy + Radiation
	————	—·—·—·—·—	————————
Number randomized	362	365	352
Any locoregional site	9.4%	13.4%	5.7%
Local	5.3%	7.1%	1.4%
Regional	4.1%	6.3%	4.3%

Figure 9.3 Cumulative incidence of locoregional and distant recurrences (A) and overall survival (B) of patients in NSABP trial B-04 in which women with clinically negative nodes were randomized to radical mastectomy, total mastectomy, or total mastectomy with radiation of the chest wall and regional lymph nodes (see Table 9.3 for definitions). Patients in the total mastectomy group who subsequently were found to have ipsilateral positive nodes that required axillary node dissection ($n = 68$) were not counted as having a regional failure unless the nodes could not be removed ($n = 1$) at this later time. Reprinted with permission from Fisher B, Jeong JH, Anderson S, et al. Twenty-five-year follow-up of a randomized trial comparing radical mastectomy, total mastectomy, and total mastectomy followed by irradiation. *N Engl J Med.* 2002;347:567–75.

lymph nodes in both studies, and most patients in these trials received adjuvant systemic therapy. The length of follow-up is too short to draw firm conclusions regarding survival. When interpreting the ACSOG Z0011 study it is important to recognize that this was designed as a non-inferiority trial with an anticipated accrual of 1,900, and that the study was stopped early because of poor accrual. However, because the local recurrence rate at 5 years is very low in both arms of both trials, it is highly unlikely that an important survival difference related to the use of ALND will eventually emerge in either (see earlier discussion). The patients contributing most of the information to these studies had relatively small tumors with good prognostic signs and nodal micrometastases, were treated with BCS and radiation, and received adjuvant systemic therapy. For such patients, ALND can and probably should be avoided.[24,25]

SUMMARY

Fifty years ago it was possible to make the case that local treatment had no effect on the survival of breast cancer patients. Since then, large randomized trials and long follow-up have established that there is, indeed, an overall survival benefit from local treatment, at least for some patients. During this same interval, however, the extent of local treatment has steadily shrunk. Extensive (and mutilating) surgery has been replaced by lumpectomy. Axillary dissections that frequently resulted in clinically important lymphedema have been replaced with sentinel lymph node biopsy and limited or no axillary surgery. Radiation therapy that included considerable normal tissue (including axillary and non-breast tissue) and required 5–6 weeks duration is being replaced with radiation techniques that spare normal tissue, limit radiation to the axilla, and may—in the near future—treat only part of the breast. Control of the disease in the breast and regional nodes is important, but the aim of local treatment today is to provide the minimum surgery and radiation that will provide optimal control.

REFERENCES

1. Fisher B, Anderson S, Bryant J, et al. Twenty-year follow-up of a randomized trial comparing total mastectomy, lumpectomy, and lumpectomy plus irradiation for the treatment of invasive breast cancer. N Engl J Med. 2002;347:1233–41.

2. Early Breast Cancer Trialists Collaborative Group. Effects of radiotherapy and of differences in the extent of surgery for early breast cancer on local recurrence and 15-year survival: an overview of the randomised trials. Lancet. 2005;366:2087–106.

3. Taghian A, Jeong JH, Mamounas E, et al. Patterns of locoregional failure in patients with operable breast cancer treated by mastectomy and adjuvant chemotherapy with or without tamoxifen and without radiotherapy: results from five National Surgical Adjuvant Breast and Bowel Project randomized clinical trials. J Clin Oncol. 2004;22:4247–54.

4. Early Breast Cancer Trialists Collaborative Group. Effect of radiotherapy after breast-conserving surgery on 10-year recurrence and 15-year breast cancer death: meta-analysis of individual patient data for 10,801 women in 17 randomised trials. Lancet. 2011;378:1707–16.

5. Hughes KS, Schnaper LA, Cirrincione C, et al. Lumpectomy plus tamoxifen with or without irradiation in women age 70 or older with early breast cancer. J Clin Oncol. 2010;28:15s (suppl: abstr 507).

6. Smith BD, Bentzen SM, Correa CR, et al. Fractionation for whole breast irradiation: an American Society for Radiation Oncology (ASTRO) evidence-based guideline. *Int J Radiat Oncol Biol Phys.* 2011;81:59–68.

7. Bartelink H, Horiot JC, Poortmans PM, et al. Impact of a higher radiation dose on local control and survival in breast-conserving therapy of early breast cancer: 10-year results of the randomized boost versus no boost EORTC 22881-10882 trial. *J Clin Oncol.* 2007;25:3259–65.

8. Whelan TJ, Pignol JP, Levine MN, et al. Long-term results of hypofractionated radiation therapy for breast cancer. *N Engl J Med.* 2010;362:513–20.

9. Werkhoven E, Hart G, Tinteren H, et al. Nomogram to predict ipsilateral breast relapse based on pathology review from the EORTC 22881-10882 boost versus no boost trial. *Radiother Oncol.* 2011;100:101–7.

10. Vaidya JS, Joseph DJ, Tobias JS, et al. Targeted intraoperative radiotherapy versus whole breast radiotherapy for breast cancer (TARGIT-A trial): an international, prospective, randomised, non-inferiority phase 3 trial. *Lancet.* 2010;376:91–102.

11. Smith BD, Arthur DW, Buchholz TA, et al. Accelerated partial breast irradiation consensus statement from the American Society for Radiation Oncology (ASTRO). *Int J Radiat Oncol Biol Phys.* 2009;74:987–1001.

12. Vaidya JS, Wenz F, Bulsara M, et al. Targeted intraoperative radiotherapy for early breast cancer: TARGIT-A trial- updated analysis of local recurrence and first analysis of survival. *Cancer Res.* 2012;72 100s.

13. Recht A, Gray R, Davidson NE, et al. Locoregional failure 10 years after mastectomy and adjuvant chemotherapy with or without tamoxifen without irradiation: experience of the Eastern Cooperative Oncology Group. *J Clin Oncol.* 1999;17:1689–700.

14. Floyd SR, Buchholz TA, Haffty BG, et al. Low local recurrence rate without postmastectomy radiation in node-negative breast cancer patients with tumors 5 cm and larger. *Int J Radiat Oncol Biol Phys.* 2006;66:358–64.

15. Recht A, Come SE, Henderson IC, et al. The sequencing of chemotherapy and radiation therapy after conservative surgery for early-stage breast cancer. *N Engl J Med.* 1996;334:1356–61.

16. Hickey BE, Francis D, Lehman MH. Sequencing of chemotherapy and radiation therapy for early breast cancer. *Cochrane Database Syst Rev.* 2006:CD005212.

17. Punglia RS, Saito AM, Neville BA, et al. Impact of interval from breast conserving surgery to radiotherapy on local recurrence in older women with breast cancer: retrospective cohort analysis. *BMJ.* 2010;340:c845-c.

18. Fisher B, Jeong JH, Anderson S, et al. Twenty-five-year follow-up of a randomized trial comparing radical mastectomy, total mastectomy, and total mastectomy followed by irradiation. *N Engl J Med.* 2002;347:567–75.

19. Xie L, Higginson DS, Marks LB. Elective regional nodal irradiation in patients with early-stage breast cancer. *Semin Radiat Oncol.* 2011;21:66–78.

20. Whelan TJ, Olivotto I, Ackerman I, et al. NCIC-CTG MA.20: an intergroup trial of regional nodal irradiation in early breast cancer. *J Clin Oncol.* 2011;29:suppl; abstr LBA1003.

21. Krag DN, Anderson SJ, Julian TB, et al. Technical outcomes of sentinel-lymph-node resection and conventional axillary-lymph-node dissection in patients with clinically node-negative breast cancer: results from the NSABP B-32 randomised phase III trial. *Lancet Oncol.* 2007;8:881–8.

22. Krag DN, Anderson SJ, Julian TB, et al. Sentinel-lymph-node resection compared with conventional axillary-lymph-node dissection in clinically node-negative patients with breast cancer: overall survival findings from the NSABP B-32 randomised phase 3 trial. *Lancet Oncol.* 2010;11:927–33.

23. Giuliano AE, Hunt KK, Ballman KV, et al. Axillary dissection vs no axillary dissection in women with invasive breast cancer and sentinel node metastasis: a randomized clinical trial. *JAMA.* 2011;305:569–75.

24. Barry JM, Weber WP, Sacchini V. The evolving role of axillary lymph node dissection in the modern era of breast cancer management. *Surg Oncol.* 2012;21:143–5.

25. Barkley C, Burstein H, Smith B, et al. Can axillary node dissection be omitted in a subset of patients with low local and regional failure rates? *Breast J.* 2012;18:23–7.

26. Lucci A, McCall LM, Beitsch PD, et al. Surgical complications associated with sentinel lymph node dissection (SLND) plus axillary lymph node dissection compared with SLND alone in the American College of Surgeons Oncology Group Trial Z0011. *J Clin Oncol.* 2007;25:3657–63.

10

ADJUVANT SYSTEMIC THERAPY

The failure of radical local treatments (Chapter 9) and early diagnosis (Chapter 2) to dramatically improve the overall survival of breast cancer patients has led gradually to the realization that metastases are well established in many patients before the primary in the breast can be detected and that initial treatment must be directed at both these distant occult, metastatic foci (micrometastases) and the local-regional disease. A lesion of < 1 cm (10^9 cells) cannot be detected reliably by physical examination or most radiologic studies (see Figure 4.3 in Chapter 4). A patient with disease apparent only in the breast and regional lymph nodes may have multiple such deposits in many different organs of the body. The larger the tumor and number of involved lymph nodes, the more likely that such deposits exist (see Chapter 6). "Adjuvant" systemic therapy, administered in addition to local surgery and radiation therapy to patients who have no identifiable metastases, is nearly identical to the systemic therapy used to treat visible, symptomatic metastases (see Chapter 12). When administered immediately after the initial diagnosis, these treatments have a greater impact on patient survival. It is thought that this is because the smaller metastatic lesions are composed of cells more sensitive to treatment and/or because the smaller size of the lesion makes it easier to eradicate these occult, metastatic deposits.

NATURE OF THE BENEFIT

While it is well established that adjuvant systemic therapy will prolong the time to recurrence and survival of breast cancer patients, it is not entirely clear whether this is because the adjuvant therapy eradicates all distant foci and "cures" some patients, reduces the size of the tumor deposits and delays recurrence and death in many patients, or cures some patients while delaying death in others. In a model, an 8% improvement in 10-year survival as a result of adjuvant therapy for a group of node-positive patients was estimated to increase the life expectancy of patients who were not cured by local treatment alone from 5.2 to 7.4 years. This assumes that the effect of the treatment is to reduce but not eradicate tumor in the majority of patients. If it is assumed, instead, that the effect of therapy is to eradicate tumors in some patients and to have no benefit for the others, an 8% survival benefit would increase the life expectancy in this small subset (~ 10% of patients) from 5.2 without adjuvant to 26 years with it.[1] While it is not possible to say that all patients live for 2.2 years longer *and* 8% will be cured, it is possible that some patients will have improved survival and a few will be cured.

Since the exact effect of adjuvant systemic therapies on micrometastases is not known, it is not correct to state that a difference in survival defines the percentage of patients who benefit. An analysis of the "number needed to treat" is similarly

Table 10.1 Proportional and Absolute Effects of Therapy in a Hypothetical Trial in Which 100 Patients Are Randomized to a Treated Group and 100 to a Control Group

	Treated	*Not Treated*
Number randomized	100	100
Deaths at 10 years	30	40
Difference in mortality		
Proportional	25%	
Absolute	10%	

inappropriate since both assume that the benefit from adjuvant systemic therapy is "all or none"—that is, that there are only two outcomes: cure or no benefit at all.

Outcomes from randomized clinical trials are usually expressed as a proportional effect, such as a reduction in the annual odds of recurrence or death, or reduction in the hazard ratio for recurrence or death, and/or an absolute effect that is the difference in survival at a specified point in time. The difference in these two ways of presenting the results of a randomized trial is illustrated in Table 10.1. Since only 40 of the 100 patients died among those randomized to no treatment, it is assumed that 60 of the patients in each arm had no need for the treatment. The 10 fewer deaths are 25% (30/40) of those who needed therapy, or 10% (10/100) of all those treated. The proportional reduction in mortality will be the same among those at high and low risk of death from breast cancer (assuming no specific interaction between therapy and the factor[s] used to define risk; see following section on Proof of Principle and Effect Size), but absolute differences will be higher in high-risk groups, such as those with positive lymph nodes.

PROOF OF PRINCIPLE AND EFFECT SIZE

Randomized trials evaluating the potential value of adjuvant ovarian ablation were initiated in 1948 and are among the first randomized trials performed in any disease. By the year 2000, about 150,000 women had been enrolled in more than 200 trials designed to evaluate the impact of adjuvant endocrine therapies, chemotherapy, and combinations of these modalities on both the time to first recurrence (disease-free survival, DFS) and overall survival (OS). Guidelines for using these therapies in the adjuvant setting have been based primarily on meta-analyses or overviews of these trials.

The first generations of randomized trials demonstrated beyond question that adjuvant systemic treatment prolongs survival. Mature results of the two most important groups of trials are shown in Figure 10.1. Five years of tamoxifen, which is effective only in patients with ER+ (ER positive) tumors, reduced mortality by 30% (proportional risk reduction = 1-RR, shown on Figure 10.1). The (absolute) difference in survival at 10 and 15 years was 7.2% and 9.2%, respectively, in a population with 44% of the patients having positive lymph nodes. Four or more cycles of an anthracycline containing chemotherapy regimen, which is more effective in ER– than ER+ tumors

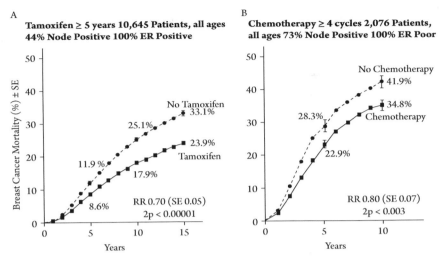

Figure 10.1 Survival plots from adjuvant tamoxifen and adjuvant chemotherapy overviews. Breast cancer mortality in a meta-analysis of all randomized trials, worldwide, in which women were randomized to receive (A) adjuvant tamoxifen or no tamoxifen (with or without the same chemotherapy in both arms, 12 trials), or (B) combination chemotherapy using an anthracycline-containing regimen or no chemotherapy (with or without adjuvant tamoxifen in both arms of the trial, 22 trials). Only patients with ER+ tumors were selected for the tamoxifen meta-analysis and ER– tumors for the chemotherapy meta-analysis, even though both ER+ and ER– tumors might have been included in the original study. The percentage of positive nodes included in these studies reflect study design and physician bias in selecting patients to enroll in the study. ER = estrogen receptor; RR = log-rank breast cancer mortality rate ratios.
Sources: Early Breast Cancer Trialists Collaborative Group. Relevance of breast cancer hormone receptors and other factors to the efficacy of adjuvant tamoxifen: patient-level meta-analysis of randomised trials. *Lancet.* 2011;378:771–84; Early Breast Cancer Trialists Collaborative Group. Comparisons between different polychemotherapy regimens for early breast cancer: meta-analyses of long-term outcome among 100,000 women in 123 randomised trials. *Lancet.* 2012;379:432–44.

(see further discussion later in this chapter), reduced mortality by 20%. The difference in survival at 10 years was 7.1% in a population with 73% of the tumors being node positive.

In general, the proportional effects of adjuvant systemic therapy are the same across groups with a different risk of recurrence based on the number of positive lymph nodes, tumor size or grade, and various measures of cellular proliferation. The proportional effect of adjuvant therapy is the same in patients with node-negative and node-positive disease, but the absolute benefit will be substantially greater for the node-positive patients. Important exceptions to this are interactions between endocrine agents and receptor status, between chemotherapy and either patient age or receptor status, and between anti-HER2 treatments and HER2 over-expression.

Absolute differences in recurrence rate or mortality are highest in patients with the highest mortality risk. This is illustrated in a study using data from an overview[4] (Table 10.2). Patients were subdivided into groups with a low (7.5%), moderate (25%), or high (50%) risk of death at 15 years without adjuvant systemic therapy. The

Table 10.2 Proportional and Absolute Benefits From Adjuvant Systemic Therapy Related
to Underlying Risk of Dying From Breast Cancer Without Treatment

Treatment	Estimated 15-Year Breast Cancer Mortality Without Treatment (%)		
	Low*	Moderate*	High*
No adjuvant treatment	12.5	25	50
	Reduction in mortality from Treatment (%)		
	Proportional	Absolute	
Tamoxifen for 5 years[a]	31	3.7	7.0	12.0
Chemotherapy[b]				
Age < 50	38	4.6	8.7	15.1
Age 50–69	20	2.4	4.4	7.4

* Risk categories: low = low risk (e.g., small size) node negative; moderate = average risk node negative;
and high = node positive disease.

[a]Effects for ER+ tumors only in trials not using chemotherapy in either arm

[b]Anthracycline containing combinations (e.g., FAC or FEC) for ~ 6 months without tamoxifen in
either arm.

Early Breast Cancer Trialists Collaborative Group. Relevance of breast cancer hormone receptors and
other factors to the efficacy of adjuvant tamoxifen: patient-level meta-analysis of randomised trials.
Lancet. 2011;378:771–84.

main factor determining risk in these studies was nodal status. Treatment with either
tamoxifen or combination chemotherapy resulted in a greater survival benefit as the
risk increased.

These benefits are well within the range that most patients who have experienced
the toxicity of chemotherapy find acceptable. In an Australian study, 104 women
who had completed treatment with CMF (cyclophosphamide, methotrexate, and
5-fluorouracil) were asked to make assumptions about the benefits from the treatment and whether under these assumptions they would still agree to undergo adjuvant CMF treatment[5] (see Table 10.3). A prolongation of life from 5 to 6 years was
sufficient to justify treatment for 77% of the women, but 5% would not repeat the
experience even with 5 years additional life. In general, patients required a larger
absolute benefit if their chances of survival without treatment were 15 years, and
this illustrates how a patient's perception of risk will likely affect her decisions.
These investigators repeated this study some years later and found that 52%–55%
of the women felt the treatment was justified if their life was prolonged for as little
as 1 day or their chance of survival at 5 years was improved by 0.1%.[6] One possible
explanation for this difference over time might be the relative toxicity of the treatment that the two patient groups received. The earlier patients all had nearly the
same regimen, and 30% were treated for 7–14 months. The latter group had several
different regimens; 54% had only 3 months of treatment with AC (doxorubicin and
cyclophosphamide).

Table 10.3 Benefits Considered by Patients Sufficient to Justify 6–12 Months of Adjuvant Chemotherapy

	Percent of patients who would take treatment if survival without treatment is			
	5 Years		15 Years	
And additional survival with treatment is		Cumulative		Cumulative
0–≤ 3 months	27	27	23	23
>3 months–1 Year	50	77	38	61
1–≤ 2 Years	12	89	13	74
2–≤ 5 Years	9	98	17	91
No increase is enough	1		9	

	Percent of patients who would take treatment if 5-year survival without treatment is			
And additional survival with treatment is	65%		85%	
< 1%	47	47	49	49
1–≤ 2%	6	53	5	54
2–≤ 5%	20	73	20	74
5–≤ 10%	9	82	9	83
10–≤ 15%	10	92	14	97
No increase is enough	2		3	

104 women were interviewed several months to > 3 years after completing from 6 months (61%) to as much as 1 year of adjuvant CMF and were asked: "Suppose that without treatment you would live 5 years. Based on your own experience of chemotherapy, what period of survival would make 6 months of initial treatment worthwhile?"

Simes RJ, Coates AS. Patient preferences for adjuvant chemotherapy of early breast cancer: how much benefit is needed? *J Natl Cancer Inst Monogr.* 2001:146–52.

ARE THERE PATIENTS WHO SHOULD NOT RECEIVE ADJUVANT SYSTEMIC THERAPY?

Even though the majority of patients with stage I or II breast cancer are cured with local treatment alone, it has not been possible to show in randomized controlled trials that there is a well-defined group of patients who will have no benefit from any form of adjuvant therapy. If nothing else, adjuvant tamoxifen will reduce the likelihood of developing a new contralateral breast cancer (see Chapter 2).

However, a relatively small fraction of breast cancer patients has a mortality rate without adjuvant treatment that is no greater than that of age-matched patients without breast cancer. These patients are mostly ≥ 60 years of age with tumors < 1 cm in diameter, low histological grade, and no involved lymph nodes.[7] It has not been possible to demonstrate that adjuvant tamoxifen reduces the mortality of ER+ tumors <

1 cm without lymph nodes because these patients already have such a good prognosis and very few events after diagnosis.[8]

The most effective chemotherapy regimens are those given for at least 6 months, and most of these have considerable toxicity. Because of this toxicity, many patients with a relatively low recurrence probability—for example, < 10%—will choose not to undergo this chemotherapy because the absolute benefit is so small. Most of these patients will be older and have small tumors and no axillary nodal involvement.

WHICH PATIENTS SHOULD RECEIVE WHICH ADJUVANT SYSTEMIC THERAPY?

Increasingly, the decision to treat and the choice of regimen are dependent on the likely benefit to be derived from the treatment. Hormone receptor (ER and PR) status, HER2 status, and molecular markers are now the determinants of the primary adjuvant systemic therapy used.

- Almost all ER+ tumors should be treated with some form of endocrine therapy.
- All HER2+ (IHC 3+ or FISH+) tumors should be treated with anti-HER2 therapy.
- All triple negative tumors (ER–, PR–, HER2–) should receive adjuvant chemotherapy.
- The source of differences in the opinions of oncologists is which patients in the first two categories should also receive adjuvant chemotherapy.

The development of new molecular markers associated with both risk of recurrence and response to therapy is slowly changing the paradigms for determining which patients will benefit from adding chemotherapy. Nonetheless, old habits die slowly, and it is still very difficult for most oncologists to consider the possibility of not using adjuvant chemotherapy therapy in all patients with positive nodes or tumors > 2 cm in diameter, even though there is now evidence that some of these patients derive no benefit from this treatment (see further discussion later in this chapter).

ER+ TUMORS: ADJUVANT ENDOCRINE THERAPY

The adjuvant endocrine therapies shown in Table 10.4 are effective only for ER+ and/or PR+ tumors. These therapies are relatively non-toxic. Recurrences are reduced while the patient is receiving the adjuvant therapy. Mortality reduction begins to appear about 5 years following the initiation of treatment and persists as long as patients have been followed in clinical trials, now more than 15 years (see Figure 10.1).

Adjuvant tamoxifen has also been shown to decrease the incidence of second, contralateral breast tumors by 30%.[4] There is likely a similar reduction in ipsilateral cancer in breasts treated with breast-conserving surgery. Similar effects by adjuvant chemotherapy are minimal or are confined to premenopausal patients where chemotherapy suppresses ovarian function, thus imparting an endocrine effect as well as a direct anti-tumor cytotoxic effect.

For postmenopausal women (often defined in study analyses as anyone aged ≥ 50) the value of adjuvant endocrine therapy was first demonstrated in studies of tamoxifen. Durations of 5 years are superior to shorter intervals, and until recently

Table 10.4 Adjuvant Endocrine Therapies

Endocrine Therapy	Route/Dose	Duration Years	Indication
Ovarian Ablation			Alternative, only for premenopausal women
Oophorectomy	Surgery	Permanent	
GNRH Agonists			
Goserelin (Zoladex®)	SQ 3.6 mg qm	5	
Leuprolide (Lupron®)	IM 3.75 mg qm	5	
Tamoxifen (Nolvadex®)	po 20 mg qd daily	10	Treatment of choice, premenopausal women Alternative for postmenopausal women
Aromatase Inhibitors			Treatment of choice, postmenopausal women only
Anastrozole (Arimidex®)	po 2 mg qd	5	
Letrozole (Femara®)	po 2.5 mg qd	5	
Exemestane (Aromasin®)	po 25 mg qd	5	
Tamoxifen/AI Sequence		7–10	Tamoxifen may be given for 2–5 years in either pre- or postmenopausal women. Patient *must* be unequivocally postmenopausal when crossed over to AI. The AI is given for 5 years

SQ: subcutaneously; po: orally; IM: intramuscularly; qd: daily; qm: monthly.(See Table 12.2 in Chapter 12 for major toxicities.)

this was the standard. In this group it reduced the annual odds of recurrence by 41%, compared to patients randomized to no tamoxifen, and reduced the annual odds of death by 31%[4] (see Table 10.5).

In more recently completed trials, 5 years of aromatase inhibitor (AI) therapy, sequential therapy with 2–3 years of tamoxifen followed by 2–3 years of an AI for a total of 5 years, and 5 years of tamoxifen followed by 5 years of an AI have all been shown to be superior to 5 years of tamoxifen in postmenopausal women[9] (Table 10.5). There is no evidence that one AI is superior to the others (Table 10.4).

Ten years of tamoxifen alone, or a sequence of 5 years of tamoxifen followed by 5 years of AI, have also been shown to be superior to 5 years of tamoxifen[9] (Table 10.5). Early randomized trials comparing 5 and 10 years of tamoxifen suggested that

Table 10.5 Incremental Benefits Derived From Adjuvant Endocrine Therapies Compared to No Endocrine Therapy or 5 Years of Tamoxifen for Postmenopausal Women With ER+ Tumors

Treatment Under Study	Control Group	No. of Patients Enrolled	No. of Trials	For Study Regimen, Proportional Reduction[a] in Rate of	
				Recurrence (%)[c]	Death (%)[c]
TAM 5 years[1,b]	No endocrine therapy	7,289	12	41	31
AI 5 yr[2]	TAM 5 years	11,163	2	14	8[d]
TAM 2–3 years → AI 2–3 years[2] (Total 5 years)	TAM 5 years	15,303	6	30	19
TAM 5 years → AI 5 years (Total 10 years)[2]	TAM 5 years	7,604	3	38	13[e]
TAM 10 years[3]	TAM 5 years	6,216	1	15[f]	NR[g]

Data are from meta-analyses of multiple trials or from a large single trial. In many of these trials patients also received chemotherapy, but if so the same chemotherapy was given to patients in both study arms. Postmenopausal was most often defined as any women aged ≥ 50.

No. = number; TAM = tamoxifen; AI = aromatase inhibitor; years = duration of treatment in years; → = sequential therapy.

[a] Reduction in annual odds or HR (hazard ratio)

[b] EBCTG trials combined ER+ and ER unknown tumors

[c] Differences in outcome highly statistically significant (≥ 0.01) except where noted

[d] $p = 0.046$

[e] p = not significant

[f] p value not reported separately for subgroup; for all menopausal groups, reduction in rate of recurrence was 16%, $p = 0.002$

[g] Mortality reduction not reported subgroup but for all menopausal groups reduction in mortality was 13%, $p = 0.01$.

[1] EBCTG (2005) Early Breast Cancer Trials Collaborative Group. Effects of chemotherapy and hormonal therapy for early breast cancer on recurrence and 15-year survival: an overview of the randomised trials. *Lancet.* 2005;365:1687–717.

[2] Aydiner (2013) Aydiner A. Meta-analysis of breast cancer outcome and toxicity in adjuvant trials of aromatase inhibitors in postmenopausal women. *Breast.* 2013;22:121–9.

[3] Davies (2013) Davies C, Pan H, Godwin J, et al. Long-term effects of continuing adjuvant tamoxifen to 10 years versus stopping at 5 years after diagnosis of oestrogen receptor-positive breast cancer: ATLAS, a randomised trial. *Lancet.* 2013;381:805–16.

there might actually be a detrimental effect from prolonged tamoxifen therapy, and in preclinical models tumors have been shown to become resistant and to even be stimulated by prolonged exposure to tamoxifen (see Chapter 12). However, two recent, very large trials comparing 5 and 10 years of tamoxifen demonstrated a significant advantage for the longer duration of treatment; the most mature of these studies is summarized in Table 10.5.

These trial data, taken together, have led most medical oncologists to conclude that AIs are the most effective and least toxic of the adjuvant therapies available for postmenopausal women. The evidence also suggests that 10 years of treatment are superior to 5 years, and sequential therapies may be more effective than only one treatment. Unfortunately, critical trials comparing 10 years of an AI with 5 years of tamoxifen, 10 years of an AI with 10 years of tamoxifen, or 10 years of a tamoxifen/AI sequence with 10 years of an AI, have not been performed. As a result, current recommendations based on evidence rather than supposition are constrained and may change in a few years as additional trial data are published.

Recommended Adjuvant Endocrine Therapy for Postmenopausal Women

All postmenopausal women with ER+ tumors should receive one of the following:

- 5 years of an AI alone
- 10 years of tamoxifen
- Sequential therapy with 2–5 years of tamoxifen, followed by 5 years of AI leading to a total treatment duration of 7–10 years.

Because direct comparisons between these three options have not yet been reported, one cannot be recommended over the others. In some cases the choice between treatments will be based on the patient's intolerance to one or the other therapy.

- Some postmenopausal women with ER+ tumors will benefit from adding chemotherapy or trastuzumab to adjuvant endocrine therapy (see further discussion later in this chapter).

For premenopausal women the value of adjuvant endocrine therapy was first demonstrated using ovarian ablation (OA, oophorectomy or ovarian radiation). In a meta-analysis of trials comparing OA with no adjuvant therapy of any type, OA reduced the annual odds of recurrence by 32% and the odds of death by 31%.[4] (Most of these studies were conducted in the 1940s and 1950s, long before ER was identified, so a large percentage of these patients were likely ER negative. Because of this, these numbers may seriously underestimate the benefit of OA in premenopausal women with ER+ tumors.) Ovarian suppression (OSup) using a GNRH agonist appears to be equally effective, but there are no direct comparisons in the adjuvant setting, and indirect comparisons are difficult because the number of patients randomized to OSup alone versus no adjuvant systemic therapy is small.[11] Another limitation of these trials of OSup, alone or in combination with tamoxifen or chemotherapy, is that in all but one of 17 such studies the duration of the OSup is only 2 years. This is probably too short in light of the demonstration that longer durations of tamoxifen are more effective than shorter. The value of 5 years of OSup is under study, and recommendations about its use in this setting may change in the near future.

Five years of adjuvant tamoxifen reduces the odds of recurrence and death by 45% and 32%, respectively, compared to no adjuvant treatment at all for premenopausal women (or those assumed to be premenopausal because of age < 50 or < 55) with ER+ tumors.[12] The value of adding tamoxifen to chemotherapy in premenopausal women may be smaller since in the meta-analysis of all trials comparing 5 years of tamoxifen with no tamoxifen (patients in both arms might have received the same chemotherapy), the reduction in the odds of recurrence was smaller: 34%[4] (see Table 10.6). Chemotherapy suppresses ovarian function in premenopausal women, and this may explain its apparently greater effect in premenopausal than postmenopausal women.

In premenopausal, as in older women, 10 years of adjuvant tamoxifen is more effective than 5 years[10] (Table 10.6).

Although an AI should never be used in premenopausal women, it has been used in women who were premenopausal at diagnosis and became menopausal during a 5-year course of adjuvant tamoxifen. In the only trial with published results, 5 years of an AI following 5 years of tamoxifen in this group substantially reduced recurrences.[13]

Studies evaluating combinations of OSup and an AI are underway, but until results of both efficacy and toxicity are available, combining these agents is not recommended. (Of course, chemotherapy is also a form of OSup. See discussion later in this chapter on the use of chemotherapy added to tamoxifen.)

Recommended Adjuvant Endocrine Therapy for Premenopausal Women

- 10 years of tamoxifen
- Sequential therapy with 5 years of tamoxifen followed by 5 years of AI, leading to a total treatment duration of 10 years. (Menopausal status should be confirmed by biochemical measurement before starting the AI since AIs may be harmful to premenopausal patients.) *goserelin, leuprolide, triptorelin + TAM /exemestane*
- Addition of a GNRH agonist to tamoxifen therapy may be advantageous. The data are inconsistent, and major groups do not recommend ovarian ablation or suppression as part of adjuvant therapy until more data are available. *High risk < 35yr ↑ benefit*

SOFT + TEXT trial →

Estrogen Receptor Level and Adjuvant Endocrine Therapy

Resistance to adjuvant endocrine therapies likely occurs in a substantial fraction (possibly > 50%) of patients with ER+ tumors, just as in the metastatic setting (see Chapter 12), but there is no widely agreed-upon method for identifying these patients. There is also evidence that the relative reduction in recurrence rate may be 10%–15% greater among those with higher quantitative measurements of ER.[2] The studies suggesting a relationship between ER level and response employed dextran-coated charcoal, not immunohistochemistry. There is no evidence of a response relationship to quantitative IHC, and there is wide variation in methods used to assess ER with IHC (see Chapter 7). Until reliable markers of endocrine resistance are found,

Table 10.6 Incremental Benefits Derived From Adjuvant Endocrine Therapies Compared to No Adjuvant Therapy at All, to No Endocrine Therapy, or to 5 Years of Tamoxifen for Premenopausal Women With ER+ Tumors

Treatment Under Study	Therapy for Control Group	No. of Patients Enrolled	No. of Trials	For Study Regimen, Proportional Reduction[a] in Rate of	
				Recurrence (%)[d]	Death (%)[d]
OA[1, b]	No adjuvant	1,294	8	32	31
TAM 5 years[2]	No adjuvant	1,327	2	45	32
TAM 5 years[1, c]	No endocrine	3,073	12	34	29
TAM 10 years[3]	TAM 5 years	630	1	19[e]	NR[f]
TAM 5 years → AI 5 years [4] (Total 10 years)	TAM 5 years	877	1	74	57[g]

Data are from meta-analyses of multiple trials or from a large single trial. In many of these trials patients also received chemotherapy, but if so the same chemotherapy was given to patients in both study arms. In most of the studies premenopausal was defined as aged < 50.

OA = ovarian ablation with oophorectomy or radiation therapy; TAM = tamoxifen; years = duration of treatment; No. = number; NR = not reported

[a] Reduction in annual odds or HR

[b] Most of these studies were conducted prior to 1960, so ER is largely unknown

[c] EBCTG trials combined ER+ and ER unknown tumors;

[d] Differences in outcome highly statistically significant (≥ 0.01) except where noted

[e] p not reported separately for subgroup; for all menopausal groups, reduction in rate of recurrence was 16%, $p = 0.002$; for subgroup, effect not statistically significant

[f] Mortality reduction not reported for subgroup, but for all menopausal groups reduction in mortality was 13%, $p = 0.01$

[g] $p = 0.31$

[1] EBCTG (2005) Early Breast Cancer Trials Collaborative Group. Effects of chemotherapy and hormonal therapy for early breast cancer on recurrence and 15-year survival: an overview of the randomised trials. *Lancet.* 2005;365:1687–717.

[2] EBCTG (1998) Early Breast Cancer Trialists Collaborative Group. Tamoxifen for early breast cancer: an overview of the randomised trials. *Lancet.* 1998;351:1451–67.

[3] Davies (2013) Davies C, Pan H, Godwin J, et al. Long-term effects of continuing adjuvant tamoxifen to 10 years versus stopping at 5 years after diagnosis of oestrogen receptor-positive breast cancer: ATLAS, a randomised trial. *Lancet.* 2013;381:805–16.

[4] Goss (2013) Goss PE, Ingle JN, Martino S, et al. Impact of premenopausal status at breast cancer diagnosis in women entered on the placebo-controlled NCIC CTG MA17 trial of extended adjuvant letrozole. *Ann Oncol.* 2013;24:355–61.

it is recommended that all patients with an unequivocally positive ER tumor be given adjuvant endocrine treatment.[14]

Adverse Events from Endocrine Therapies

Generally the side effects from adjuvant endocrine treatment are mild, but in spite of this and the observation that non-adherent patients have a poorer survival, up to 20% of patients discontinue therapy within the first year, and 31%–73% in various studies discontinue therapy by the end of the fifth year.[15] Up to 20% switch their regimen from an AI to tamoxifen, or vice versa.

Most premenopausal and many postmenopausal women (up to 80% altogether) will experience hot flashes, more often with AIs than tamoxifen. Menstrual irregularities, including amenorrhea in many patients receiving prolonged courses, occur with tamoxifen in premenopausal patients. All age groups have reported vaginal discharge and sexual dysfunction. Often a patient will report cognitive changes, such as increased forgetfulness, with all forms of endocrine therapy, but their frequency and importance are not certain.

Tamoxifen is associated with a significantly increased incidence of endometrial cancer. The incidence and mortality associated with 5 years of treatment is 1.6% and 0.2%, respectively, and for 5–14 years, 3.1% and 0.4%.[10] This increase is not seen with AIs, where the OR (odds ratio) relative to tamoxifen = 0.34, $p < 0.001$, in a meta-analysis.[16] Routine pre- or post-treatment screening with ultrasound and/or biopsy is not recommended.

With prolonged tamoxifen use, there is an increased incidence of venous thrombosis that has been reported to be 2.8% in a pooled analysis of large randomized trials.[16] The OR for venous thrombosis with AIs is 0.55 ($p < 0.001$).

Tamoxifen increases bone mineral density and leads to a decreased incidence of fractures. In contrast, the removal of circulating estrogens with AIs has the opposite effect, and the incidence of bone fractures is 47% higher after prolonged AI treatment compared to tamoxifen.[16] Although the use of a bisphosphonate or denosumab will reduce AI-induced bone loss, these agents are not routinely recommended for all patients who receive an AI because of potential toxicities, such as necrosis of the jaw (see Chapter 12). A baseline bone mineral density study is recommended, and a bone-target agent should then be initiated, using the criteria and regimens outlined in Table 10.7.[17] A follow-up bone density study should be obtained at 1–2 years. The reasonable or safe duration of treatment is not established.

Musculoskeletal complications (MSCs) characterized as arthralgia, myalgia, morning stiffness, and decreased grip strength occur in about 50% of patients who take AIs but not other endocrine therapies.[18] Most patients on AIs have none of these symptoms. Patients more likely to experience this toxicity are those who have joint pain prior to starting an AI, are obese, have previously been treated with hormones (e.g., HRT), and have been given adjuvant chemotherapy, especially with a taxane. Although there is no evidence that the incidence of MSCs is higher with any one AI, symptomatic patients have been shown to have less pain when switched to another AI. NSAIDs are commonly used but have not been formally evaluated. Recently it was shown in a randomized trial that regular exercise could reduce symptoms in 20% of

Table 10.7 Guidelines for Use of Bone-Targeted Agents for Cancer Treatment-Related Bone Loss: Treatments Include Ovarian Suppression From Chemotherapy or LHRH-Agonists in Premenopausal Women and Aromatase Inhibitors Postmenopausal Women

Bone-targeted agents are indicated for bone mineral density (BMD) scores of

T score ≥ −2 or −2.5

T score < −1 to < −2.0 in patients with > 1 non-BMD risk factor

Bone-targeted therapy indicated regardless of BMD score with ≥ 2 of these non-BMD risk factors:

- Prior fragility fracture of vertebrae or hip
- Oral corticosteroid use > 6 months
- History smoking or excess alcohol use
- Age > 65
- Low BMI (20 kg/m²)

Bone target therapy regimens are the same or nearly the same as those used to treat osteoporosis, but the doses are lower and the intervals longer than those used to treat patients with metastatic bone lesions:

Drug	Route	Dose	Frequency
Zoledronic acid	Intravenous	4 mg	Every 6 months
Ibandronate	Oral	150 mg	Monthly
Risedronate	Oral	35 mg	Weekly
Alendronate	Oral	70 mg	Weekly
Denosumab	Subcutaneous	60 mg	Every 6 months

Calcium and vitamin D supplements are usually used as follows:

- Elemental calcium: 1200–1500 mg for post- and 1200 mg for premenopausal women.
- Vitamin D3 400–2000 units depending in part on evidence of deficiency

These are a composite from guidelines promulgated by various international groups, including ASCO, the St. Gallen conference, Swiss Guidelines, and ad hoc international expert panel.

Aapro MS, Coleman RE. Bone health management in patients with breast cancer: Current standards and emerging strategies. *Breast.* 2012;21:8–19.

patients.[19] If nothing else is effective, the patient may be switched to tamoxifen since the benefits will be substantially greater than no adjuvant therapy at all.

The chances of developing cardiovascular (CV) disease are greater with AIs than tamoxifen. This seems to be related to the duration of treatment. Five years of AI therapy increase the odds by 30% ($p = 0.01$) in a meta-analysis of trials comparing first-line AI with tamoxifen.[16] In the pivotal trial comparing anastrozole and tamoxifen, the incidence of ischemic CV disease in patients with a prior history of ischemic CV disease was 17% for the AI and 10% for tamoxifen, a point the FDA highlighted in the product insert. Tamoxifen reduces serum cholesterol, but it has not been shown to decrease the incidence or mortality from cardiovascular disease compared to placebo.

ADJUVANT CHEMOTHERAPY

Adjuvant chemotherapy has been shown to benefit almost all groups of patients, but not necessarily to the same degree. Its effects on recurrence and death are nearly twice as great in younger women (most of whom are premenopausal) than older women[4] (see Figure 10.2).

- In younger women the effects of chemotherapy are about the same in those with ER+ and ER– tumors.

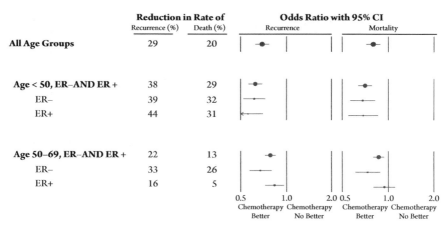

Figure 10.2 Overviews of trials evaluating combination chemotherapy compared to no adjuvant therapy at all in younger and older women and in those with ER– or ER+ tumors. No tamoxifen therapy was given to patients on either arm of these early studies even if ER+, in contrast to most later trials. The chemotherapy regimens were most often 6 or 12 months of CMF-based treatment, or about 6 months of anthracycline-based treatment with combinations such as FAC or FEC, although some involved other agents (e.g., vincristine, melphalan).
Source: Early Breast Cancer Trials Collaborative Group. Effects of chemotherapy and hormonal therapy for early breast cancer on recurrence and 15-year survival: an overview of the randomised trials. *Lancet.* 2005;365:1687–717.

- In older women (most of whom are postmenopausal) adjuvant chemotherapy has about the same benefit in those with ER− tumors as it does in younger women.
- However, in older women with ER+ tumors adjuvant chemotherapy has a much smaller effect on recurrence and a non-significant effect on mortality (Figure 10.2).

These data suggest that chemotherapy has less effect on ER+ tumors. There are a number of factors to explain this; one of the most likely is that ER+ cells more slowly multiply (see Chapter 4) and are thus less sensitive to the effects of cytotoxics that are expressed primarily when the cell attempts division. In premenopausal women, chemotherapy usually suppresses ovarian function, and in this way it exerts both a direct cytotoxic and endocrine effect on cells. This may explain the observation that chemotherapy is equally effective in ER− and ER+ tumors in premenopausal but not postmenopausal women.

There are no other factors that have reproducibly been shown to predict benefit from adjuvant chemotherapy. The proportional effects are not different in patients subsets defined by tumor size or nodal status.

Evolution of Chemotherapy Regimens: CMF and Anthracyclines

Until adjuvant chemotherapy had definitely been shown to prolong survival, it was difficult to justify giving toxic therapy to asymptomatic patients, many of whom were at very little risk of recurrence following local therapy. For this reason, the first regimens were single injections of therapy, given at the time of mastectomy, with the goal of eradicating cells released into the bloodstream as a result of surgical perturbation of the primary. Subsequently, single agents were administered for 2–4 weeks, and one trial utilizing short courses of daily oral cyclophosphamide demonstrated a survival benefit. Prolonged administration of a single drug, especially melphalan for 1–2 years, resulted in greater benefit. However, increasingly it was apparent that adjuvant systemic therapy was effective because it reduced the size of well-established, albeit occult, lesions, many of which were only slightly below the size of measurable metastatic lesions ($\geq 10^6$ cells) and that the drug regimens most effective for treating metastases would also impart the largest survival benefits when administered as adjuvant therapy. These combination chemotherapy regimens were shown in multiple trials and in meta-analyses of these studies to be superior to single agents (see Figure 10.3). There is no longer justification for the routine use of single agents in the management of early breast cancer.

The first chemotherapy regimen shown to prolong survival in the adjuvant setting was CMF, in which cyclophosphamide was administered orally on days 1–14 of a 28-day cycle ("poCMF")[26] (Table 10.8). Subsequently, CMF variations have been developed that utilize intravenous cyclophosphamide ("ivCMF"). The only direct comparison of oral CMF with an intravenous variant was conducted in the metastatic setting, where the oral regimen was shown to significantly improve response rate, time to progression, and overall survival compared to the variant, but poCMF was also more toxic.[27] Cyclophosphamide has also been used both orally and intravenously in combination with anthracyclines, and in this setting, too, the oral cyclophosphamide appears to be substantially more effective.[3] Trials comparing newer regimens with

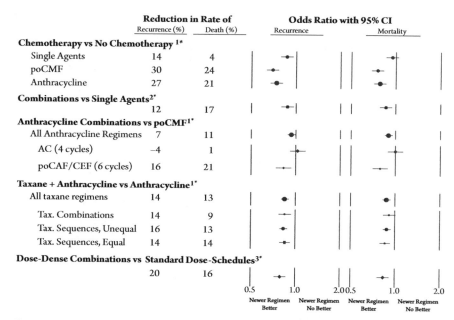

	Reduction in Rate of		**Odds Ratio with 95% CI**	
	Recurrence (%)	Death (%)	Recurrence	Mortality
Chemotherapy vs No Chemotherapy [1]*				
Single Agents	14	4		
poCMF	30	24		
Anthracycline	27	21		
Combinations vs Single Agents[2]*				
	12	17		
Anthracycline Combinations vs poCMF[1]*				
All Anthracycline Regimens	7	11		
AC (4 cycles)	−4	1		
poCAF/CEF (6 cycles)	16	21		
Taxane + Anthracycline vs Anthracycline[1]*				
All taxane regimens	14	13		
Tax. Combinations	14	9		
Tax. Sequences, Unequal	16	13		
Tax. Sequences, Equal	14	14		
Dose-Dense Combinations vs Standard Dose-Schedules[3]*				
	20	16		

0.5   1.0   2.0   0.5   1.0   2.0

Newer Regimen Better   Newer Regimen No Better   Newer Regimen Better   Newer Regimen No Better

Figure 10.3 Overviews of adjuvant chemotherapy trials evaluating various chemotherapy regimens. *In contrast to Figure 10.2, most of these trials allowed patients with ER+ tumors to receive endocrine therapy in addition to the chemotherapy as long as the same endocrine therapy was used on both arms of the study.

poCMF = oral cyclophosphamide (C) with methotrexate (M) and 5-fluorouracil (F); poCAF/ CEF = oral with F & either doxorubicin (A) or epirubicin (E); Tax. = taxane; Equal and unequal = relative durations of therapy for taxane containing arm compared to the non-taxane arm.

1 EBCTCG 2012 Early Breast Cancer Trialists Collaborative Group. Comparisons between different polychemotherapy regimens for early breast cancer: meta-analyses of long-term outcome among 100,000 women in 123 randomised trials. *Lancet*. 2012;379:432–44.

2 EBCTCG 1992 Early Breast Cancer Trialists' Collaborative Group. Systemic Treatment of Early Breast Cancer by Hormonal, Cytotoxic, or Immune Therapy: 133 Randomised Trials Involving 31,000 Recurrences and 24,000 Deaths Among 75,000 Women. *Lancet*. 1992;339:1–15, 71–85.

3 Meta-analysis based on Citron (2003), Swain (2013), Moebus (2010), Venturini (2005), Burnell (2010), and Baldini (2003). Citron ML, Berry DA, Cirrincione C, et al. Randomized trial of dose-dense versus conventionally scheduled and sequential versus concurrent combination chemotherapy as postoperative adjuvant treatment of node-positive primary breast cancer: first report of Intergroup Trial C9741/Cancer and Leukemia Group B Trial 9741. *J Clin Oncol*. 2003;21:1431–9. Swain SM, Tang G, Geyer CE, Jr., et al. Definitive results of a phase III adjuvant trial comparing three chemotherapy regimens in women with operable, node-positive breast cancer: the NSABP B-38 trial. *J Clin Oncol*. 2013;31:3197–204. Moebus V, Jackisch C, Lueck HJ, et al. Intense dose-dense sequential chemotherapy with epirubicin, paclitaxel, and cyclophosphamide compared with conventionally scheduled chemotherapy in high-risk primary breast cancer: mature results of an AGO phase III study. *J Clin Oncol*. 2010;28:2874–80. Venturini M, Del Mastro L, Aitini E, et al. Dose-dense adjuvant chemotherapy in early breast cancer patients: results from a randomized trial. *J Nat Cancer Inst*. 2005;97:1724–33. Burnell M, Levine MN, Chapman JA, et al. Cyclophosphamide, epirubicin, and Fluorouracil versus dose-dense epirubicin and cyclophosphamide followed by paclitaxel versus doxorubicin and cyclophosphamide followed by paclitaxel in node-positive or high-risk node-negative breast cancer. *J Clin Oncol*. 2010;28:77–82. Baldini E, Gardin G, Giannessi PG, et al. Accelerated versus standard cyclophosphamide, epirubicin and 5-fluorouracil or cyclophosphamide, methotrexate and 5-fluorouracil: a randomized phase III trial in locally advanced breast cancer. *Ann Oncol*. 2003;14:227–32.

Table 10.8 Most Effective and Recommended Cytotoxic Drug Regimens to Use as Adjuvant Therapy

Regimens	Cycle Length (Weeks)	Doses (mg/m^2) and Schedule of Each Drug in Regimen					No. of Cycles	Therapy Duration (Months)
		C	M	A or E	F	Taxane P^a or D^b		
poCMF (standard)	4	100 po d1–14	40 iv d1 & d8	–	600 iv d1 & d8	–	6	6
poCAF	4	100 po d1–14	–	A: 30 iv d1 & d8	600 iv d1 & d8		6	6
poCEF	4	75 po d–1–14		E: 60 iv d1 & d8	500 iv d1 & d8		6	6
AC →T**	3/1*	600 iv d1		A: 60 iv d1		P: 80 iv d1	4/12	6
TAC**	3	500 iv d1		A: 50 iv d1		D: 75 iv d1	6	6
DD AC →T^c,**	2/2	600 iv d1		A: 60 iv d1		P: 175 iv d1	4/4	4

DD Dose Dense; po = orally; iv = intravenously; d = day; No. = number.

→ Sequential regimen: all cycles of the drugs before the arrow are administered before drug(s) after arrow.

* AC portion given every 3 weeks and T (paclitaxel) administered weekly

^{a} P = paclitaxel. To prevent hypersensitivity reactions with P, premedicate with dexamethasone, diphenhydramine, and ranitidine or famotidine

^{b} D = docetaxel. To prevent hypersensitivity reactions with D, premedicate with dexamethasone

^{c} DD regimen has high incidence of febrile neutropenia; G-CSF required with each cycle of therapy.

** AC→T, TAC, and DD AC→T have never been compared to either poCAF or poCEF, the most effective anthracycline regimens. See text regarding the implications of this.

(See Table 12.7 in Chpater 12 for toxicities associated with each drug.)

ivCMF may erroneously overestimate the benefit of the newer therapy if it is assumed that the poCMF and ivCMF are equivalent.

The second generation of adjuvant trials added an anthracycline, doxorubicin or epirubicin, to one or more of the CMF drugs. This further reduces the odds of recurrence by 7% and odds of death by 11% compared with poCMF. However, not all anthracycline combinations provide additional benefit. The use of intravenous doxorubicin with intravenous cyclophosphamide (AC) every 3 weeks for 4 cycles is very popular because of its short duration and limited toxicity. However, it has no advantage over poCMF. It is often assumed that it is at least equivalent, but this, too, is incorrect since it was not evaluated in an appropriately powered non-inferiority trial.[28] Either poCAF or poCEF is the optimal anthracycline regimen to use; in the meta-analysis of trials using these combinations the reduction in odds of recurrence and mortality was 16% and 21%, respectively[3] (Figure 10.3).

Taxanes and Dose-Dense Regimens

Taxanes (T) have recently been added to an anthracycline either in combination (e.g., TAC) or in sequence (e.g., AC→T) (Table 10.8). Overall these regimens improve outcomes over anthracycline combinations, reducing the odds of recurrence and mortality by 14% and 13%, respectively[3] (Figure 10.3). The earliest of the taxane trials randomized patients to either 4 cycles of AC followed by 4 cycles of T, or only 4 cycles of AC. The superior outcomes from using the taxane regimen in these trials could have been due either to the more prolonged course of treatment or the addition of the taxane, but a meta-analysis comparing trials using taxanes in sequences in which the two arms were of unequal duration, as in the original trial, or of identical duration fail to show a difference. The sequential regimens appear to be as effective as but are somewhat less toxic than combinations in which the taxane and anthracycline are given together in each cycle.

It is not clear that paclitaxel is superior to docetaxel.[29] However, weekly paclitaxel is significantly more effective in reducing recurrence and improving survival than paclitaxel given every 3 weeks. The opposite is true for docetaxel, which seems to be most effective when given every 3 weeks.

There are as yet very limited data on substituting a taxane for an anthracycline. One study randomized 1,016 women with early breast cancer to 4 cycles of either a combination of docetaxel and intravenous cyclophosphamide (DC) or AC.[30] The HR for recurrence and death was significantly reduced by 26% and 31% by DC. However, this regimen cannot be accepted yet for routine practice since it is not clear that it is as effective or better than the most effective anthracycline or taxane regimens already established.[28]

In dose-dense regimens the drugs already shown to be effective are administered more intensely, usually at 2-week rather than at 3-week intervals.[20] One of these regimens is shown in Table 10.8. The number of published trials evaluating dose-dense therapy is small with varying design and the follow-up is still short, but an overview of 5 dose-dense trials suggests that these might further increase disease-free and overall survival by 20% and 16%[20–25] (Figure 10.3).

It should be noted that none of the taxane regimens and only one of the dose-dense regimens were compared to the most effective anthracycline regimens: poCAF or poCEF. However, in one trial, 2,104 patients were randomized to either poCEF, DD EC→T (dose-dense epirubicin + cyclophosphamide followed by paclitaxel) or AC→T for 6 months.[24] The poCEF was very significantly superior to AC→T and roughly equal to the DD EC→T. The results of this very large study by a major group of investigators suggests that the relative value of taxane or dose-dense treatment for early breast cancer is not fully settled.

Adjuvant Chemotherapy in ER+ Patients

In a number of trials, adding adjuvant chemotherapy to adjuvant tamoxifen in postmenopausal women with ER+ tumors added no benefit at all.[31,32] However, in the Oxford overviews, the addition of chemotherapy to tamoxifen leads to about the same proportional decrease in odds of recurrence and death as the use of chemotherapy in ER+ patients who do not receive tamoxifen.[4] This apparent contradiction may be due to a number of factors, including the fact that the overview divided patients by age rather than menopausal status, so some of the women aged 50–69 were actually premenopausal, a group in which chemotherapy affects endocrine function as well as being directly cytotoxic (see earlier discussion). In addition, the overviews are taken from trials conducted at numerous places over the entire globe, and the quality of the ER determinations may be quite variable (see Chapter 7).

The most likely explanation for the discordance between individual trial results and the overview is that there is a subset of patients with ER+ tumors who respond to chemotherapy and another for whom it provides no advantage. This has been demonstrated in post hoc analyses of two independent randomized trials comparing tamoxifen alone or tamoxifen plus chemotherapy in those with ER+ tumors (see Figure 10.4). Recurrence scores (RS) were determined using the 21-gene recurrence score assay (see Chapter 7) on all blocks with adequate tissue. On the basis of the RSs the ER+ tumors were divided into those with a low risk (< 18% chance), high risk (≥ 31%), or intermediate risk of recurring.[33,34] Then the effect of adding chemotherapy in each risk category was determined. There was no benefit from adding chemotherapy to tamoxifen in the low-risk group, which constituted 54% of the node-negative and 40% of the node-positive patients, but there was a highly significant benefit from adding chemotherapy in high-risk patients (25% and 32% of node-negative and node-positive patients, respectively). Randomized trials designed to further evaluate the 21-gene RS assay and other gene profiling tests (Chapter 7) are underway, especially for those in the intermediate RS categories and in node-positive patients, but the evidence available from these retrospective analyses of prospective randomized trials is sufficiently compelling to justify the use of these assays before deciding to use chemotherapy (in addition to endocrine therapy) in postmenopausal women with an ER+ tumor, especially those with node-negative tumors where over half of patients might be harmed by the use of toxic therapy that is almost certainly not likely to provide any kind of benefit.

The decisions to use chemotherapy or to use endocrine therapy are independent of each other. These modalities are additive but *not* synergistic. In fact, they may be antagonistic; the inhibition of tumor cell turnover by endocrine therapy may decrease the cells' sensitivity to a cytotoxic drug. It has been shown in randomized trials that using chemotherapy and tamoxifen in sequence is more effective than using them

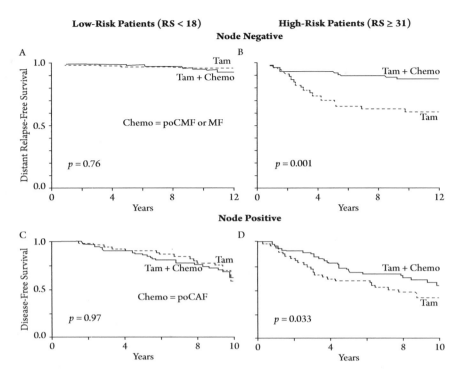

Figure 10.4 Adding chemotherapy to tamoxifen as adjuvant therapy for patients with ER+ tumors further defined as low-risk or high-risk using the 21-gene recurrence score assay. A and B are post-hoc analyses of a trial (NSABP B-20) in which 2,363 patients with node-negative tumors were randomized to receive either tamoxifen alone or tamoxifen plus chemotherapy using either poCMF or MF. C and D are post hoc analyses of a trial (SWOG-8814) in which 1,477 patients with node-positive tumors were randomized to receive either tamoxifen alone or tamoxifen plus poCAF chemotherapy. Adequate tissue in blocks was available to determine recurrence score (RS) in 353 of the node negative and 367 of the node-positive patients; patients were placed in low-, intermediate-, and high-risk groups with cut points at 18 and 31. (Only results from the low- and high-risk groups are shown here). In the node-negative study, 54.2% were in the low-risk category and 25.2% in the high-risk category. In the node-positive trial, 63% of tumors were 2–5 cm in size and 62% had 1–3 positive nodes; the proportion with an RS in the low- and high-risk categories was 39.8% and 32.2%. Reprinted with permission from Paik S, Tang G, Shak S, et al. Gene expression and benefit of chemotherapy in women with node-negative, estrogen receptor-positive breast cancer. *J Clin Oncol.* 2006;24:3726–34; and Albain KS, Barlow WE, Shak S, et al. Prognostic and predictive value of the 21-gene recurrence score assay in postmenopausal women with node-positive, oestrogen-receptor-positive breast cancer on chemotherapy: a retrospective analysis of a randomised trial. *Lancet Oncol.* 2010;11:55–65.

concomitantly.[35] This may be true for radiotherapy and tamoxifen as well. As a general rule, all chemotherapy and radiotherapy are completed first, usually within 6 months of diagnosis, and endocrine therapy is then administered for 5 to 10 years.

Although chemotherapy affects endocrine function in premenopausal women and has a much greater effect on ER+ tumors in pre- than in postmenopausal women (see earlier discussion), premenopausal patients, especially those under age 40, clearly benefit from having endocrine therapy added to the chemotherapy.[36]

Adverse Events from Chemotherapy

Most cytotoxic therapies are associated with multiple side effects, the most common being anorexia, fatigue, nausea, vomiting, diarrhea, alopecia, rash, and bone marrow suppression resulting in myelosuppression and, less often, thrombocytopenia. The specific symptoms, their frequency, and severity will vary depending on the cytotoxic regimen used. Although patients without clinically evident metastases and prior treatment tolerate these regimens better than those with advanced disease, the toxicity profile for the most commonly used regimens are the same in both settings. Details for the side effects of specific drugs and regimens are provided in Chapter 12.

Chemotherapy-associated cognitive dysfunction, often referred to as "chemobrain," is a well-established entity that occurs in many or even most patients while receiving chemotherapy; in some patients it may persist for as long as 20 years after completion of chemotherapy. The most common symptoms are memory lapses for recent events, names, common words and dates, difficulty completing tasks as quickly and in as orderly a fashion equal to that prior to the cancer diagnosis, and a decreased ability to multi-task. Between 20% and 40% of patients have been found to have symptoms or objective evidence of cognitive dysfunction *prior to any treatment*—surgery or chemotherapy; 17%–75% have decline in cognitive function during chemotherapy; and 60% have dysfunction or even develop it for the first time after completion of chemotherapy.[37] Post-therapy symptoms may slowly disappear or persist for years or even decades. Subjective complaints occur more frequently than objective signs and are often associated with depression, anxiety, coping issues, and cancer-related fatigue. The underlying mechanisms for objective findings are unknown, but it is hypothesized that either cancer causes neurological impairment or that there are shared risks for cancer and cognitive dysfunction. Neuroimaging studies (e.g., MRI) have demonstrated reductions in gray matter volume and white matter connectivity during the time when patients are receiving chemotherapy, and these changes correlate with objective cognitive dysfunction. Chemobrain has been reported with most forms of chemotherapy but may be more frequent with FAC (5-fluorouracil, doxorubicin, and cyclophosphamide). Severe encephalopathy has been reported on rare occasions with methotrexate, 5-fluorouracil, and cisplatin. In longitudinal studies it has been shown that there is a cumulative increase in cognitive dysfunction with each additional course of treatment. There is less certainty about the impact of endocrine therapy, but there are reports that SERMs may induce cognitive impairment. Interventions that have been shown in numerous studies, including a few randomized trials, to be beneficial include cognitive rehabilitation (patients meeting as individuals or in groups with trained clinicians to improve memory and attention), cognitive training (more focused exercise, often using computer programs, to improve mental processing speed for time-order judgment, spatial match, and narrative memory tasks), increased physical activity using breathing exercises and/or yoga, and neurofeedback using EEG, functional near-infrared spectroscopy, or real-time fMRI.[37] Pharmacologic interventions have generally not been shown to be effective, but the studies are limited in number, small, and often of suboptimal design.

The incidence of symptomatic cardiomyopathy (congestive heart failure, CHF) has been reported to range from 0.5% to 1.5% in the first 5 years following adjuvant treatment with cumulative doses of 240–360 mg/m^2 of doxorubicin or 240–720 mg/m^2 of epirubicin.[28] However, this may underestimate the true incidence of cardiotoxicity that will become clinically important as follow-up lengthens, patients age, or the anthracycline is combined with other drugs. The frequency of systolic dysfunction, defined by a substantial fall in left ventricular ejection fraction, may be as high as four times the incidence of CHF.[38] When an anthracycline is combined with trastuzumab, the incidence of cardiotoxicity is increased by about 4-fold[28] (see Chapter 12). Limiting the cumulative dose of the anthracycline is the most important method for avoiding cardiotoxicity. Dexrazoxane may also be used for this purpose.

Since most cytotoxic agents are mutagens, it is surprising that the frequency of second tumors following adjuvant chemotherapy is relatively small. The overall incidence is about 1 in 20.[38] The most common secondary, non-breast cancers are acute myeloid leukemia (AML) and myelodysplastic syndrome (MDS). AML typically appears 5 years after treatment with an alkylating agent, such as cyclophosphamide. In a meta-analysis of 19 studies the cumulative incidence of AML/MDS was 0.37 (95% CI, 0.13%–0.61%) 8 years after completion of standard dose cyclophosphamide plus epirubicin.[38]

Premenopausal women commonly experience amenorrhea while receiving chemotherapy. The frequency varies with the age of the patient, the specific chemotherapy regimen used, and the duration of treatment.[38] For example, four cycles of AC induces amenorrhea in 57%–63% of women aged > 40, but only 13% of those aged 30–40. In contrast, classic CMF using oral cyclophosphamide induces amenorrhea in 76%–96% of those aged > 40 and 31%–38% of those aged 30–40. For younger women, menses usually return sometime after the completion of chemotherapy, but the older the patient, the more likely that amenorrhea will be permanent. Amenorrheic patients usually experience all the symptoms of menopause, and hot flashes can be particularly troublesome. Fertility returns with menses (or even before the resumption of a regular menstrual cycle). It is generally accepted that women can safely become pregnant after completion of adjuvant chemotherapy, but the data are limited and somewhat inconsistent. Chemotherapy given entirely before gestation is not likely to be associated with birth defects, but there may be increased complications associated with the pregnancy or reduced birth weight.[38]

HER2+ TUMORS: ADJUVANT SYSTEMIC THERAPIES

Prior to trastuzumab, patients with HER2+ tumors had the worst prognosis among all patient subsets defined by various prognostic factors. The use of adjuvant trastuzumab has changed that, and now appropriately treated patients with HER2+ tumors are among those with the best prognosis.

Six very large randomized trials in the adjuvant setting were started shortly after the drug was initially introduced. In all cases, trastuzumab was used with a chemotherapy regimen that usually included an anthracycline, a taxane, and cyclophosphamide, but the actual regimens differed considerably (see Table 10.9). In most of the studies, trastuzumab was administered along with part or all of the chemotherapy and then as a single agent for some time after the chemotherapy was complete. In all cases the initial dose of trastuzumab was larger than subsequent doses; the most popular dose schedule used in US and European trials differed in both dose and schedule (Table 10.9).

The overall effect of adding trastuzumab to chemotherapy is as large or larger than any other adjuvant intervention previously evaluated: a 40% reduction in the

Table 10.9 Adjuvant Trastuzumab Trials: Design of Individual Trials and Results of a Meta-Analysis of Eight Studies

TRIAL	SCHEMA Arm 1*	SCHEMA Arm 2	SCHEMA Arms 3 & 4*	Trastuzumab Dose	Chemotherapy Doses
NSABP B-31	AC→PH→H	AC→P		4 mg/kg 1st dose → 2 mg/kg weekly	AC 60/600 mg/m² q 3 X 4 cycles; P 175 mg/m² q3 X 4 cycles;
NCCTG N9831	AC→PH→H	AC→P	AC→P→H	Same as NSABP	AC 60/600 mg/m² q 3 X 4 cycles; P 80 mg/m² weekly X 12 cycles;
HERA	Chemo→H	Chemo	Chemo→H[a]	8 mg/kg 1st dose → 6 mg/kg 3-weekly	Chemo: any approved regimen for at least 4 cycles; maximum A = 360 or E = 720 mg/m²
BCIRG 006	AC→DH→H	AC→P	DCarboH →H	NA	AC 60/600 mg/m² q 3 X 4 cycles; D 100 mg/m² q3 X 4 cycles; DCarbo 75/75 mg/m² q3 X 6 cycles.
FinHer	DH[b]→FEC	D→FEC	V in place of D	Same as NSABP	D 100 mg/m² q3 X 3 cycles; V 25 mg/m² d 1, 8 & 15 q 3 X 3 cycles; FEC 600/60/600 mg/m² q 3 X 3 cycles
PACS-04	FEC	FEC→H	ED in place of FEC	Same as HERA	FEC 500/100/500 mg/m² q 3 X 6 cycles; ED 75/75 mg/m² q 3 X 6 cycles
Meta-analysis[c]	Number of Patients 11,991	Recurrence 40% p < 0.00001	Reduction in Hazard of Recurrence	Death 34% p < 0.00001	Death p < 0.00001

H = trastuzumab; A = doxorubicin; C = cyclophosphamide; P = paclitaxel; D = docetaxel; Carbo = carboplatin; V = vinorelbine; E = epirubicin; Chemo = chemotherapy regimen chosen by primary physician from approved list; q3 = every 3 weeks; d = day (of cycle); NA = not available

* H alone administered for a total of 52 weeks except as noted

[a] H administered for 104 weeks

[b] H administered for 9 weeks

[c] Meta-analysis includes 6 trials above + 2 randomized neoadjuvant studies not shown.

From Moja L, Tagliabue L, Balduzzi S, et al. Trastuzumab containing regimens for early breast cancer. *Cochrane Database Syst Rev.* 2012;4:CD006243.

proportional risk of recurrence and a 34% reduction in the risk of death. This is with a median follow-up of 18–65 months at the times the results of these studies were reported.

Key points to consider in using anti-HER2 therapies in the adjuvant setting are the following:

- Most patients with HER2+ tumors should be treated with trastuzumab plus chemotherapy. The patients enrolled in the pivotal trials were at high risk of recurrence either because of nodal involvement (> 80%) or tumor size. However, about half of them had ER+ tumors.
- The one group not well represented in trials were those with HER2+ tumors of < 1 cm in size. These patients have an increased risk of recurrence, and there is no reason to expect that they will derive less benefit from adjuvant trastuzumab than other groups. The NCCN has concluded that any HER2+ tumor > 0.5 cm should be considered for adjuvant trastuzumab, as well as smaller tumors with pN1m (axillary nodes ≤ 2 mm).[40]
- The criteria for HER2+ defined in guidelines developed by the American Society of Clinical Oncology (ASCO) and the American College of Pathologists (ACP) are either 3+ immunohistochemical staining for HER2 in > 10% of invasive tumor cells, a FISH amplification ratio of ≥ 2.0 using a dual HER2/CEP17 probe, or a FISH amplification ratio of < 2.0 using a dual HER2/CEP17 probe with an average gene copy number per cell of > 6.[41]
- Trastuzumab should be administered for 1 year, the duration of therapy most often used in pivotal trials. In the HERA trial patients were randomized to either 1 or 2 years of trastuzumab; there was no advantage for the longer duration. The FinHer study utilized only 9 week of trastuzumab, and this appeared to be beneficial. The one reported randomized trial comparing 12 and 6 months of adjuvant trastuzumab failed to show that the 6-month arm was non-inferior.[42]
- Trastuzumab significantly improves disease-free and overall survival whether given concommitantly with chemotherapy (usually a taxane but not with an anthracycline) or sequentially after chemotherapy (usually including an anthracycline) has been completed. However, one direct comparison and a meta-analysis based on whether trastuzumab was given sequentially or concurrently suggest that concurrent chemotherapy and trastuzumab *might* eventually prove superior.[39,42,43]
- In general, the chemotherapy regimen should include an anthracycline and a taxane. This was true for most of the studies shown in Table 10.9 and it is less certain that other regimens would be as effective in this setting. In BCIRG 006, trastuzumab was combined with docetaxel and carboplatin (DCarboH) and was compared with trastuzumab combined with AC followed by docetaxel (AC→DH). (Table 10.9; this study has not been published yet.) Outcomes with DCarboH were not significantly worse than with AC→DH, but because BCIRG 006 was not designed as a non-inferiority trial one cannot conclude that DCarboH is equivalent to AC→DH.[28] However, there was significantly less cardiotoxicity with DCarboH. Congestive heart failure occurred in 0.7% of the patients who received AC-P without trastuzumab, 2% of those given AC→DH, and 0.4% of those on DCarboH. These data suggest that DCarboH is sufficiently effective that it can be selected as a

reasonable alternative to an anthracycline-containing regimen for patients at higher than average risk of cardiotoxicity from trastuzumab.
- Anti-HER2 drugs other than trastuzumab have not yet been shown in randomized trials to be effective in this setting. In a trial with 3,161 patients with HER2+ tumors, lapatinib was shown to be no better than placebo.[44]
- Patients with HER2+ tumors that are also ER+ should be given endocrine therapy alone with trastuzumab after the completion of adjuvant chemotherapy using the principles for selecting therapy just described. This was the policy in the pivotal trials described in Table 10.9. It is generally not appropriate to substitute endocrine therapy for chemotherapy in HER2+ patients (see Chapter 12), but patients with very small tumors (< 1 cm) might be an exception to this rule.

GENERAL PRINCIPLES IN USING ADJUVANT SYSTEMIC THERAPIES

- First determine the patient's likelihood of recurrence within the next 10 years. Although the degree of toxicity that a patient is willing to accept for a given treatment benefit is highly variable, most patients with a risk under 10%–15% are unlikely to accept chemotherapy. More patients in this risk category will accept the toxicity of endocrine therapy, but some patients will find even this unacceptable with a risk of recurrence < 10%.
- ER and HER2 should be measured on all patients, both as a factor in determining risk and in choosing specific adjuvant systemic therapies.
- All patients with ER+ tumors with sufficient risk should receive endocrine therapy.
- All patients with ER– tumors with sufficient risk should receive chemotherapy with at least poCAF or poCEF for 6 months or, alternatively, one of the taxane or dose-dense regimens.
- All patients with HER2+ tumors > 1 cm in size should receive a combination of chemotherapy using an anthracycline, a taxane and trastuzumab.
- If a postmenopausal patient with an ER+ tumor is thought to be of sufficiently high risk to receive chemotherapy as well as endocrine therapy, obtain a gene-profiling study to more accurately estimate risk and the likelihood of benefiting from chemotherapy prior to finalizing the decision.

REFERENCES

1. Haybittle JL. Life expectancy as a measurement of the benefit shown by clinical trials of treatment for early breast cancer. *Clin Oncol.* 1998;10:92–4.
2. Early Breast Cancer Trialists Collaborative Group. Relevance of breast cancer hormone receptors and other factors to the efficacy of adjuvant tamoxifen: patient-level meta-analysis of randomised trials. *Lancet.* 2011;378:771–84.
3. Early Breast Cancer Trialists Collaborative Group. Comparisons between different polychemotherapy regimens for early breast cancer: meta-analyses of long-term outcome among 100,000 women in 123 randomised trials. *Lancet.* 2012;379:432–44.

4. Early Breast Cancer Trials Collaborative Group. Effects of chemotherapy and hormonal therapy for early breast cancer on recurrence and 15-year survival: an overview of the randomised trials. *Lancet.* 2005;365:1687–717.

5. Simes RJ, Coates AS. Patient preferences for adjuvant chemotherapy of early breast cancer: how much benefit is needed? *J Natl Cancer Inst Monogr.* 2001:146–52.

6. Duric VM, Stockler MR, Heritier S, et al. Patients' preferences for adjuvant chemotherapy in early breast cancer: what makes AC and CMF worthwhile now? *Ann Oncol.* 2005;16:1786–94.

7. Christiansen P, Bjerre K, Ejlertsen B, et al. Mortality rates among early-stage hormone receptor-positive breast cancer patients: a population-based cohort study in Denmark. *J Nat Cancer Inst.* 2011;103:1363–72.

8. Griggs JJ, Hayes DF. Do all patients with breast cancer require systemic adjuvant therapy? *J Nat Cancer Inst.* 2011;103:1350–1.

9. Aydiner A. Meta-analysis of breast cancer outcome and toxicity in adjuvant trials of aromatase inhibitors in postmenopausal women. *Breast.* 2013;22:121–9.

10. Davies C, Pan H, Godwin J, et al. Long-term effects of continuing adjuvant tamoxifen to 10 years versus stopping at 5 years after diagnosis of oestrogen receptor-positive breast cancer: ATLAS, a randomised trial. *Lancet.* 2013;381:805–16.

11. Early Breast Cancer Trialists Collaborative Group. Use of luteinising-hormone-releasing hormone agonists as adjuvant treatment in premenopausal patients with hormone-receptor-positive breast cancer: a meta-analysis of individual patient data from randomised adjuvant trials. *Lancet.* 2007;369:1711–23.

12. Early Breast Cancer Trialists Collaborative Group. Tamoxifen for early breast cancer: an overview of the randomised trials. *Lancet.* 1998;351:1451–67.

13. Goss PE, Ingle JN, Martino S, et al. Impact of premenopausal status at breast cancer diagnosis in women entered on the placebo-controlled NCIC CTG MA17 trial of extended adjuvant letrozole. *Ann Oncol.* 2013;24:355–61.

14. Wolff AC, Dowsett M. Estrogen receptor: a never ending story? *J Clin Oncol.* 2011;29:2955–8.

15. Murphy CC, Bartholomew LK, Carpentier MY, et al. Adherence to adjuvant hormonal therapy among breast cancer survivors in clinical practice: a systematic review. *Br Cancer Res Treat.* 2012;134:459–78.

16. Amir E, Seruga B, Niraula S, et al. Toxicity of adjuvant endocrine therapy in postmenopausal breast cancer patients: a systematic review and meta-analysis. *J Nat Cancer Inst.* 2011;103:1299–309.

17. Aapro MS, Coleman RE. Bone health management in patients with breast cancer: Current standards and emerging strategies. *Breast.* 2012;21:8–19.

18. Niravath P. Aromatase inhibitor-induced arthralgia: a review. *Ann Oncol.* 2013;24:1443–9.

19. Irwin ML, Cartmel B, Gross C, et al. Randomized trial of exercise vs. usual care on aromatase inhibitor-associated arthralgias in women with breast cancer: the hormones and physical exercise (HOPE) study. *Cancer Res.* 2013;73:S3–03.

20. Citron ML, Berry DA, Cirrincione C, et al. Randomized trial of dose-dense versus conventionally scheduled and sequential versus concurrent combination chemotherapy as postoperative adjuvant treatment of node-positive primary breast cancer: first report of Intergroup Trial C9741/Cancer and Leukemia Group B Trial 9741. *J Clin Oncol.* 2003;21:1431–9.

21. Swain SM, Tang G, Geyer CE, Jr., et al. Definitive results of a phase III adjuvant trial comparing three chemotherapy regimens in women with operable, node-positive breast cancer: the NSABP B-38 trial. *J Clin Oncol.* 2013;31:3197–204.

22. Moebus V, Jackisch C, Lueck HJ, et al. Intense dose-dense sequential chemotherapy with epirubicin, paclitaxel, and cyclophosphamide compared with conventionally scheduled chemotherapy in high-risk primary breast cancer: mature results of an AGO phase III study. *J Clin Oncol.* 2010;28:2874–80.

23. Venturini M, Del Mastro L, Aitini E, et al. Dose-dense adjuvant chemotherapy in early breast cancer patients: results from a randomized trial. *J Nat Cancer Inst.* 2005;97:1724–33.

24. Burnell M, Levine MN, Chapman JA, et al. Cyclophosphamide, epirubicin, and Fluorouracil versus dose-dense epirubicin and cyclophosphamide followed by paclitaxel versus doxorubicin and cyclophosphamide followed by paclitaxel in node-positive or high-risk node-negative breast cancer. *J Clin Oncol.* 2010;28:77–82.

25. Baldini E, Gardin G, Giannessi PG, et al. Accelerated versus standard cyclophosphamide, epirubicin and 5-fluorouracil or cyclophosphamide, methotrexate and 5-fluorouracil: a randomized phase III trial in locally advanced breast cancer. *Ann Oncol.* 2003;14:227–32.

26. Bonadonna G, Brusamolino E, Valagussa P, et al. Combination chemotherapy as an adjuvant treatment in operable breast cancer. *N Engl J Med.* 1976;294:405–10.

27. Engelsman E, Klijn JC, Rubens RD, et al. "Classical" CMF versus a 3-weekly intravenous CMF schedule in postmenopausal patients with advanced breast cancer: an EORTC Breast Cancer Co-operative Group Phase III Trial (10808). *Eur J Cancer.* 1991;27:966–70.

28. Henderson IC. Can we abandon anthracyclines for early breast cancer patients? *Oncology (Williston Park).* 2011;25:115–24, 27.

29. Sparano JA, Wang M, Martino S, et al. Weekly paclitaxel in the adjuvant treatment of breast cancer. *N Engl J Med.* 2008;358:1663–71.

30. Jones S, Holmes FA, O'Shaughnessy J, et al. Docetaxel with cyclophosphamide is associated with an overall survival benefit compared with doxorubicin and cyclophosphamide: 7-year follow-up of US Oncology Research Trial 9735. *J Clin Oncol.* 2009;27:1177–83.

31. Aebi S, Sun Z, Braun D, et al. Differential efficacy of three cycles of CMF followed by tamoxifen in patients with ER-positive and ER-negative tumors: long-term follow up on IBCSG Trial IX. *Ann Oncol.* 2011;22:1981–7.

32. Henderson IC, Berry DA, Demetri GD, et al. Improved outcomes from adding sequential paclitaxel but not from escalating doxorubicin dose in an adjuvant chemotherapy regimen for patients with node-positive primary breast cancer. *J Clin Oncol.* 2003;21:976–83.

33. Paik S, Tang G, Shak S, et al. Gene expression and benefit of chemotherapy in women with node-negative, estrogen receptor-positive breast cancer. *J Clin Oncol.* 2006;24:3726–34.

34. Albain KS, Barlow WE, Shak S, et al. Prognostic and predictive value of the 21-gene recurrence score assay in postmenopausal women with node-positive, oestrogen-receptor-positive breast cancer on chemotherapy: a retrospective analysis of a randomised trial. *Lancet Oncol.* 2010;11:55–65.

35. Albain KS, Barlow WE, Ravdin PM, et al. Adjuvant chemotherapy and timing of tamoxifen in postmenopausal patients with endocrine-responsive, node-positive breast cancer: a phase 3, open-label, randomised controlled trial. *Lancet.* 2009;374:2055–63.

36. Aebi S, Gelber S, Castiglione-Gertsch M, et al. Is chemotherapy alone adequate for young women with oestrogen-receptor- positive breast cancer? *Lancet.* 2000;355:1869–74.

37. Wefel JS, Kesler SR, Noll KR, et al. Clinical characteristics, pathophysiology, and management of noncentral nervous system cancer-related cognitive impairment in adults. *CA Cancer J Clin*. 2015;65:123–38.

38. Azim HA, Jr., de Azambuja E, Colozza M, et al. Long-term toxic effects of adjuvant chemotherapy in breast cancer. *Ann Oncol*. 2011;22:1939–47.

39. Moja L, Tagliabue L, Balduzzi S, et al. Trastuzumab containing regimens for early breast cancer. *Cochrane Database Syst Rev*. 2012;4:CD006243.

40. National Comprehensive Cancer Network. NCCN clinical practice guidelines in oncology: breast cancer. Version 1.2014. (Accessed December 27, 2013, at http://www.nccn.org/professionals/physician_gls/PDF/breast.pdf.)

41. Wolff AC, Hammond ME, Hicks DG, et al. Recommendations for human epidermal growth factor receptor 2 testing in breast cancer: American Society of Clinical Oncology/College of American Pathologists clinical practice guideline update. *J Clin Oncol*. 2013;31:3997–4013.

42. Pinto AC, Ades F, de Azambuja E, et al. Trastuzumab for patients with HER2 positive breast cancer: delivery, duration and combination therapies. *Breast*. 2013;22 Suppl 2: S152–5.

43. Perez EA, Suman VJ, Davidson NE, et al. Sequential versus concurrent trastuzumab in adjuvant chemotherapy for breast cancer. *J Clin Oncol*. 2011;29:4491–7.

44. Goss PE, Smith IE, O'Shaughnessy J, et al. Adjuvant lapatinib for women with early-stage HER2-positive breast cancer: a randomised, controlled, phase 3 trial. *Lancet Oncol*. 2013;14:88–96.

11

NEOADJUVANT THERAPY AND
LOCALLY ADVANCED OR
INFLAMMATORY BREAST CANCER

Systemic therapy is increasingly being used before surgery and radiotherapy as the primary treatment for breast cancer. This is commonly referred to as neoadjuvant therapy (NAT). The aims of NAT, *none of which has yet been shown with proper randomized clinical trials to be entirely achievable,* are the following:

- Improve survival of newly diagnosed breast cancer patients
- Improve local control after breast-conserving surgery (BCS)
- Predict which patients will benefit from new therapies or new treatment strategies using relatively small trials with short follow-up.

NEOADJUVANT OR PRIMARY SYSTEMIC THERAPY

The rationale for using NAT is strong.

- Local therapies alone are of questionable value in prolonging the survival of patients with T3, T4, N2, or N3 lesions. In some cases these patients are technically inoperable, and most of them develop distant metastases even with extensive surgery and radiotherapy (see Chapter 4). Since metastases in these locally advanced breast cancers have occurred by the time of diagnosis, the use of systemic therapy along with local therapy offers them the best hope currently available for an improved outcome.
- The use of early systemic therapy (i.e., adjuvant therapy) soon after surgical removal of the primary tumor prolongs patient survival to a greater extent than employing it first when distant metastases have appeared (see Chapter 10). Theoretical considerations and evidence from preclinical models support the idea that drug resistance mutations occur over a short period of time and that delay in the initiation of systemic therapy will reduce its effectiveness because of drug resistance.[1] It makes sense, then, that employing systemic therapy even earlier—before surgery—might impart an even greater survival benefit.
- In mouse models of breast cancer, distant metastases begin to proliferate when the primary tumor is removed. The use of chemotherapy before removing the primary tumor substantially reduced this proliferation, and preoperative hormone therapy blocked it[2] (see Figure 11.1).
- The probably of recurrence following any surgery and especially BCS increases with the size of the tumor. Although the acceptable size for BCS varies among surgeons,

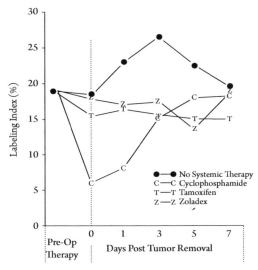

Figure 11.1 C3H mouse model showing effects of neoadjuvant endocrine or chemotherapy on tumor labeling indices (LI). In this CH3 mouse tumor model, tumors were injected into both the right and left legs. After growth was established, the larger of the two tumors (the "primary") was removed and the labeling index in the smaller tumor was measured on days 1, 3, 5, and 7. Animals were given either no systemic therapy, a single intraperitoneal dose of cyclophosphamide 5 days before removal of the primary, a single dose of goserelin (Zoladex®) 14 days prior to tumor inoculation, or tamoxifen daily starting the day of inoculation and continuing throughout the experiment. (For more on LI, see Chapter 7.)
Reprinted with permission from Fisher B, Saffer E, Rudock C, et al. Effect of local or systemic treatment prior to primary tumor removal on the production and response to a serum growth-stimulating factor in mice. *Cancer Res.* 1989;49:2002–4.

it is usually < 4 cm (see Chapter 9). The overall and complete clinical response rates of primary breast cancers to chemotherapy have been reported to be 70%–90% and 20%–35%, respectively. This suggests that using chemotherapy to first reduce the size of <u>larger tumors will increase the number of patients who may reasonably be treated with BCS <u>*without an unacceptable increase in local recurrence rate*</u>.

- Adjuvant chemotherapy is quite toxic, and adjuvant endocrine therapy durations are very prolonged. It is also certain that a substantial percentage of patients do not benefit from these treatments, but we have only limited ability to predict who those patients are (see Chapter 10). It is plausible that if the primary tumor does not respond, distant micrometastases will not respond either. Possibly non-responding patients are best served by either discontinuing ineffective systemic therapy to avoid toxicity or switching to more effective systemic therapy.

RESPONSE TO NEOADJUVANT CHEMOTHERAPY

Between 60% and 95% of tumors will respond to neoadjuvant chemotherapy (NACT).[3] This is substantially higher than the response rates to the same regimens in patients with distant metastases (see Chapter 12). This may be in part because assessment of soft tissue responses in one organ of an asymptomatic patient is so much easier than assessment of multiple metastatic sites in very symptomatic patients. The clinical complete response (cCR) and pathological complete response (pCR) rates are much lower, 7%–40% and 10%–15%, respectively. Clinical responses are used to reassess whether a patient's tumor has shrunk sufficiently to do breast-conserving surgery (BCS), but it has not been shown to be prognostic for longer term outcomes to the same extent as pCR. (See later in this chapter for full discussion of pCR definitions and interpretation.)

Determining pCR requires removal of breast tissue (or even the whole breast) and surgical assessment of nodes. A method for more accurately assessing response that is less invasive than surgery is badly needed. Digital mammography (DM), ultrasound (US), and MRI are often used for this purpose. Using pooled data from six trials, these radiological procedures were shown to be more accurate than clinical breast exam (CBE), (74%, 79%, and 84% vs. 57%, respectively).[4] The overall positive predictive value of the four approaches was about the same, but the negative predictive value was better, albeit far from sufficiently better, for MRI than the others (DM 41%, US 44%, and MRI 65% vs. CBE 31%). These early studies probably underestimate the full potential of MRI since it may also be used to measure functional properties of the tumor, such as pharmacokinetic parameters associated with transfer of gadolinium between intravascular and extravascular space or signal-enhancement ratios for contrast wash-in and wash-out.[5] Dynamic contrast-enhanced and diffusion-weighted imaging MRI are newer techniques undergoing prospective evaluations in the neoadjuvant setting.[6] Outside the trial setting, however, the role of MRI in the routine management of neoadjuvant therapy is unclear and is not yet recommended for routine assessment of response to NACT.

OPERABLE BREAST CANCER: EFFECT OF NEOADJUVANT CHEMOTHERAPY ON SURVIVAL

Trials in which patients with operable tumors were randomized to either neoadjuvant or adjuvant chemotherapy have failed to demonstrate a disease-free or overall survival benefit for NACT. Fourteen trials (5,500 patients) evaluating this comparison were identified for a meta-analysis. (Eight of these trials that were smaller and included less than a third of the patients compared NACT plus adjuvant chemotherapy after surgery to adjuvant chemotherapy alone. These trials are described as having a "sandwich design.") Disease-free and overall survival was an endpoint in 10 of the trials.[7] The median follow-up in these trials ranged from 24 to 124 months (see Table 11.1). In most of these studies, the duration of neoadjuvant and adjuvant therapy was identical. Two-thirds of the patients came from three studies of this type: the NSABP (32% of the patients) used 3 months of AC (doxorubicin + cyclophosphamide) before or after surgery; the EORTC (15% of patients) used 3 months of FEC (5- fluorouracil + epirubicin + cyclophosphamide); and ECTO (20% of patients) used 6 months of AT (doxorubicin + paclitaxel) followed by CMF (cyclophosphamide + methotrexate + 5-fluorouracil). The HR (hazard ratio) for overall survival was 0.98 and disease-free survival was 0.97. There was not much heterogeneity in the results from the trials; no

Table 11.1 Meta-Analysis of Randomized Trials Evaluating Neoadjuvant Therapy

Endpoint	Number of Patients/Trials	HR (95% CI) for Neoadjuvant Relative to Adjuvant Study Arm
Overall survival	4,620/ 10	0.98 (0.89–1.09)
Neoadjuvant design	3,808/ 6	1.00 (0.88–1.13)
Sandwich design	812/ 4	0.89 (0.68–1.16)
Disease-free survival	4,510/ 10	0.97 (0.89–1.00)
Frequency of local recurrence	3,257/ 8	1.13 (0.88–1.46)
After breast conserving surgery	1,830/ 4	1.13 (0.82–1.54)
After mastectomy	1,427/ 4	1.14 (0.75–1.75)
Time to local recurrence		
All studies	5,041/ 11	1.21 (1.02–1.43)[a]
All patients had surgery	4,198/ 8	1.12 (0.92–1.37)
Some patients had no surgery*	843/ 3	1.45 (1.06–1.97)[b]

Two trial designs were employed in these studies: preoperative versus postoperative chemotherapy ("neoadjuvant design") or preoperative plus postoperative versus postoperative chemotherapy ("sandwich design"). Not all trials had the same endpoints.

* ~ one-third of patients had radiotherapy without surgery after tumor regression

HR = hazard ratio; CI = confidence interval.

[a] p = 0.03

[b] p = 0.02

No other effects are statistically significant.

From Mieog JS, van der Hage JA, van de Velde CJ. Neoadjuvant chemotherapy for operable breast cancer. *Br J Surg.* 2007;94:1189–200; and Mieog JS, van der Hage JA, van de Velde CJ. Preoperative chemotherapy for women with operable breast cancer. *Cochrane Database Syst Rev.* 2007:CD005002 and Mieog JS, van der Hage JA, van de Velde CJ. Neoadjuvant chemotherapy for operable breast cancer. *Br J Surg.* 2007;94:1189–1200.

individual study found a significant disease-free or overall survival difference between NACT and adjuvant alone.

EFFECT ON LOCAL CONTROL OF OPERABLE BREAST CANCERS

A major concern in the use of NAT is whether the delay in the initiation of definitive local treatment will increase the frequency of uncontrolled or recurrent disease in the breast, on the chest wall, or in regional nodes. The risk of local disease recurring while patients are receiving NACT is less than 5%.[3,9] In these patients NAT can almost always be stopped and local therapy promptly initiated, but it is not certain whether such patients have identical long-term control.

The frequency of and time to locoregional recurrence *as a first event* were endpoints in 8 and 11 randomized trials, respectively. As long as some form of surgery was used, no significant increase in the local recurrence rate or decrease in the time to local recurrence following NAT was seen in the individual trials. However, in the meta-analysis of these trials there was a non-significant trend favoring the adjuvant therapy.[8] The local recurrence rate was 5.9% with adjuvant and 8.2% with NACT ($p = 0.35$). A 13% increase in the risk of recurrence was not significantly different in trials using mastectomy or BCS (see Table 11.1). The HR (hazard ratio) for time to local recurrence was significantly greater for patients on the neoadjuvant arms of these studies. However, the authors of the meta-analysis noted that in some of the trials, patients were given radiotherapy without tumor excision or node dissection, and in one of these trials the local recurrence rate was higher in patients who had radiation therapy only. They hypothesized that these trials may have inappropriately biased the results against neoadjuvant chemotherapy, and when the trials in which all patients had some form of surgery were analyzed separately the HR was no longer significant (Table 11.1).

The importance of these increased recurrence rates is not yet clear and probably will not be for some time. There is no evidence that they have affected survival in these trials, but the follow-up in some of them is as short as 2 years. An accurate estimate of local recurrence rate at 5 years will provide better insight into the safety of neoadjuvant chemotherapy. (See Chapter 9 on the relationship between local recurrence at 5 years and long-term survival.) Most of these trials substituted neoadjuvant for adjuvant therapy; it is plausible that using both pre- and postoperative chemotherapy (i.e., sandwich design) is more effective. The number of patients enrolled in sandwich trials is too small to compare the two strategies with available data.

ENABLING BREAST-CONSERVING THERAPY

Tumor size with a cut point of either 4 or 5 cm is the criterion used most often to choose between BCS and mastectomy, but this varies between institutions and surgeons. It will also vary between patients treated by the same surgeon since the patient's willingness to accept an increased risk of local recurrence in order to retain her breast will often influence this decision.

Neoadjuvant chemotherapy shrinks tumor size in the vast majority of treated patients. In the NSABP B-18 trial, 80% of all patients treated with NACT had tumor shrinkage, and in 36% all clinical evidence of tumor within the breast disappeared.[10] For patients with clinically palpable nodes, the overall and complete clinical response rates were 79% and 44%. This means that many tumors that do not meet criteria for BCS before will do so after completion of NACT.

The frequency with which surgeons actually change their surgical approach based on response to therapy is suggested by the results of two of the large randomized neoadjuvant trials (see Table 11.2). The actual surgery changed from that planned prior to the chemotherapy in 18% of patients; in 12% this was from planned mastectomy to BCS, and in 6% it was from planned BCS to mastectomy. However, the NSABP reported that BCS was planned for only 3% of those with a tumor ≥ 5 cm, but after preoperative chemotherapy 22% of them had BCS.[11] This suggests that about 1 in 5 patients deemed inappropriate for BCS therapy will be able to select this option after NACT.

It is not clear that patients treated with BCS after downstaging do as well as BCS patients who did not have NACT. In the NSABP study the ipsilateral breast tumor

Table 11.2 Comparison of Surgery Planned Before and Actual Surgery Employed After Neoadjuvant Therapy

Change in Surgery After Neoadjuvant Therapy	Frequency	
Planned → Actual	Number of Patients	%
No change in treatment		82
BCS → BCS	498	47
Mastectomy → Mastectomy	376	35
Treatment changed		18
Mastectomy → BCS	126	12
BCS → Mastectomy	66	6

Pooled results from two randomized trials in which physicians indicated which surgery they would perform prior to use of neoadjuvant therapy. This is compared to the actual surgery after completion of neoadjuvant. In the two trials, 87% and 70% of the patients had tumors < 5 cm.

BCS = breast-conserving surgery.

From Wolmark N, Wang J, Mamounas E, et al. Preoperative chemotherapy in patients with operable breast cancer: nine-year results from National Surgical Adjuvant Breast and Bowel Project B-18. J Natl Cancer Inst Monographs 2001:96–10 and van der Hage JA, van de Velde CJ, Julien JP, et al. Preoperative chemotherapy in primary operable breast cancer: results from the European Organization for Research and Treatment of Cancer trial 10902. J Clin Oncol. 2001;19:4224–37.

recurrence rate was 15.9% and 9.9% ($p = 0.04$) for these two groups, respectively, but these differences were not statistically significant after an adjustment for patient age and initial clinical tumor size.[11] In the EORTC trial the survival of the downstaged BCS patients was worse than that of BCS patients who did not need NACT: HR = 2.53 (95% CI, 10.02–6.25).[12]

OTHER NEOADJUVANT THERAPIES: HORMONAL AND ANTI-HER2

Both hormonal and anti-HER2 therapies are used commonly in the neoadjuvant setting, but there are no clinical trials comparing neoadjuvant with adjuvant using these treatments. However, clinical trials using these modalities have addressed secondary questions, such as whether an aromatase inhibitor (AI) is superior to tamoxifen, which AI is most effective, or whether dual anit-HER2 treatments are superior to a single agent.[13,14] From adjuvant therapy trials (see Chapter 10) it is known that longer durations of hormonal therapy are more effective than shorter. Thus when neoadjuvant hormonal therapy (NAHT) is given, it is for more prolonged periods than NACT. Most NAHT trials have used 3–4 months of treatment, and eight trials have used durations of 6 months or longer, including one in which patients received NAHT for 12 months before surgery.[13] The median time to an objective response was 3.9 months and to maximum response 4.2 months, with one-third of the patients reaching maximum response only after 6 months of treatment. Longer duration of treatment increases the chance that a patient will progress before local therapy is instituted; in two studies this was observed to be 10% and 5% after 4 and 6 months, respectively.[15]

In patients with HER2+ tumors neoadjuvant trastuzumab is always given with NACT for the same duration as the NACT.[16] However, in contrast to most of the NACT studies, the trastuzumab neoadjuvant trials had a sandwich design, with trastuzumab used as adjuvant therapy following local treatment, usually for 1 year.

The relationship between pCR (or other measures of tumor response) and clinical endpoints such as disease-free or overall survival has not been studied systematically for hormonal and anti-HER2 agents. An important exception to that is the NOAH trial comparing trastuzumab with no trastuzumab in HER2+ patients with locally advanced and inflammatory cancer. The pCR rate was 35% and 15%, respectively, for trastuzumab plus NACT and NACT alone. The pCR odds ratio was 3.04 and the HR for EFS was 0.59.[17] The correlation between pCR rates and outcomes in the NOAH trial is better than in any of the NACT trials.

A cross-comparison of two randomized trials, one neoadjuvant and the other adjuvant, that used the same design and the same endocrine therapies—tamoxifen, anastrozole, or a combination of both drugs—failed to demonstrate a correlation between response rate during the NAHT and disease-free survival outcomes in the adjuvant study.[18] In the neoadjuvant study, IMPACT, the clinical response rate was not significantly different in the three arms (pCR rate was not determined). In the adjuvant study, ATAC, anastrozole was significantly better than tamoxifen alone or the combination.

As with NACT trials, NAHT studies are providing new insight into the biological effects of these therapies, and they are likely to have profound effects on clinical practice. In "window trials," patients receiving NAHT undergo FNA biopsies of their tumors for Ki-67 (see Chapter 7) measurements prior to initiation of treatment and again after 2 and 12 weeks of therapy.[19] In the IMPACT trial, described earlier, there was greater suppression of Ki-67 in the anastrozole than the tamoxifen arms. In this comparison the Ki-67 change predicted the outcomes of the ATAC trial better than clinical response. However, Ki-67 suppression with anastrozole was not better than the combination of anastrozole plus tamoxifen, in contrast to the findings in the adjuvant trial. A somewhat more sophisticated approach combines the Ki-67 response with other variables independently associated with relapse and survival (tumor size, node, and ER status) following NAHT to obtain a "preoperative endocrine prognostic index" (PEPI).[20] In several trials PEPI has outperformed clinical or Ki-67 responses in predicting outcomes from randomized NAHT trials.

Another example of new biological insights is the observation that there is no difference in response to NAHT and NACT in luminal cancers with a low Ki-67, while NACT is more effective than NAHT in luminal cancers with high Ki-67 or in luminal B cancers.[21,22]

Only one therapy has been specifically approved as a neoadjuvant therapy. This is the combination of pertuzumab, trastuzumab, and docetaxel, which was shown in a randomized neoadjuvant trial that enrolled 417 HER2+ patients to induce pCR in 39% of the patients compared to pCR rates of 22%, 18%, and 11% in the non-pertuzumab, non-trastuzumab, and non-docetaxel arms, respectively.[14]

WHAT CAN WE LEARN FROM A PCR?

Patients with a pathological complete response (pCR) following NACT chemotherapy have a significantly longer event-free and overall survival than patients who have a response less than a pCR or no response at all[23] (see Figure 11.2).

The likelihood of a pCR is low (13%–22%), but how low will depend on how pCR is defined (see Table 11.3). The definition used varies from one study to another. It is more difficult to achieve a pCR in both the breast and axillary lymph nodes than in breast alone, or if elimination of DCIS as well as invasive cancer is required. However, when the definition of pCR is more stringent, there is a greater difference in the event-free and overall survival of patients with a pCR compared to less than a pCR.

The likelihood of achieving a pCR also varies in patient subsets defined by tumor grade, hormone receptor (HR), and HER2 status[23] (Table 11.4). The pCR rates in the patients with HR+ tumors treated with NACT were low, especially those with low-grade HR+ tumors (intrinsic subtype luminal A), and the differences in the survival of the pCR and no pCR patients in HR+ groups were not statistically significant, even when trastuzumab was used in the HR+/HER2+ patients. Adding trastuzumab to HER2+ patients substantially increased the pCR rate; in those with HER2+/HR– tumors the proportional reduction in mortality was 92%! Younger patients, especially those < 35, are more likely and those with invasive lobular histology less likely to have a pCR in response to NACT, but there is no difference in patient groups defined by tumor size or clinical nodal status pre-therapy.[23,24] These studies of neoadjuvant therapy provide some of the most compelling evidence we have that there is a very large difference in the responsiveness of tumors to chemotherapy and that many patients with HR+ tumors derive very little benefit.

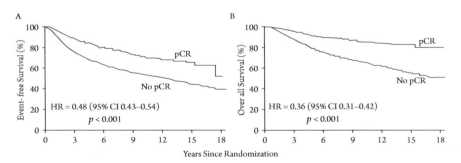

Figure 11.2 Event-free and overall survival of patients with a pathological complete response (pCR) or not following neoadjuvant chemotherapy. Pooled data from 12 randomized trials (11,955 patients) comparing neoadjuvant with no neoadjuvant chemotherapy (+/- trastuzumab in some HER2+ patients). Lesions were T2 in 61% and T4d (inflammatory) in 4% of patients; 46% had clinically involved nodes, 30% HR–, 17% HR+, and the remainder HR unknown. HER2 status was largely unknown since it was measured in only four trials. 10% were triple negative. Median follow-up was 5.4 years. pCR was defined as ypT0/is ypN0 (see text).

HR = hazard ratio.

Reprinted with permission from Cortazar P, Zhang L, Untch M, et al. Pathological complete response and long-term clinical benefit in breast cancer: the CTNeoBC pooled analysis. *Lancet.* 2014;384:164–72.

Table 11.3 Pathological Complete Response (pCR): Likelihood and Effect on Survival From a Pooled Analysis of 12 Randomized Trials Comparing Neoadjuvant With No Neoadjuvant Chemotherapy in Patients With Operable Breast Cancers

Definition of pCR	Likelihood of pCR (%)	HR (95% CI) for Survival of pCR versus no pCR	
		Event-Free	Overall
ypT0 ypN0	13	0.44 (0.39–0.51)	0.36 (0.30–0.44)
ypT0/is ypN0	18	0.48 (0.43–0.54)	0.36 (0.31–0.42)
ypT0/is	22	0.60 (0.55–0.66)	0.51 (0.45–0.58)

ypT0 ypN0 = no invasive or in situ (is) cancer in breast and axillary nodes.

ypT0/is ypN0 = no invasive cancer in breast and axillary nodes irrespective of DCIS.

ypT0/is = no invasive cancer in breast irrespective of DCIS or nodal involvement.

DCIS = ductal carcinoma in situ; HR = hazard ratio; CI = confidence interval. From Cortazar P, Zhang L, Untch M, et al. Pathological complete response and long-term clinical benefit in breast cancer: the CTNeoBC pooled analysis. *Lancet.* 2014;384:164–72.

Theoretically, patients who do not respond to the first couple of cycles of a neo-adjuvant therapy might benefit from crossover to a more effective regimen (i.e., response-guided therapy). This strategy has been evaluated in a number of trials with mixed results. The largest of these studies treated 2,072 patients with 2 cycles of chemotherapy and then randomized non-responders either to continue the same regimen or to crossover to a different chemotherapy combination, each for 4 additional cycles.[25] Responders were randomized to continue the same regimen for either 4 or 6

Table 11.4 Histologic Grade, Molecular Characteristics and Likelihood of Achieving a pCR and Improved Survival from a Pooled Analysis of 12 Randomized Trials Comparing Neoadjuvant with no Neoadjuvant Chemotherapy in Patients with Operable Breast Cancers

Tumor Grade and Molecular Characteristics	Likelihood of pCR (%)	HR (95% CI) for Survival of pCR versus no pCR
HR+, HER2−, grade 1or 2	7.5	0.47 (0.21–1.07)[a]
HR+, HER2−, grade 3	16.2	0.29 (0.13–0.65)
HER2+, HR+, trastuzumab	30.9	0.56 (0.23–1.37)[a]
HER2+, HR+, no trastuzumab	18.3	0.57 (0.31–1.04)[a]
HER2+, HR−, trastuzumab	50.3	0.08 (0.03–0.22)
HER2+, HR−, no trastuzumab	30.2	0.29 (0.17–0.50)
Triple negative (see chapter VII)	33.6	0.16 (0.11–0.25)

HR: hormone receptor.

[a] Reduction in HR for pCR not statistically significant.

Drom Cortazar P, Zhang L, Untch M, et al. Pathological complete response and long-term clinical benefit in breast cancer: the CTNeoBC pooled analysis. *Lancet.* 2014;384:164–72.

additional cycles. There was no difference in the primary endpoint: pCR rate. There was a significant difference favoring response-guided therapy in the secondary end-points of disease-free survival and overall survival, but this survival benefit was significant only for those with HR+ tumors. These apparently discordant results between the primary and secondary endpoints and the counterintuitive effect in the HR+ subsets have led many experts to be cautious about accepting these data as a guideline for practice, especially in light of negative results from other, albeit smaller, trials evaluating the use of response to NAT as a determinant of future therapy.[26,27]

NEOADJUVANT THERAPY, LOCOREGIONAL RECURRENCE, AND LOCAL THERAPY

Neoadjuvant therapy should not be used instead of local treatment. There are a number of randomized trials in which patients, usually elderly or debilitated, were randomized to either tamoxifen alone or surgery (alone or with tamoxifen, depending on the trial.)[3] In all cases, the survival of the two groups was essentially the same, but the locoregional recurrence (LRR) rate was substantially higher in the tamoxifen alone arm.

The pathological response to neoadjuvant therapy is also a better predictor of LRR than the patient's initial clinical stage, and this could reasonably affect the decision to use adjuvant radiotherapy following mastectomy in patients who initially present with stage II disease.[28] (Radiation is recommended for all patients treated with BCS and those with locally advanced breast cancer—see further discussion later in this chapter). Among patients with pathologically negative nodes (ypN0) following NACT, those with less than a pCR in the breast have 2.2-fold greater likelihood of an LRR than those with a pCR (ypT0).[29] However, patients who are ypT0 with one or more positive nodes after NACT have a 4.5-fold greater likelihood of LRR. Patients with any pathologically involved lymph nodes after NACT for a stage II cancer have a 10 year LRR probability > 10%, while those with a pCR and negative nodes have a LRR rate < 5%. Based on this, adjuvant radiation therapy is recommended for all patients with residual nodal involvement. It may be reasonable to withhold adjuvant radiotherapy from those who are ypT0 ypN0, or ypT0/is ypN0 after NAT, but this is not yet standard. For those who are ypN0 who have some residual disease in the breast, most radiation therapists will nuance their decision using other factors known to increase risk of LRR, such as younger age, extent of residual disease, close margins, lymphatic or vascular invasion, and triple negative status.[28,30]

PCR AS A SURROGATE FOR APPROVING NEW DRUGS

Although a patient's response to neoadjuvant therapy has meaning for that patient, it is less clear what can be inferred from a pCR rate regarding the general value of a treatment or treatment strategy, either for all patients or for a defined group of patients. The FDA has undertaken an extensive analysis of this question in collaboration with investigators of 12 large randomized trials.[23] To be a suitable surrogate, there needs to be a tight correlation between increasing pCR and outcome measures, such as disease-free and overall survival, for all patients randomized in the trial. Figure 11.3A illustrates the ideal relationship between pCR and EFS. Data from 10 randomized neoadjuvant trials

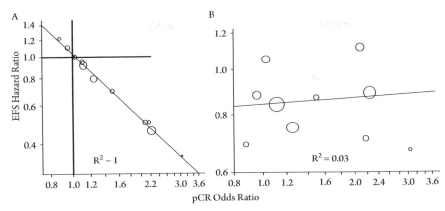

Figure 11.3 Trial-level correlation between pathological complete response (pCR) and event-free survival. Each circle represents one randomized trial plotted at the intersection of the EFS (event-free survival) hazard ratio and the pCR odds ratio for the neoadjuvant versus adjuvant study arms of that trial. A: Simulated data illustrating the curve that might be obtained if pCR were a suitable surrogate for EFS. B: Actual data from the 10 randomized trials included in an FDA analysis.
Reprinted with permission from Cortazar P, Zhang L, Untch M, et al. Pathological complete response and long-term clinical benefit in breast cancer: the CTNeoBC pooled analysis. *Lancet.* 2014;384:164–72.

are plotted in Figure 11.3B. The ideal coefficient of determination is 1.0. The observed is 0.03 for EFS and 0.24 for overall survival (OS data not shown). There are a number of potential reasons for this lack of correlation. One is that the tumors undergoing a pCR may be one subtype that occurs as the predominant subtype in only a small percentage of all the tumors in the study. Other tumors with different subtypes may also respond to therapy but to varying degrees, thus obscuring the relationship between pCR and EFS or OS. This may change in the future with the use of targeted therapy in patients with similar tumors (see the results from the Noah trial described earlier). Another example may be the use of NACT in women aged < 50 where, at least in one of the major studies, there is a significant or near-significant overall survival favoring neoadjuvant over adjuvant therapy.[31] The authors of the FDA analysis concluded that pCR following neoadjuvant chemotherapy is not yet suitable as a surrogate for new drug approval, and by extension it should not generally be used yet for determining practice policies without a prospective trial evaluating any hypotheses generated by a neoadjuvant study.

INOPERABLE LOCALLY ADVANCED BREAST CANCER

When staging systems were introduced in the 1940s, surgeons concluded that many locally advanced breast cancers (LABCs) were technically inoperable and that extensive surgical procedures did not prolong the survival of patients in this group.[32] LABC was defined as a tumor with at least one of these characteristics: size > 5 cm with clinically suspicious lymph nodes, tumor extension to skin or underlying muscles, axillary lymph nodes that were matted together, supraclavicular or infraclavicular nodes, or inflammatory breast cancer. This encompasses patients with stage IIIA, IIIB, and IIIC tumors—a very heterogeneous group. Patients who are stage IIIA only by virtue of size ≥ 5 cm and positive nodes are included in many operative series (including almost all the trials included in Table 11.1) and have a prognosis only slightly worse than those in stage IIB. Stage IIIB includes those with tumors attached to skin and/or underlying muscle that are very difficult to control locally but that may be associated with a relatively long survival, as well as those with inflammatory breast cancer, the most aggressive of all breast tumors and invariably associated with short survival. The overall 5-year survival of patients with stage IIB, IIIA, IIIB, and IIIC in the US National Cancer Data Base in 2001–2002 were 74%, 67%, 41%, and 49%[33] (see Chapter 6). Comparisons of recurrence rates (local or distant) and survival between non-randomized groups of patients with LABC are generally not informative since differences in treatment outcomes are more likely a result of differences in patient mix than in the treatment administered.

With widespread use of screening mammography, patients present less often at this advanced stage, but LABC, excluding IBC, still accounts for 4.6% of breast cancers diagnosed in the United States today.[34]

The local recurrence rate after surgery alone for LABC is very high. Even with a radical mastectomy, it was 46% (with a 6% overall survival) at 5 years.[9] The results with radiotherapy alone were no better: 46% and 72% in two series.

Adding systemic therapy reduces local recurrence rates and improves the survival of patients with LABC. The definitive trial demonstrating this was conducted by the EORTC between 1979 and 1985.[35] Patients were randomized to receive radiation alone or radiation followed by either hormone therapy, chemotherapy, or a combination of these modalities (see Figure 11.4). Adding systemic therapy significantly reduced both the frequency of local recurrence and increased the duration of local control. Overall survival was also improved, but this was statistically significant only for hormone therapy. (This difference between the survival benefit from hormonal and chemotherapy may be due to the fact that patients randomized to chemotherapy were mostly postmenopausal and ER+, groups for which chemotherapy is relatively less effective; see Chapter 10.)

Neither this trial nor any other trial in patients with LABC demonstrates that the use of systemic therapy first (i.e., as neoadjuvant therapy) is superior in any way to adjuvant therapy following local therapy.

Local control of disease and overall survival are not significantly different when chemotherapy (or chemohormonal therapy in those with ER+ tumors) is combined with either surgery or radiation therapy in patients with LABC. This has been evaluated in three randomized trials in which chemotherapy was given both preoperatively and postoperatively.[36] In one trial, the local recurrence rate following mastectomy or radiation therapy was 42% and 55% ($p = 0.43$), respectively; in another trial, local recurrences rates were 30% and 31%. There was no significant difference in disease-free or overall survival. However, all three of these studies were small with very limited statistical power.

Using all three modalities—chemotherapy, mastectomy, and radiation therapy—gives the best local control. Three hundred thirty-two patients with LABC (53% with IIIA and 40% with IIIB tumors) who were free of disease after mastectomy, axillary dissection, and 6 months of adjuvant chemohormonal therapy were randomized to receive radiation therapy to the chest wall and regional lymph nodes or

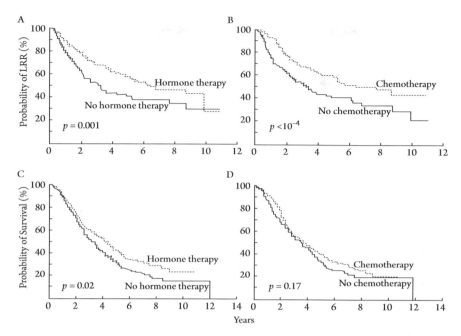

Figure 11.4 Locally advanced breast cancer (LABC) treated with radiation alone or radiation plus systemic therapy. In this EORTC trial 410 patients with LABC were randomized to treatment with breast radiotherapy alone or radiotherapy followed by either hormone therapy (HT) (ovarian irradiation + prednisolone for 5 years for premenopausal women or tamoxifen for 5 years for postmenopausal women), chemotherapy (CT) (classic CMF for 1 year), or both types of systemic therapy. There was no requirement for surgery other than biopsy, and only 5 patients received a mastectomy. Median follow-up was 8 years. Key tumor/patient characteristics: 14% had inflammatory and 38% had T4 lesions; 31% had N2 or N3 nodes; 72% had ER+ tumors and 62% were postmenopausal. Local recurrences were reduced from 59% to 48% with CT and from 61% to 47% with HT. Analyzed as a 2 x 2 trial. A & B: Time to locoregional recurrence (LRR) comparing 2 arms with hormone therapy (A) or 2 arms with chemotherapy (B) to the 2 arms without hormone therapy or 2 arms without chemotherapy. C & D: Same analysis with survival as endpoint.
Reprinted with permission from Bartelink H, Rubens RD, van der Schueren E, et al. Hormonal therapy prolongs survival in irradiated locally advanced breast cancer: a European Organization for Research and Treatment of Cancer Randomized Phase III Trial. *J Clin Oncol.* 1997;15:207–15.

to observation with radiation therapy given only if and when there was evidence of locoregional recurrence.[37] There was no difference in the time to recurrence (local or distant) in the two treatment arms, but only 15% of the patients given radiation therapy had a local recurrence as the first site of recurrence, compared to 25% of those not given radiation. The uncontrolled local disease rate at the time of death was 30% and 40% for those given and not given radiation, respectively (statistical significance not reported).

The standard of care for patients with LABC is neoadjuvant chemotherapy, mastectomy, postoperative radiotherapy, and, in most cases, additional adjuvant chemotherapy (plus hormonal therapy if ER+) after completion of local treatment.

BCS is commonly used for patients with stage IIIA disease (see earlier discussion under operable tumors) but only judiciously in those with IIIB and IIIC tumors.[38] It is almost never used in those with T4 lesions.

INFLAMMATORY BREAST CANCER

This very aggressive form of breast cancer was first described as a diffuse enlargement of the breast with overlying erythematous changes, warmth, and edema (peau d'orange) of the skin *but no palpable mass*. Invasive ductal carcinoma, usually high grade, infiltrates breast stroma diffusely and may or may not form a mass.[39] There is increased angiogenesis and lymphangiogenesis.[40] Inflammatory breast cancers (IBCs) are more commonly HER2+ tumors and uncommonly luminal A, but there is not a defining molecular characteristic.[34] IBC constitutes 2.5% of breast cancers diagnosed in the United States. The incidence is higher in African Americans. The average age of diagnosis, 55, is younger than that of other breast cancers.

Prior to 1974, when most patients received only local treatments, IBC was considered uniformly fatal with a 5-year survival of < 5% and a median survival of 15 months.[41] This has changed with the widespread use of systemic therapy for IBC. Today the 15-year survival rate is between 20% and 30%. A recent comparison of survival changes over the last 20 years was demonstrated using the SEER database.[41] Two-year breast cancer–specific survival significantly increased over four 5-year intervals. In the period 1990–1995, it was 62%; 1996–2000, 67%; 2001–2005, 72%; and 2005–2010, 76% ($p < 0.0001$). These changes in survival coincided with periods in which systemic therapy of IBC was improved with the addition of the taxanes, long-term aromatase therapy for ER+ patients, and anti-HER2 therapies.

Because of very rapid local recurrences following mastectomy alone, its use as the sole or primary treatment of IBC is contraindicated. However, mastectomy with lymph node dissection and adjuvant radiation therapy following successful neoadjuvant therapy is associated with improved local control.[39] It is as important to achieve negative surgical margins in patients with IBC as it is for other types of breast cancer (see Chapter 9). BCS is not indicated because of the diffuse nature of the disease in most patients. Sentinel lymph node biopsy is not considered sufficiently accurate to use for avoiding full dissection in patients with IBC.[34] Patients who do not respond to neoadjuvant chemotherapy should be treated with radiation therapy (including electron beam to the chest wall because of dermal tumor emboli) and then should be considered for mastectomy. There are no randomized trials from which to draw firm conclusions about the impact of these local treatments on long-term survival.

KEY POINTS IN USING NEOADJUVANT THERAPIES FOR OPERABLE AND INOPERABLE TUMORS

- The only group for which NAT is clearly the treatment of choice is inflammatory breast cancer. This may eventually prove true for women aged < 50 and those with triple negative cancers.
- There is no group for which NAT is contraindicated, including all patients with tumors ≥ 2 cm who would be candidates for adjuvant therapy.

- NAHT is as effective as or more effective than NACT in patients with HR+ (especially luminal A or luminal tumors with low Ki-67).
- In patients with HER2+ tumors, neoadjuvant trastuzumab added to chemotherapy is much more effective than NACT alone.
- NAT makes some tumors suitable for BCS that are initially thought to be better treated with mastectomy. However, this may come at the cost of a small increase in LRR.
- Response or failure to respond to NAT cannot yet be used reliably to omit either surgery or radiotherapy.
- In using neoadjuvant chemotherapy
    - it has not been shown that the optimal regimens to use in the neoadjuvant setting are any different from those used as adjuvant therapy (see Chapter 10);
    - it is not clear that there is an advantage in adding adjuvant chemotherapy after surgery if 4–6 months of preoperative chemotherapy have been given (however, adjuvant endocrine and anti-HER2 therapy should be used);
    - MRI should not be used outside of a trial to assess response or guide therapeutic decisions outside a clinical trial;
    - there is no evidence that non-responding patients benefit from crossover to another regimen.
- Neoadjuvant therapy is a powerful research tool that has provided proof of principle for hypotheses generated in other settings, such as the relatively poor response of HR+ tumors to chemotherapy, and promises to be a source of new hypotheses that can then be more intelligently tested in the adjuvant setting.
- Maximum local control and best survival for patients with LABC and IBC are achieved with a combination of NAT (either NACT, NAHT or both), surgery, and radiation therapy.

REFERENCES

1. Goldie JH, Coldman AJ. A mathematic model for relating the drug sensitivity of tumors to their spontaneous mutation rate. *Cancer Treat Rep.* 1979;63:1727–33.
2. Fisher B, Saffer E, Rudock C, et al. Effect of local or systemic treatment prior to primary tumor removal on the production and response to a serum growth-stimulating factor in mice. *Cancer Res.* 1989;49:2002–4.
3. Shannon C, Smith I. Is there still a role for neoadjuvant therapy in breast cancer? *Crit Rev Oncol Hematol.* 2003;45:77–90.
4. Croshaw R, Shapiro-Wright H, Svensson E, et al. Accuracy of clinical examination, digital mammogram, ultrasound, and MRI in determining postneoadjuvant pathologic tumor response in operable breast cancer patients. *Ann Surg Oncol.* 2011;18:3160–3.
5. Hylton N. Magnetic resonance imaging of the breast: opportunities to improve breast cancer management. *J Clin Oncol.* 2005;23:1678–84.
6. McLaughlin S, Mittendorf EA, Bleicher RJ, et al. The 2013 Society of Surgical Oncology Susan G. Komen for the Cure Symposium: MRI in breast cancer: where are we now? *Ann Surg Oncol.* 2014;21:28–36.
7. Mieog JS, van der Hage JA, van de Velde CJ. Neoadjuvant chemotherapy for operable breast cancer. *Br J Surg.* 2007;94:1189–1200.

8. Mieog JS, van der Hage JA, van de Velde CJ. Preoperative chemotherapy for women with operable breast cancer. *Cochrane Database Syst Rev.* 2007:CD005002.

9. Lee MC, Newman LA. Management of patients with locally advanced breast cancer. *Surg Clin North Am.* 2007;87:379–98, ix.

10. Fisher B, Brown A, Mamounas E, et al. Effect of preoperative chemotherapy on local-regional disease in women with operable breast cancer: findings from National Surgical Adjuvant Breast and Bowel Project B-18. *J Clin Oncol.* 1997;15:2483–93.

11. Wolmark N, Wang J, Mamounas E, et al. Preoperative chemotherapy in patients with operable breast cancer: nine-year results from National Surgical Adjuvant Breast and Bowel Project B-18. *J Natl Cancer Inst Monographs.* 2001:96–102.

12. van der Hage JA, van de Velde CJ, Julien JP, et al. Preoperative chemotherapy in primary operable breast cancer: results from the European Organization for Research and Treatment of Cancer trial 10902. *J Clin Oncol.* 2001;19:4224–37.

13. Charehbili A, Fontein DB, Kroep JR, et al. Neoadjuvant hormonal therapy for endocrine sensitive breast cancer: a systematic review. *Cancer Treat Rev.* 2014;40:86–92.

14. Kumler I, Tuxen MK, Nielsen DL. A systematic review of dual targeting in HER2-positive breast cancer. *Cancer Treat Rev.* 2013.

15. Mathew J, Agrawal A, Asgeirsson KS, et al. Primary endocrine therapy in locally advanced breast cancers: the Nottingham experience. *Breast Cancer Res Treat.* 2009;113:403–7.

16. Valachis A, Mauri D, Polyzos NP, et al. Trastuzumab combined to neoadjuvant chemotherapy in patients with HER2-positive breast cancer: a systematic review and meta-analysis. *Breast.* 2011;20:485–90.

17. Gianni L, Eiermann W, Semiglazov V, et al. Neoadjuvant chemotherapy with trastuzumab followed by adjuvant trastuzumab versus neoadjuvant chemotherapy alone, in patients with HER2-positive locally advanced breast cancer (the NOAH trial): a randomised controlled superiority trial with a parallel HER2-negative cohort. *Lancet.* 2010;375:377–84.

18. Smith IE, Dowsett M, Ebbs SR, et al. Neoadjuvant treatment of postmenopausal breast cancer with anastrozole, tamoxifen, or both in combination: the Immediate Preoperative Anastrozole, Tamoxifen, or Combined with Tamoxifen (IMPACT) multicenter double-blind randomized trial. *J Clin Oncol.* 2005;23:5108–16.

19. Dowsett M, Smith IE, Ebbs SR, et al. Short-term changes in Ki-67 during neoadjuvant treatment of primary breast cancer with anastrozole or tamoxifen alone or combined correlate with recurrence-free survival. *Clin Cancer Res.* 2005;11:951s–8s.

20. Ellis MJ, Tao Y, Luo J, et al. Outcome prediction for estrogen receptor-positive breast cancer based on postneoadjuvant endocrine therapy tumor characteristics. *J Nat Cancer Inst.* 2008;100:1380–8.

21. Alba E, Calvo L, Albanell J, et al. Chemotherapy (CT) and hormonotherapy (HT) as neoadjuvant treatment in luminal breast cancer patients: results from the GEICAM/2006-03, a multicenter, randomized, phase-II study. *Ann Oncol.* 2012;23:3069–74.

22. Ades F, Zardavas D, Bozovic-Spasojevic I, et al. Luminal B breast cancer: molecular characterization, clinical management, and future perspectives. *J Clin Oncol.* 2014;32:2794–803.

23. Cortazar P, Zhang L, Untch M, et al. Pathological complete response and long-term clinical benefit in breast cancer: the CTNeoBC pooled analysis. *Lancet.* 2014;384:164–72.

24. von Minckwitz G, Untch M, Blohmer JU, et al. Definition and impact of pathologic complete response on prognosis after neoadjuvant chemotherapy in various intrinsic breast cancer subtypes. *J Clin Oncol.* 2012;30:1796–804.

25. von Minckwitz G, Blohmer JU, Costa SD, et al. Response-guided neoadjuvant chemotherapy for breast cancer. *J Clin Oncol.* 2013;31:3623–30.

26. Telli ML. Insight or confusion: survival after response-guided neoadjuvant chemotherapy in breast cancer. *J Clin Oncol.* 2013;31:3613–5.

27. Schott AF, Hayes DF. Defining the benefits of neoadjuvant chemotherapy for breast cancer. *J Clin Oncol.* 2012;30:1747–9.

28. Bellon JR, Wong JS, Burstein HJ. Should response to preoperative chemotherapy affect radiotherapy recommendations after mastectomy for stage II breast cancer? *J Clin Oncol.* 2012;30:3916–20.

29. Mamounas EP, Anderson SJ, Dignam JJ, et al. Predictors of locoregional recurrence after neoadjuvant chemotherapy: results from combined analysis of National Surgical Adjuvant Breast and Bowel Project B-18 and B-27. *J Clin Oncol.* 2012;30:3960–6.

30. Smith BD. Using chemotherapy response to personalize choices regarding locoregional therapy: a new era in breast cancer treatment? *J Clin Oncol.* 2012;30:3913–5.

31. Rastogi P, Anderson SJ, Bear HD, et al. Preoperative chemotherapy: updates of National Surgical Adjuvant Breast and Bowel Project Protocols B-18 and B-27. *J Clin Oncol.* 2008;26:778–85.

32. Haagensen CD, Stout AP. Carcinoma of the breast. III. Results of treatment, 1935–1942. *Ann Surg.* 1951;134:151–72.

33. *AJCC Cancer Staging Manual.* 7th ed. New York: Springer; 2010.

34. Chia S, Swain SM, Byrd DR, et al. Locally advanced and inflammatory breast cancer. *J Clin Oncol.* 2008;26:786–90.

35. Bartelink H, Rubens RD, van der Schueren E, et al. Hormonal therapy prolongs survival in irradiated locally advanced breast cancer: a European Organization for Research and Treatment of Cancer Randomized Phase III Trial. *J Clin Oncol.* 1997;15:207–15.

36. Shenkier T, Weir L, Levine M, et al. Clinical practice guidelines for the care and treatment of breast cancer: 15. Treatment for women with stage III or locally advanced breast cancer. *Can Med Assoc J.* 2004;170:983–94.

37. Olson JE, Neuberg D, Pandya KJ, et al. The role of radiotherapy in the management of operable locally advanced breast carcinoma: results of a randomized trial by the Eastern Cooperative Oncology Group. *Cancer.* 1997;79:1138–49.

38. Macdonald SM, Harris EE, Arthur DW, et al. ACR appropriateness criteria locally® advanced breast cancer. *Breast J.* 2011;17:579–85.

39. Robertson FM, Bondy M, Yang W, et al. Inflammatory breast cancer: the disease, the biology, the treatment. *CA Cancer J Clin.* 2010;60:351–75.

40. Breast cancer and depot-medroxyprogesterone acetate: a multinational study. WHO Collaborative Study of Neoplasia and Steroid Contraceptives. *Lancet.* 1991;338:833–8.

41. Dawood S, Lei X, Dent R, et al. Survival of women with inflammatory breast cancer: a large population-based study. *Ann Oncol.* 2014;25:1143–51.

12

MANAGEMENT OF METASTATIC DISEASE

Once it is metastatic, breast cancer is considered an "incurable disease" in that most (but not all) of these patients will eventually die as a result of the cancer. However, a substantial percentage of patients with metastases have many years of active and meaningful life. Specific anti-cancer therapies palliate symptoms more effectively with fewer side effects than analgesics alone. Because recurrence, even a local recurrence on the chest wall, is evidence of more widespread metastases that will eventually become symptomatic, systemic therapies, such as endocrine and chemotherapy, are most commonly used, but there is a role for both surgery and radiotherapy in the management of metastases as well. Most patients with distant metastases will receive some form of therapy for the remainder of their lives.

OUTCOMES FROM THERAPY

Treatment of metastases often prolongs survival, but it is difficult to demonstrate this. This is because most patients with metastatic breast cancer receive multiple different treatments over the course of the disease, and each contributes varying amounts of survival benefit.

Response rates (RR) are the most easily measured endpoint and the most reliable evidence of a drug's biological effect. Using RECIST (Response Evaluation Criteria in Solid Tumors) criteria, a partial response (PR) indicates that treatment has caused at least a 30% reduction in the sum of the longest diameter(s) of target lesions selected prior to initiation of treatment; a complete response (CR) indicates that all target lesions have disappeared, and overall response rate (ORR) is the sum of PR and CR. These criteria are helpful in determining the relative efficacy of treatments in randomized trials, but a response does not necessarily mean that a patient has had a clinical benefit. For example, a patient may have a totally asymptomatic pulmonary metastasis that disappears while receiving systemic therapy. Since there were no symptoms prior to treatment, it is hard to argue that there is a clinical benefit from eradicating the lesions in this patient, and the response is not necessarily associated with better survival. Responses usually appear gradually over 2–4 months but sometimes only after 9–12 months. For this reason patients are usually kept on a systemic therapy until there is progressive disease (PD), defined in RECIST as at least a 20% increase in the sum of the target lesion diameters.

This definition of PD may lead to a patient being removed from therapy prematurely. This is because it is difficult to accurately measure a 20% change in tumor size, whether based on physical examination of soft tissues, such as lymph nodes, or a CT scan of the lung, where lesion size and location are easily affected by the depth of a patient's breath at the time of exam. These measurement problems may be compounded by an inadequate duration of exposure to treatment before the first evaluation. It is not uncommon for a patient's *baseline* measurement of target lesions to be made 2–3 weeks prior to the initiation of treatment. Several weeks after starting a new treatment, the patient may have new or more intense symptoms. These could be a result of disease progression, toxicity from the therapy, and/or anxiety relating to the uncertainty of her disease status. A new evaluation of metastases ordered at this point and compared with the baseline is likely to underestimate potential treatment benefit because the patient was not on therapy for much of the time interval from the baseline to the follow-up measurement; any small progression seen at that point could be a result of progression *before* treatment was begun. Treatment should *not* be discontinued under these circumstances.

Unless a patient's symptoms cannot be adequately controlled,

- the first evaluation for response should not be performed until the patient has completed 3 months of treatment, and
- there is evidence of progression on two evaluations performed a month apart.

These rules are particularly important when evaluating non-toxic treatments since premature discontinuation of these could cost the patient many months or even years of tumor control with minimal symptoms.

Disease stabilization for periods of 3–6 months has been shown to be as closely associated as response rate with improved patient survival and quality of life (QofL), especially in patients receiving endocrine therapy. This is reflected in the clinical benefit rate (CBR), which is the sum of ORR and the percentage of patients with disease stabilization.

Progression-free survival (PFS) and time to progression (TTP) measure the interval from the initiation of treatment to tumor progression (or, in the case of PFS, tumor progression or death), whether that occurs without a response or after a transient response. Time to treatment failure (TTF) is to time to discontinuing treatment for any reason, including disease progression, death, or toxicity. These measures have little meaning outside the context of a randomized trial. However, since PFS and TTP are usually shorter with each treatment in a sequence of different therapies, an increase in the PFS/TTP compared to that achieved with the last therapy may be evidence of therapeutic effect. Most medical oncologists and patients feel that increasing PFS/TTP is a desirable goal of therapy and will almost always select the drug shown to induce a significantly better PFS in a randomized trial. The FDA has generally not accepted improved PFS as evidence of a clinical benefit unless the drug has minimal toxicity.

When initially elevated, serum markers such as CA15-3, CA 27.29, and CEA are useful adjuncts in determining a patient's response to therapy, especially with sites of metastases, such as bone, that cannot be easily evaluated. However, these markers should never be the sole basis for determining whether to stop or continue treatment because they may increase transiently before decreasing in response to an effective therapy (see Chapter 7). High levels of circulating tumor cells (CTCs; see Chapter 4) at the start of treatment and after the first course of chemotherapy are prognostic for a worse survival compared with those without a high baseline CTC or those whose CTC level falls with chemotherapy. However, switching those with a persistently high CTC after the first cycle of chemotherapy to a different regimen has not been shown to improve survival.[1]

CHOOSING AMONG THERAPIES FOR METASTATIC BREAST CANCER

Most patients with metastases will receive multiple forms of therapy, both in combination and sequentially. At each decision point, the potential for a therapy to relieve symptoms, restore organ function, and prolong survival must be balanced against the toxicity of the treatment and the patient's net quality of life. In general, more toxic therapies are associated with a higher likelihood of response but not necessarily with a greater survival benefit or quality of life. Factors that should be considered at each therapeutic decision point to individualize therapy for each patient are shown in Table 12.1.

Table 12.1 Factors Used in Selecting the Optimal Treatment for an Individual Patient

Factor	Implications for Selection of Therapy
Extent of metastases, specific organs involved	More extensive disease usually requires systemic therapy. Bone and soft tissue are particularly responsive to endocrine therapy. Liver and lung may require chemotherapy. See text on "visceral crisis."
Disease-free interval (DFI)	Longer DFI is associated with responsiveness to endocrine therapy.
Age, comorbidities, performance status (PS)	Older patients and those with poor PS are often less tolerant of toxic therapies
Molecular markers: ER, PR, HER2	ER+ tumors should almost always be treated with endocrine therapy alone; HER2+ tumors should be treated with anti-HER2 therapy, usually combined with another form of systemic therapy.
Menopausal status	Optimal endocrine therapy differs for pre- and postmenopausal women
Prior therapy and response	Response to one endocrine therapy is usually an indication for using another. Tumor growth on chemotherapy usually precludes further use of that class of drugs.
Symptoms and the need for palliation	Toxicity is the most important criterion in selecting therapy for asymptomatic or minimally symptomatic patients since the toxicity of treatment without palliation of symptoms may result in decreased quality of life
Potential morbidity of disease: death, fracture, organ failure	Therapeutic efficacy is the most important criterion for patients with life- or organ-threatening disease
Patient attitudes	Either toxicity or therapeutic efficacy may become the most important criterion depending on patient's desire to maximize quality or duration of life.

There are several ways in which physicians often shortchange their patients.

- Hippocrates stated that "dire diseases require dire remedies," and both physicians and patients usually consider cancer a dire disease. However, this may lead to the assumption that cancer patients need "aggressive" (usually synonymous with "toxic") therapy. For breast cancer, this is usually not true.
- Because metastatic breast cancer is viewed as a systemic disease, it is often assumed that systemic therapy is *always* required. There are numerous situations in which radiation therapy or surgery alone may suffice. These are usually patients with a long disease-free interval (DFI) and a single or very few clinically apparent sites of metastases.
- Because surgery and radiotherapy are generally more effective in eradicating any particular metastatic lesion, they are often given in combination with systemic therapy, but in some cases this may increase toxicity and compromise the ability to deliver the systemic therapy without improving survival or palliation. For example, radiotherapy may compromise the bone marrow and the ability to give cytotoxic therapies. Surgically removing an asymptomatic breast tumor in a patient with multiple distant metastases may delay the initiation of more effective treatments and needlessly subject the patient to the risks of anesthesia.
- Patients, non-oncology physicians, and even cancer specialists are understandably repelled by the toxicities of cancer therapy. In addition, it is easy to underestimate the life expectancy of breast cancer patients. This may lead to premature referral to hospice care that does not include specific anti-cancer therapy or the use of inappropriate use of analgesics alone.

LOCAL THERAPY FOR LOCAL RECURRENCES OR PATIENTS PRESENTING WITH STAGE IV DISEASE

A recurrence of cancer within a breast previously treated with breast-conserving therapy and not involving overlying skin or underlying chest wall structures is usually managed as a new primary.

Mastectomy does not remove every breast cell, and very small foci of remaining normal tissue may become cancerous with time. These lesions are usually distinguished from metastatic breast cancer by the presence of an in situ component in the biopsy specimen. These recurrences are also treated as new cancers with surgical excision alone or with radiotherapy if none was administered at the time of the first cancer diagnosis.

If a chest wall or regional recurrence involves skin, lymph nodes, or muscle, it is generally metastatic. Local recurrences may occur several or many years after the original diagnosis, and in some cases this is the only evidence of metastases. Conventional wisdom is that these lesions are hematogenously spread metastases and always a harbinger of metastases at distant sites,[2] but it is also possible that some of them are oligometastatic, which means that they are isolated recurrences with little or no capability of metastasizing further and might be treated as if they were primary tumors.[3] (The same reasoning has been applied to isolated metastases in other organs including lung, liver, and brain.)[4] There are no established rules for distinguishing metastatic from oligometastatic lesions, but a patient with a low histological grade, no lymph node involvement at the time of initial diagnosis, and an isolated lesion after a long DFI may have a long interval before the appearance of the next metastasis. For these relatively uncommon patients, treatment with local therapy alone may be reasonable. In one study, the 5-year PFS for a group like this was 53% and the OS 66%.[5] Such patients are often given systemic therapy ("pseudoadjuvant therapy") after completion of the local treatment, but no randomized trials have demonstrated either a PFS or OS advantage from doing so.

Local recurrences that appear synchronously with distant recurrences should initially be treated with systemic therapy. If there is a good response, any remaining local tumor can later be removed surgically or, if there is a CR, it can be consolidated with radiotherapy.

Some forms of local recurrence, such as peau d'orange (see Chapter 4) or large ulcerating lesions, are very difficult to control, even with intensive local therapy coupled with systemic therapy. Isolated local recurrences that are symptomatic but refractory to all forms of conventional therapy are sometimes treated with full thickness chest wall excision, re-irradiation, hyperthermia with or without additional radiation, or systemic therapies known to localize in skin (e.g., pegylated liposomal doxorubicin).

Responses to these very aggressive therapies are often very transient. On the other hand, refractory isolated local recurrences often smolder for years without the development of distant metastases or life-threatening progression; these patients suffer primarily from the constant presence of the disease and its potential threat.

Patients who initially present with stage IV disease and who also have a painful, ulcerating, bleeding, infected, or fungating primary are conventionally treated with a toilet mastectomy, which does not include lymph node dissection. Recently completed randomized trials failed to demonstrate any survival advantage from surgical removal of the primary in this setting. Patients can reasonably be treated first with systemic therapy and have toilet mastectomy performed later if symptoms persist and the response to systemic therapy is incomplete.

ENDOCRINE THERAPY: THE TREATMENT OF CHOICE FOR ER+ TUMORS

Almost all breast cancer patients with ER+ tumors should receive one or several forms of endocrine therapy over the course of their disease, even if the ER value is relatively low. Possible exceptions to this fundamental principle are those whose tumors clearly grew while receiving prior endocrine treatment, or those with relatively low ER levels *and* evidence of rapidly growing disease (see discussion of visceral crisis later in this chapter).

Endocrine therapy is both cytocidal and cytostatic: it results in tumor cell death and slows or stops tumor cell growth. Somewhere between 30% and 50% of patients with ER+ tumors not previously treated with endocrine therapy will have a PR or CR depending on the level of endocrine sensitivity[6] and the sites of disease under evaluation. A larger percentage of patients will undergo stabilization of disease for > 6 months. In previously untreated patients the CBR is between 50% and 75%. Responses are gradual in onset, so patients should be treated for a minimum of 3 months unless the signs of progression are both unequivocal and unacceptably symptomatic. The median duration of an objective response to the first endocrine therapy is 1.5–2 years, with the longest response durations in excess of 3.5 years. The median PFS or TTP is 7–15 months. Median survival averages 3.5–4 years, but a substantial number of patients among those in the half surviving over 4 years will make it to 8–12 years. Response is usually associated with a high quality of life because symptoms are alleviated while the toxicity of endocrine therapy is generally very mild. Endocrine treatment is usually continued until the tumor begins to grow again, but some patients respond repeatedly to the same therapy by alternating 6–12 months of treatment with intervals of no therapy.[7]

The first successful use of endocrine therapy was oophorectomy in 1896, and this is still one of the most effective therapies for premenopausal women (see Table 12.2). Responding patients often experience relief from bone pain within 24 hours, and this treatment is usually available even in areas of the world with very limited medical resources. Ovarian suppression with radiotherapy is equally effective but slower in onset; today it is uncommonly used but may be an "incidental treatment" when radiotherapy is administered to bone lesions in the spine or pelvis. Tamoxifen (see discussion later in this chapter) appears to be as effective as oophorectomy, but it has been difficult to conduct adequate randomized trials to compare various forms of endocrine treatment in premenopausal women. There are four small trials that compared tamoxifen and oophorectomy. Together they enrolled only 220 patients, but a meta-analysis ruled out a survival advantage of 25% or more for ovarian ablation.[8] Underpowered trials suggest that GNRH agonists are as effective as other forms of endocrine treatment for premenopausal women, and they have the advantage of being reversible. Goserelin is most commonly used.

Tumor "flare" has been described with many forms of endocrine therapy, including estrogens, androgens, and tamoxifen (and occasionally with chemotherapy as well). Within 24 hours following oophorectomy, patients with painful bone metastases may have hypercalcemia. More often, flare is manifest by increased bone pain lasting several weeks after the initiation of treatment. Less often there will be a transient increase in the size of measurable lesions, the appearance of erythema around skin lesions, transient changes in liver function studies or tumor markers, such as CA 15-3, or the appearance of new lesions on bone scans. These changes occur within a month of starting treatment. Flare can be observed on a fluorodeoxyglucose PET/CT scan. A 12% increase in uptake at 24 hours has been termed a "metabolic flare," and it has been shown to be predictive of benefit from endocrine therapy.[9] Since patients with flare, no matter how documented or manifest, are more likely to experience tumor regression than those without flare, treatment following flare should be continued for at least 3 months unless flare symptoms are life-threatening (e.g., severe hypercalcemia). Flare is particularly associated with the GNRH agonists, which cause a transient increase in both gonadotrophins and estrogen.

The aromatase enzyme converts androstenedione, which is normally produced in the ovary and adrenal gland, to estrone and estradiol. This occurs in fatty tissue throughout the body and in breast tissues, and this is the main source of estrogen in postmenopausal women. At one time, oophorectomy combined with adrenalectomy or hypophysectomy was a very effective form of endocrine treatment, but these operations have now been replaced by third-generation aromatase inhibitors (AIs): anastrozole, letrozole, and exemestane. None of these suppresses adrenal function, and they are remarkably well tolerated, their main side effects being arthralgias and myalgias

Table 12.2 Endocrine Therapies With Route, Dose/Schedule and Important or Dose-Limiting Toxicities

Category Therapeutic Group Drug	Route/Dose	Important or Dose-Limiting Toxicities, Comments
Ovarian Ablation, Premenopausal Women		Menopausal symptoms, hot flashes, possible osteopenia. All therapies in this category, including GNRH agonists, are effective only in premenopausal patients.
Oophorectomy	Surgery	Requires hospitalization, irreversible, but very inexpensive and available in areas with limited medical resources.
Radiation ablation of ovaries	Radiotherapy	Pelvic bone marrow suppression may complicate later chemotherapy. Slower onset of response than oophorectomy
Medical ovarian suppression with GNRH agonists		Transient increase in gonadotrophins and estrogen may lead to initial tumor flare (see text). There are depot, long-acting forms of some of these agents.
Goserelin (Zoladex®)	SQ 3.6 mg monthly	Injection often painful.
Leuprolide (Lupron®)	IM 3.75 mg monthly	FDA approved for prostate but not breast cancer. More depot forms available than other GNRH agonists.
Buserelin (Suprefact®)	SQ and nasal spray	Not FDA approved for breast cancer in US but often used in European breast cancer trials.
Triptorelin (Trelstar Depot®)	IM 3.75 mg monthly	Not yet FDA approved for breast cancer in US but in trials
Postmenopausal Estrogen Suppression		Postmenopausal symptoms. Osteopenia/osteoporosis
Adrenalectomy and oophorectomy or hypophysectomy	Surgery	Surgical removal of adrenal or pituitary gland. Requires lifelong corticosteroid support. Very effective but no longer used because AIs are less toxic and the effects are reversible.
Aromatase Inhibitors (AI's):		Arthralgias, myalgias. Effective only in postmenopausal women
Anastrozole (Arimidex®)	PO 2 mg daily	Non-steroidal aromatase inhibitor
Letrozole (Femara®)	PO 2.5 mg daily	Non-steroidal aromatase inhibitor
Exemestane (Aromasin®)	PO 25 mg daily	Steroidal aromatase inhibitor

	Dose	Comments
Estrogen or tamoxifen withdrawal		Very effective treatment, not commonly used today because it is perceived as "no therapy" by patients
Hormone Addition		
Estrogen (or high-dose estrogen)		Used today only after response and failure to SERMs, SERDs, AIs, or ovarian ablation.
Estradiol (generic)	PO 2 mg tid	Dose-related nausea, vomiting, fluid retention. Effective only in postmenopausal women
		Numerous published dose schedules including ethinyl estradiol 1 mg tid, and premarin 3.5 mg tid
Progestin		Increases appetite, fluid retention, and causes weight gain independent of fluid retention.
Megestrol acetate (Megace®)	PO 50 mg qid	
Medroxyprogesterone acetate (Provera®)	PO 500 mg bid	May also be given IM
Androgen		
Fluoxymesterone (Halotestin®)	PO 10 mg bid	Masculinization. Less effective than estrogen, but provides better sense of "well-being" than other endocrine therapies.
SERM (Selective estrogen receptor modulator)		
Tamoxifen (Nolvadex®)	PO 20 mg daily	Thromboembolic events, uterine cancer; decreases bone demineralization and improves lipid profile. Effective in pre- and postmenopausal women.
Toremefine (Fareston®)	PO 60 mg daily	May prolong QT interval. Never shown to have an advantage in efficacy or toxicity compared to tamoxifen.
SERD (Selective estrogen receptor down-regulators)		
Fulvestrant (Faslodex®)	IM 500 mg on days 1,15, 29 and then monthly*	Limited toxicity. Most trials used a smaller dose until it was found recently that this was suboptimal.

SQ = subcutaneously; PO = orally; IM = intramuscularly; bid = twice daily; tid = three times daily; qid = 4 times daily.

in up to 50% of patients (as many as 20% of patients discontinue AIs because of the arthralgias) and an exacerbation of postmenopausal symptoms, such as hot flashes. AIs do not suppress ovarian aromatase and should never be used in premenopausal women. Exemestane is a steroidal analogue of androstenedione and binds irreversibly to the aromatase, while the other two AIs are non-steroidal and bind reversibly. Direct comparisons of the three AIs are limited, but in general there appears to be little difference in either efficacy or toxicity. Letrozole has been shown to induce greater estrogen suppression, but it is not clear that this is associated with increased efficacy.

Non-physiologic or "high-dose" estrogens, which cause considerable nausea/ vomiting and fluid retention, were first shown to induce regression of metastatic breast cancer deposits in 1944, and for almost 3 decades this was the first treatment administered to postmenopausal breast cancer patients with recurrent disease. Physiologic doses of estrogen and progesterone will stimulate tumor cell proliferation, but there is no evidence of a dose effect among the much higher doses that have been used to treat breast cancer.[9] Progestins eventually replaced estrogens because they caused less nausea and vomiting. Androgens are also effective anti–breast cancer therapy, but they were shown in randomized trials to be less effective than estrogens.

Tamoxifen is a triphenylethylene that was originally developed to stimulate ovulation in infertile women and later was found to be an effective breast cancer treatment. Although referred to as an "anti-estrogen," tamoxifen has both estrogen agonist and antagonist activity, and while it suppresses the growth of breast cancer cells it has an estrogenic effect on bone and blood lipids. Tamoxifen binds to ER at the same site as estrogen, inactivates the AF2 (activating function-2) but not the AF1 domain on the receptor, and *partially* inactivates transcription and reduces the rate of tumor cell division. Thus it is classified as a selective estrogen receptor modulator (SERM). Its agonist effects may be a result of binding of non-genomic, membrane associated ER (see Figure 7.1 in Chapter 7). In animal models, prolonged exposure to tamoxifen results in prolonged suppression of cell growth and apoptosis, but eventually these effects are reversed, and continued tamoxifen exposure stimulates tumor cell growth. A randomized trial comparing tamoxifen with DES (diethylstilbestrol) in postmenopausal women initially demonstrated equal efficacy and reduced toxicity with tamoxifen. This established tamoxifen as the preferred endocrine therapy, but long-term follow-up demonstrated that DES was associated with a modest but statistically significant better overall survival.[10] The primary toxicities of tamoxifen are relatively uncommon thromboembolic events and a small but significant increase in uterine cancer.

Fulvestrant has only estrogen antagonist effects, and in preclinical models tamoxifen-resistant tumors will respond to fulvestrant.[11] In contrast to tamoxifen, fulvestrant inactivates both AF1 and AF2, downgrades ER, and totally inactivates transcription. It is classified as a selective estrogen receptor down-regulator (SERD) and is often referred to as a "pure antiestrogen." In the clinic it has been difficult to determine the optimal dose, but the CONFIRM trial[12] (see Table 12.3) strongly suggests that a higher dose is superior to that initially approved by the FDA and used in early clinical trials, which demonstrated that fulvestrant was about as effective as but not necessarily more effective than tamoxifen. Fulvestrant has induced remission in tumors resistant to tamoxifen, but in general it appears to be more effective against tamoxifen-sensitive than tamoxifen-resistant tumors.[6] After several loading doses 2 weeks apart, it is given intramuscularly monthly. This route of administration is considered a disadvantage by some patients.

Table 12.3 Outcomes From Selected Randomized Endocrine Therapy Trials Illustrating Likely Overall Response Rates (ORR), Clinical Benefit Rates (CBR), Progression-Free Survival (PFS) or Time to Progression (TTP), and Overall Survival (OS)

Trials of "first-line" therapy in patients who have had no endocrine therapy for metastatic disease and have had at least a 12-month interval from the completion of adjuvant endocrine therapy.

Trial Name	Study Arms	Number of Patients	ORR (%)	CBR (%)	Median PFS or TTP (Months)	Median OS (Months)
Meta-analysis[a]	Tamoxifen	2650	25	49		
	Any AI		33[††]	60[††]		
N. American & Target Trial[b]	Tamoxifen	1021	27	52	7.0	40.1
	Anastrozole		29	57	8.5	39.2
Europe Multicenter[c]	Tamoxifen	907	21	38	6.0	30
	Letrozole		32[††]	50[††]	9.4[††]	34
EORTC[d]	Tamoxifen	371	31	67	5.8	43.3
	Exemestane		46[†]	75	9.9	37.2
FIRST[e]	Anastrozole	205		67	13.1	
	Fulvestrant 500			73	23.4[†]	
SWOG S0226[f]	Anastrozole	707	22	70	13.5	41.3
	Anastrozole + Fulvestrant 500/250**		27	73	15.0[†]	47.7[†]
FACT[g]	Anastrozole	514	34	55	10.2	37.8
	Anatrozole + Fulvestrant 500/250**		32	55	10.8	38.2

(continued)

Table 12.3 Continued

Trials of "second-line" therapy in patients who have had responded to first-line endocrine therapy for metastatic disease and then progressed.

Trial Name	Study Arms	Number of Patients	ORR (%)	CBR (%)	Median PFS or TTP (Months)	Median OS (Months)
CONFIRM[h]	Fulvestrant 250	736	10	40	5.5	22.3
	Fulvestrant 500		9	46	6.5[+]	26.4
BOLERO-2[i]	Exemestane	724	0.4		3.2	HR = 0.77 (95%
	Exemestane + Everolimus		9.5[++]		7.8[++]	CI, 0.57–1.04)
GINECO[j]	Tamoxifen 20	111	14	42	4.5	HR = 0.45 (95%
	Tamoxifen + Everolimus		13	61[+]	8.6[+]	CI, 0.24–0.81
SoFEA[k]	Exemestane	723	4	27	3.4	21.6
	Fulvestrant 500/250**		8	32	4.8	19.4
	Fulvestrant** + Anastrozole		8	34	4.4	20.2
EFFECT[l]	Exemestane	693	7	32	3.7	
	Fulvestrant** 500/250		7	32	3.7	
Arimidex Study Group[m]	Megestrol acetate	516	12	40	4.6	22.5
	Anastrozole*		13	42	4.8	26.7[+]

Outcomes from these trials are factored into the sequence of endocrine therapies shown in Figure 12.2. Doses are those shown in Table 12.1 except when otherwise noted for fulvestrant trials in the study arms column.

+ Significant at some level of $p < 0.05$ and > 0.001 ++ Significant at some level of p <0.001

AI = aromatase inhibitor

* This was a three-arm study but only the comparison of anastrozole 1 mg, the FDA-approved dose, and megestrol acetate are shown.

** Loading dose of 500 mg on days 0 or 1 and followed by 250 mg on day 14 and then monthly. Other fulvestrant dose/schedules employed the same dose during both loading and in subsequent months.

[a] Xu HB, *Clin Breast Cancer* 2011 [Bibliography Ref #16]

[b] Nabholtz, JM, *Eur J Cancer* 2003 [Bibliography Ref #18]

[c] Mouridsen H, *J Clin Oncol* 2003 [Bibliography Ref #19]

[d] Paridaens RJ, *J Clin Oncol* 2008 [Bibliography Ref #20]

[e] Robertson JF, *Br Cancer Res Treat* 2012 [Biblio Ref #21]

[f] Mehta RS, *N Engl J Med* 2012 [Bibliography Ref #22]

[g] Bergh J, *J Clin Oncol* 2012;30:1919–25. [Biblio Ref #23]

[h] Di Leo A, *J Clin Oncol* 2010 [Bibliography Ref #12]

[i] Baselga J, *N Engl J Med* 2012 [Bibliography Ref #24]

[j] Bachelot T, *J Clin Oncol* 2012 [Bibliography Ref #25]

[k] Johnston SR, *Lancet Oncol* 2013;14:989–98. [Biblio Ref #26]

[l] Chia S, *Clin Oncol* 2008 [Bibliography Ref #27]

[m] Buzdar AU, *Cancer* 1998 [Bibliography Ref #28]

ENDOCRINE THERAPY SEQUENCES

One of the most important facets of endocrine therapy is the sequence of responses that may be obtained from sequential administration of different types of endocrine therapy. This was first observed when postmenopausal women were treated with pharmacological doses of estrogen. Tumors that shrank invariably regrew after some months or years, but simply discontinuing the estrogen administration at the time of regrowth caused about one-third of them to once again regress. When these tumors began growing again after 6 to 12 months, another remission could often be achieved by further reducing circulating estrogen levels through either adrenalectomy or hypophysectomy. In some patients, additional responses were obtained by adding progestins, then androgens, and finally estrogens again. Generally, only patients who respond to one endocrine treatment respond to a subsequent form of hormone therapy, so the endocrine cascade was discontinued whenever the patient failed to have any response at all to an endocrine treatment.

Laboratory studies suggest that sequential responses occur because breast cancer cells adapt to different levels of circulating and intratumoral estrogen[13,14] (see Figures 12.1 and 7.1). This is not a result of clonal selection. It is postulated that similar phenomena

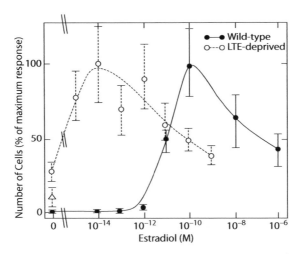

Figure 12.1 Growth stimulation and inhibition (apoptosis) from various concentrations of estradiol applied either to wild-type MCF-7 cells or MCF-7 cells grown without estradiol for long periods (LTE-deprived cells). The amount of estradiol needed to stimulate growth of LTE-deprived cells is much lower than that required to stimulate wild-type MCF-7 cells, as is the higher estradiol concentration required to suppress growth by causing apoptosis. When grown in estradiol again or passaged through a nude mouse with estradiol pellets, the LTE-deprived cells regain the biological properties of the wild type. These estradiol effects are rapid, cause up-regulation of ERα, and use non-genomic, plasma-membrane mediated pathways to activate the MAP kinase, PI-3 kinase, and mTOR pathways. Results expressed as percentage (%) of maximum response. Apoptosis was confirmed in additional experiments.
Sources: Masamura S, Santner SJ, Heitjan DF, et al. Estrogen deprivation causes estradiol hypersensitivity in human breast cancer cells. J Clin Endocrinol Metab. 1995;80:2918–25; Santen RJ, Song RX, Masamura S, et al. Adaptation to estradiol deprivation causes up-regulation of growth factor pathways and hypersensitivity to estradiol in breast cancer cells. Adv Exp Med Biol. 2008;630:19–34.

occur in the clinic.[13] Breast cancers in postmenopausal, but not premenopausal, women respond to high-dose estrogen therapy; presumably this is because the cancer cells in the postmenopausal woman have been deprived of physiological sources of estrogen in the years leading up to the initiation of the treatment, and are hypersensitive to estrogen and apoptose in response to high doses of estrogen. Surgical oophorectomy lowers estradiol levels in a premenopausal woman from approximately 200 pg/ml to 10 pg/ml, and this estrogen deprivation induces tumor regression for 12–18 months, at which time the breast cancers have adapted and begin to grow on the lower levels of estrogen produced by aromatases. Treatment with an aromatase inhibitor further reduces estradiol levels in women without functioning ovaries to 1–2 pg/ml and induces an additional regression.

A therapy shown in a randomized trial to be more efficacious will generally be used earlier in the endocrine cascade (see Table 12.3 and Figure 12.2). AIs have been shown in five to six independent trials and in an overview of these trials with > 2,600 patients to induce a significantly higher ORR and CBR and longer PFS than tamoxifen in patients who have not had prior endocrine therapy for their metastases.[15,16,18-21] (This therapy would be classified as "first line" even though adjuvant endocrine therapy might have been previously given to some patients.) The FDA has given only the non-steroidal AIs (NS-AIs, anastrozole and letrozole) a first-line indication, but the available evidence suggests that exemestane is probably equally effective in this setting.[17] A combination of an AI and fulvestrant is also a first line option (see section later in this chapter on Endocrine Therapy in Combination).

Patients who progress within 6 months *without* any evidence of an objective response are usually switched to cytotoxic agents as their next form of systemic therapy since their chance of responding to another endocrine treatment is very low. However, if they have had a response or prolonged stable disease, they should be given a "second-line" endocrine therapy[12, 24-28] (see bottom half of Table 12.3). The kind of response that might be expected from second-line treatment are illustrated by the EFFECT trial in which all patients had responded and then progressed while receiving a first-line NS-AI. The overall response rate to the second-line therapy was low, but 32% of patients on each arm had clinical benefit, and the median duration of response was 13.5 and 9.8 months for those who did respond to fulvestrant or exemestane, respectively.[27] Patients treated initially with exemestane have a reasonable chance of responding secondarily to an NS-AI. Randomized trials comparing suboptimal doses of fulvestrant with an AI showed no advantage for either as a second-line treatment, but this may change when optimal doses of fulvestrant are evaluated in this setting.

On rare occasions, patients respond sequentially to or remain stable on as many as seven endocrine treatments and continue for years with few symptoms from breast cancer and almost no toxicity from therapy.

If a patient progresses while receiving adjuvant endocrine treatment, it is impossible to assess whether she has an endocrine-sensitive tumor. By convention, if the DFI on adjuvant endocrine therapy is < 12 months, it is assumed that the tumor has limited or no endocrine sensitivity, and chemotherapy is usually used first line. However, if the patient has a particularly high ER value, a limited number of metastases confined primarily to bone and soft tissue, and few symptoms, it is reasonable to try endocrine treatment first, in which case an AI is used if the adjuvant endocrine therapy was tamoxifen. If the adjuvant therapy was an AI, a different AI might be used. Another option following adjuvant AI or sequential tamoxifen followed by an AI is fulvestrant.

ENDOCRINE THERAPY IN COMBINATION

Combinations of endocrine and chemotherapy usually result in a higher RR or longer TTP, but no survival advantage and increased toxicity compared to using the endocrine therapy alone. Because this deprives the patient of the high quality of life that often ensues from endocrine therapy, combinations with chemotherapy are generally contraindicated.

Recently combing several endocrine therapies with different mechanisms of action has proven beneficial. In a meta-analysis of four trials that randomized 506 premenopausal patients either to an LHRH agonist alone or the same plus tamoxifen, the RRs were 30% and 39% ($p = 0.03$), respectively.[29] This small difference in RR was associated with a 30% ($p = 0.0003$) improvement in PFS and a 22% ($p = 0.02$) improvement in overall survival (OS) for those randomized to the combination.

Some physicians have combined LHRH agonists with an AI in premenopausal women, but there are insufficient data to conclude that this is safe or more efficacious than standard treatments.

The rationale for combining an aromatase inhibitor and fulvestrant in postmenopausal women comes from preclinical studies, such the one shown in Figure 12.1, that demonstrate increased sensitivity to endocrine therapies with changes in estrogen levels. Fulvestrant, in particular, is more efficient in a low-estrogen environment; in addition, it reduces cross-talk between ER and growth-factor signaling.[22] The results of clinical trials comparing these two in combination have shown mixed results[22,23], but in the largest of these trials (SWOG S0226 with 707 patients), those randomized to anastrozole plus fulvestrant had a slightly better RR and significantly better PFS and OS than those on anastrozole alone (Table 12.3). The FACT trial showed no difference in outcome. At present, the use of an AI alone remains the treatment of choice for first line endocrine therapy.

There is considerable evidence that resistance to endocrine therapy is a result of or at least associated with estrogen-independent signaling through the PI3k/Akt pathway, of which mTOR is a part (Figure 7.1 in Chapter 7), and this provided the rationale for combining an AI, exemestane, with an mTOR inhibitor, everolimus.[24] All patients in the BOLERO-2 trial had tumors that had progressed during prior AI therapy. The RR to the combination was significantly improved and PFS more than double ($p < 0.001$) that achieved with the AI alone (Table 12.3). There was a 23% reduction in short-term mortality ($p = $ NS). However, the benefits were achieved with a substantial increase in treatment-related toxicity. Patients given the combination were five times more likely to have discontinued treatment because of signs and symptoms such as stomatitis, anemia, dyspnea, hyperglycemia, fatigue, and pneumonitis.[24] Similar results were obtained when everolimus plus tamoxifen was compared to tamoxifen in the GINECO trial[25] (Table 12.3). These are important results because of their implications for new combinations of endocrine therapy and other agents that target signal transduction pathways. However, because of the toxicity and the absence of evidence that this improves outcomes for first-line patients, everolimus combinations should be reserved for those whose disease has been demonstrated in the clinic to be resistant (see Figure 12.2). This is likely to change soon.

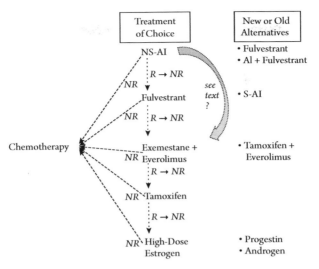

Figure 12.2 Sequence of endocrine therapies given to a postmenopausal woman with metastatic breast cancer.
NR = no response of any kind; R→NR = response followed by progression; NS-AI = non-steroidal aromatase inhibitor; S-AI = steroidal AI.

CHEMOTHERAPY: TREATMENT FOR ENDOCRINE INSENSITIVE TUMORS

There are few, if any, tumor types that respond to so many different types of cytotoxic treatments. *Although this group of drugs is associated with varied and often severe side effects, the appropriate use of these drugs is more effective than pain medications alone or with other support therapy in most symptomatic patients.* Formal quality of life (QofL) studies have repeatedly demonstrated that the most effective agents are associated with a better QofL even if they are more toxic. The results of one such study are shown in Table 12.4. Patients were randomized to a relatively non-toxic single agent or a more toxic combination, CMFP.[30] The response rate and median time to progression were higher for CMFP, but it caused much more non-hematological toxicity. However, when patients and physicians were independently queried using standard QofL instruments, the more effective but more toxic regimen was associated with better quality of life.

Either a single agent or a combination of cytotoxic drugs should be given to symptomatic patients whose tumors are ER negative or who have had one or more endocrine therapies without evidence of response or stabilization during the last one. If the patient has not previously received chemotherapy for metastases and has an interval of a year or more since the completion of adjuvant chemotherapy, the likelihood of having a PR or CR is between 35% and 55%[31] (see Table 12.5). The CBR with response or disease stabilization for at least 3–4 months is 75%–80%, and the average TTP is 5 to 8 months. Median survival from the time chemotherapy is begun will be about 19–22 months, with 50%–60% of that survival time occurring after the patient's tumor begins to regrow and first-line chemotherapy is discontinued.

Table 12.4 Effectiveness, Toxicity, and Quality of Life Outcomes From a Trial in Which Breast Cancer Patients With Metastases Not Previously Treated With Cytotoxic Drugs Were Randomized to Receive Either Mitoxantrone or the Combination of CMFP (Cyclophosphamide, Methotrexate, 5-Fluorouracil, and Prednisone)

	Mitoxantrone	CMFP	p value
Effectiveness Outcomes			
Overall response rate	25%	39%	
Median PFS (months)	3.9	5.6	0.02
Median OS (months)	11.6	10.1	0.81
Toxicity			
At least one grade 3 non-hematological toxic episode	8%	27%	0.0001
Treatment-related deaths	2%	6%	
Stomatitis: any degree	18%	48%	<0.001
Grade 3–4	1%	11%	
Nausea and vomiting	73%	72%	0.82
Alopecia	45%	69%	< 0.001
Diarrhea	10%	29%	< 0.001
Anemia	45%	62%	0.001
Relative Quality of Life Scores			
Mood		+ 6.1	0.04
Nausea and vomiting		+ 7.3	0.03
"Feeling sick"		+ 6.5	0.02
Hair loss	+20.5		< 0.01
GLQ-8 Uniscale score by patient	No difference		0.53
Global QofL Score by patient*		+1.7	0.18
Subset QofL Score by patient*		+2.4	0.03
Spitzer QL-score by physician	No difference		0.20

Quality of life (QofL) was assessed prior to randomization and again at each 12-week interval until patient death. Scores reflect changes in QofL between the baseline and first 12-week assessment. [Lee CK, *Springerplus* 2013] [In Bibliography, ref #30]

* A global quality of life (QofL) score, derived using a regression function, was a weighted combination of the measured global QofL scale (GLQ-8) and all individual LASA QofL (except sexual interest) items. A subset QofL score was a weighted combination of only individual LASA (linear analogue self-assessment) QofL (except sexual interest) items.

If the patient has previously had chemotherapy for metastases or has recurred within a year following adjuvant chemotherapy, the benefits from chemotherapy given as second line will be smaller[32] (Table 12.5).

The effect of chemotherapy on survival is difficult to demonstrate. There are no trials randomizing patients with metastases to active therapy or best supportive care

Table 12.5 Clinical Outcomes From the Use of Chemotherapy in Metastatic Breast Cancer Patients Who (A) Had Not Previously Been Treated With Chemotherapy for Metastatic Disease or (B) Who Had Previously Received Both an Anthracycline and a Taxane

A. Outcomes from First-Line Therapy

Meta-analysis of 3,953 patients in 11 randomized trials that compared an anthracycline, alone or in combination with non-taxane drugs, and a taxane, alone or in combination with an anthracycline. Fifty-eight percent of the patients had ER+ tumors and 41% had received some form of adjuvant chemotherapy. [Piccart-Gebhart MJ, Burzykowski T, Buyse M, et al. Taxanes alone or in combination with anthracyclines as first-line therapy of patients with metastatic breast cancer. J Clin Oncol. 2008;26:1980–6.]

	Combination Regimen Trials 8 trials, 3,034 patients		Single Agent Trials 3 trials, 919 patients	
	Anthracycline	Taxane	Anthracycline	Taxane
Overall response rate (%)	46	57[a]	38	33
Complete response rate (%)	10	6	6	4
Disease control rate (%)	80	84	76	73
Median progression-free survival (mos)	6.9	7.7[b]	7.2	5.1
Median overall survival (mos)	19.2	19.8	18.6	19.5
Time from progression to death (mos)	10.9	10.5	11.6	12.5

B. Outcomes from Second-Line Therapy

Systematic review of 19 observational and randomized trials that evaluated single agent capecitabine or vinorelbine (two studies included both) in 1,810 patients, > 80% of whom had previously been treated with both an anthracycline and taxane. Results are either ranges or weighted averages based on the number of studies. [Oostendorp LJ, Stalmeier PF, Donders AR, et al. Efficacy and safety of palliative chemotherapy for patients with advanced breast cancer pretreated with anthracyclines and taxanes: a systematic review. Lancet Oncol. 2011;12:1053–61]

	Capecitabine 10 trials, 1,404 patients	Vinorelbine 9 trials, 406 patients
Overall response rate range (%)	9–32	13–35
Disease control rate (%)	57	49
Median progression-free survival (mos)	4.2	3.8
Median overall survival (mos)	13.5	12.6

[a] p < 0.001 for comparison with anthracycline without taxane regimen

[b] p = 0.031 for comparison with anthracycline regimen.

Disease control rate = overall response plus stable disease.

Mos = months.

for the remainder of their lives, and patients randomized to less effective regimens in a trial are usually given multiple other treatments after disease progression. The effect of these second-line treatments obscures any survival benefits imparted by the more effective regimen in first line. However, there appears to be a survival benefit even when chemotherapy is administered to patients with very advanced and relatively refractory disease. This was demonstrated in a large trial that randomized patients to a new, active agent, eribulin, or physician's choice (see Figure 12.3). The difference in median survival was 2.5 months.[33]

Simply citing median PFS and OS values to patients oversimplifies their situation and may lead them to make inappropriate decisions regarding treatment or lifestyle. An alternative is to describe a number of possible outcomes that includes a best- and worst-case scenario.[34] This is illustrated in Table 12.6. The pooled median survival of 13,083 patients enrolled in first-line chemotherapy trials was 21.7 months, but the 10% with the worst survival lived an average of 6.3 months and the 10% with the best survival averaged 55.8 months. While the outcomes from this overview might apply to most patients about to start first-line chemotherapy, a patient could obtain a more accurate appraisal of her situation by looking at PFS or OS data from a trial enrolling patients with her particular characteristics. A best-case and worst-case scenario would

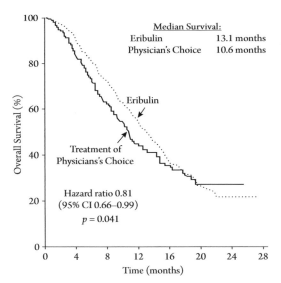

Figure 12.3 Overall survival of 762 women with very advanced and refractory disease randomized in ratio of 2:1 to eribulin or the physician's choice. Patients had received 2–5 prior chemotherapy regimens (46% had 4 or more) that included at least an anthracycline and a taxane and had progressed within 6 months of their last chemotherapy; 51% had metastases to 3 or more organs, and 60% had liver metastases. On the physician's choice arm, 96% received chemotherapy with vinorelbine (25%), gemcitabine (19%), capecitabine (18%), a taxane (15%), an anthracycline (10%), or other agents (10%). The ORR for eribulin and physician's choice, respectively, were 13% and 7% ($p = 0.028$), the CBR's were 23% and 17%, PFSs were 3.6 and 2.2 months ($p = 0.002$), and median OSs were 13.1 months (95% CI, 11.8–14.3) and 10.6 (95% CI, 9.3–12.5).

With permission from Cortes J, O'Shaughnessy J, Loesch D, et al. Eribulin monotherapy versus treatment of physician's choice in patients with metastatic breast cancer (EMBRACE): a phase 3 open-label randomised study. *Lancet*. 2011;377:914–23.

Table 12.6 Worst- and Best-Case Overall Survival Following First-Line Chemotherapy for 13,083 Metastatic Breast Cancer Patients Enrolled in 36 Clinical Trials Between 1999 and 2009

Outcome	Group Percentile	Observed (Months)	Interquartile Range	Multiple of Median
Median overall survival		21.7	18.2–24	
Alternative overall survival scenarios				
Worst-case	90th	6.3	4.8–7.5	0.25
Lower typical	75th	11.9	9.9–13.2	0.5
Upper typical	25th	36.2	31.1–41.3	2.0
Best-case	10th	55.8	47.5–60.2	3.0

Most of the patients were postmenopausal; about half had ER+ tumors and two-thirds had visceral metastases. OS and PFS curves were generated from pooled data, and the median, 90th, 75th, 25th, and 10th percentile values were determined. Using these observations, a multiple of the median that might be applied to other trial data was generated.

Data from Kiely BE, Soon YY, Tattersall MH, et al. How long have I got? Estimating typical, best-case, and worst-case scenarios for patients starting first-line chemotherapy for metastatic breast cancer: a systematic review of recent randomized trials. J Clin Oncol 2011;29:456–63.

then be derived by applying the multipliers shown in the last column of Table 12.6 ("multiple of median") to the survival data generated in the trial.

Among those who respond, the median time to a response to chemotherapy is about the same as the time to a response to endocrine therapy: about 3 months (see discussion of "visceral crisis" later in this chapter). This suggests that cytotoxic therapies should also be administered for *at least 3 months* unless there is unequivocal evidence of tumor growth. (see earlier discussion).

CYTOTOXIC DRUGS AND THEIR SIDE EFFECTS

This list of agents commonly used to treat metastatic breast cancer is very long. Differences in effectiveness are real but relatively small, while side effects vary considerably in both frequency and severity (see Table 12.7). The decision to use one rather than another agent or combination of drugs is highly individualized and depends on the balance between potential benefits and toxicity appropriate for each individual patient. Patient concerns about toxicity, patient age, symptoms, tumor growth rate, comorbidities, prior therapies, and the response to prior therapies should all be considered when choosing a specific regimen.

Since most of these drugs target cellular mechanisms involved in cell division, it is not surprising that the most common side effects are in organs characterized by high growth rates: the bone marrow, GI tract (nausea, vomiting, stomatitis, diarrhea), and hair follicles. The anthracyclines doxorubicin and epirubicin lead to total baldness within a couple of weeks after the first dose, while the alkylating agents, antimetabolites, antifolates, platinums, and mitomycin cause gradual hair thinning or no hair loss at all. Nausea and vomiting can be substantially reduced or blocked with a variety of

Table 12.7 Commonly Used or Historically Important Cytotoxic Drugs

Category Drug Abbreviation	Route/Dose When Used Alone	**Prior Therapy	Important or Dose-Limiting Toxicities, Comments
Alkylating Agents			
Cyclophosphamide (Cytoxan®) C	PO 50–100 mg daily IV 400 mm² qd X 5, monthly		Myelosuppression, thrombocytopenia, anemia, mild vomiting, alopecia, leukemia. Used in CMF, CAF, other combinations.
Melphalan (Alkeran®) [a] L-PAM	PO 6 mm² qd X 5, q 6 wks		Infrequent use today; early adjuvant therapy.
Thiotepa [a]	IV 0.2–0.4 mg/kg monthly		Less toxic than other alkylators. Infrequent used today but used in ABMT regimens.
Antimetabolites, Antifolates			
Methotrexate M	IV 25 mm² twice weekly		Limited alopecia. Stomatitis. Most used in combination regimens. Stomatitis, mild vomiting, renal toxicity
5-fluorouracil F	IV 500 mm² weekly or Continuous IV 200-300 mg/day X 21 of 28 days	1,2	Bolus used in combinations. Continuous IV less toxic but with more stomatitis and PPE. Effective in very refractory tumors.
Capecitabine (Xeloda®) X	PO 825–1250 mm² BID d1-d14 q 3 wks.	1,2	PPE related to peak dose. Diarrhea. Lower dose may be as effective and less toxic, but PPE still occurs. Often used as single agent because of excellent toxicity profile.
Gemcitabine (Gemzar®) G	IV 800–1200 mm² over 30 minutes d1, d8, d15 monthly	1,2	Neutropenia, pulmonary toxicity rarely severe.
Pemetrexed (Alimta®) [a]	IV 500 mm² q3wks or IV 600mm² q 2wks	1,2,3	Neutropenia, neuropathy. Folic acid and vitamin B12 given with drug. Limited use.

	Dose/Schedule		Comments
Anthracyclines, Anthraquinones			
Doxorubicin (*Adriamycin*®) A	IV 60–75 mm^2 q 3 wks *or* IV 20 mm^2 weekly		All are cardiotoxic related to cumulative dose. Severe vomiting and alopecia. Moderate myelosuppression. Weekly less cardiotoxic.
Epirubicin (*Ellence*®) E	IV 60–90 mm^2 q 3 wks		Less cardiotoxic (see text). No alopecia.
Pegylated liposomal doxorubicin (*Doxil*®)[a]	IV 35–50 mm^2 monthly		PPE related to cumulative dose. Much less vomiting, myelosuppression, alopecia than other anthracyclines. Less cardiotoxicity.
Mitoxantrone[a] (*Novantrone*®) N	IV 12–14 mm^2 q 3 wks		Less cardiotoxicity, nausea, vomiting, and alopecia than bolus anthracyclines.
Taxanes			
Paclitaxel (*Taxol*®) T or P	IV 175 mm^2 q 3 wks. *or* IV 80 mm^2 weekly	1	Sensory peripheral neuropathy; neutropenia; mild to moderate alopecia. Weekly dose/schedule more efficacious. Used alone and in many combinations.
Docetaxel (*Taxotere*®) T or D	IV 80–100 mm^2 q 3 wks *or* IV 40 mm^2 weekly X 6, then rest 2 wks	1	3-weekly dose/schedule more efficacious. Used alone and in many combinations.
Nab-paclitaxel (*Abraxane*®)	IV 100 or 150 mm^2 d1, d8, d15 each month *or* IV 260 mm^2 q 3 wks.	1,2	Less neutropenia than other taxanes, higher doses tolerated. Weekly dose/schedule more efficacious than 3-weekly and superior to 3-weekly docetaxel.
Other Agents Targeting Microtubules			
Vinorelbine (*Navelbine*®)[a]	IV 25 mm^2 weekly	1,2	Neutropenia. Very little neuropathy. Compared with taxanes, less active but much better tolerated, especially in combinations.
Ixabepilone (*Ixempra*®)	IV 40 mm^2 over 3 hours q 3 wks	1,2,	Neuropathy; severe myelosuppression. PPE. Effective in very advanced disease.
Eribulin (*Halaven*®)	IV 1.4 mm^2 d1 & d8 q 3 wks	1,2,3	Severe neutropenia; neuropathy; alopecia, Effective in very advanced disease.

Table 12.7 Continued

Category Drug Abbreviation	Route/Dose When Used Alone	**Prior Therapy	Important or Dose-Limiting Toxicities, Comments
Topoisomerase Inhibitors			
Irinotecan (Camptosar®)[a]	IV 100 mm² weekly X 6, then rest X 2	1,2	Neutropenia, nausea, vomiting. Diarrhea can be severe. Limited activity.
Platinums			Very active as first-line agents but not in those with chemotherapy resistance. Possible role in BRCA-1 positive and HER2 positive tumors, including some triple negative.
Cisplatin (Platinol®)[a]	IV 100 mm² q 4 weeks or IV 75 mm² q 3 weeks or IV 30 mm² qd X 4 q 3 weeks		Marked nausea/vomiting, nephrotoxicity, ototoxicity
Carboplatin (Paraplatin®)[a]	IV 400 mm² or AUC 6–7 q 4 weeks		Myelosuppression, less nausea/vomiting, less nephrotoxicity than cisplatin. Dose usually adjusted for glomerular filtration rate.
Miscellaneous			
Mitomycin C (Mutamycin®)[a]	IV 20 mm² q 6 weeks		Few side effects but causes delayed myelosuppression that can be severe and prolonged. Used only in very advanced disease.

Doses are the usual starting dose when the drug is used alone; doses used in subsequent treatment cycles or are adjusted on the basis of toxicity, especially myelosuppression. Doses are usually lower when the drug is used in a combination (see Table 12.8).

[a] Not approved by the FDA for breast cancer

** Prior therapy codes: drug shown to have at least limited activity after prior treatment with or clear resistance to an anthracycline (1), a taxane (2), capecitabine (3)

mm² = mg/m²; q = every; ABMT = autologous bone marrow (or stem cell) transplant; PPE = palmar-plantar erythrodysesthesia (hand-foot syndrome).

anti-emetics, and for this reason nausea/vomiting is a less important factor in choosing drugs. At recommended doses, these drugs, whether used alone or in combination, do not generally require the use of G-CSF.

Several drug classes are associated with unique toxicities. Anthracyclines cause a cardiomyopathy that is related to the cumulative dose. Epirubicin may be less cardiotoxic than doxorubicin, but since it is not clear what the equi-effective doses are, it has not been established that there is a difference in cardiotoxicity at equi-effective doses of these two drugs. Doxorubicin administered weekly or by continuous infusion, instead of a bolus every 3 weeks, is less cardiotoxic, as are non-pegylated and pegylated liposomal doxorubicin, the latter having pharmacokinetics similar to a continuous infusion. Mitoxantrone, an anthraquinone, is less cardiotoxic, but its efficacy relative to the anthracyclines is uncertain. Cardiotoxicity from these agents can be reduced by concomitant administration of dexrazoxane.

Drugs with prolonged circulation or very long half-lives are associated with palmar-plantar erythrodysesthesia (hand-foot syndrome, PPE). These include continuous infusions of doxorubicin or 5-fluorouracil, capecitabine, and pegylated liposomal doxorubicin. The pain and less common desquamation may be dose limiting for these drugs, but this toxicity can be reduced or avoided by changes in dose schedule. For this reason, many oncologists avoid the FDA-approved doses of capecitabine and administer instead 825 or 1,000 mg/m^2 twice daily for 14 days of a 3-week cycle.[35]

Sensory neuropathies that may persist long after treatment is stopped are dose limiting for the taxanes and most other agents that target the microtubules. More frequent administration, such as weekly paclitaxel or nab-paclitaxel, is associated with both increased efficacy and neurotoxicity.[36]

The most frequently used drugs seem to be the most toxic. It is often perceived that these are the most effective, and in some cases there are data to justify that conclusion. However, it is uncommon for one drug or drug combination to improve survival substantially and significantly more than another. A more toxic therapy may lead to a better QofL for some patients (see earlier discussion), but it is possible to choose drugs or to design regimens that are quite effective but with limited alopecia, nausea, vomiting, diarrhea, stomatitis, and fatigue. This is accomplished either by using lower doses or choosing single agents rather than combinations. Cytotoxic drugs with a favorable overall toxicity profile include lower doses of capecitabine, vinorelbine, pegylated liposomal doxorubicin, daily (or every other day) oral cyclophosphamide, and mitomycin C.

SELECTING AND USING THE MOST EFFECTIVE CHEMOTHERAPY AGENTS AND COMBINATIONS

Patients with metastases that have never been treated before fall into three categories based on their prior exposure to cytotoxics:

1. No prior chemotherapy of any type or completion of prior adjuvant chemotherapy > 12 months before relapse using a regimen without either an anthracycline or a taxane
2. Prior adjuvant chemotherapy that included an anthracycline and/or taxane and was completed > 12 months before relapse

3. Prior adjuvant chemotherapy that included an anthracycline and a taxane and was completed < 12 months before relapse.

Patients in the first group will usually be treated with an anthracycline, a taxane, or a combination that includes one or both of these drugs. This is because each of these has been shown in randomized trials to improve PFS and OS compared to earlier "standard chemotherapy regimens"[31,37] (Table 12.5).

Patients in the second group are usually treated with a taxane alone or a taxane combination that does not include an anthracycline. These patients still have anthracycline-responsive tumors, but as the cumulative dose of anthracycline exposure increases, the risk of cardiotoxicity also increases substantially. (An anthracycline might still be considered for these patients later when their tumors have been proven resistant to non-cardiotoxic agents.)

It is assumed that patients in the third group are resistant to both an anthracycline and a taxane, and they are treated with one of the drugs that have been shown to induce objective responses in resistant tumors (see Prior Therapy column of Table 12.7). The FDA has specifically approved only three drugs for resistant tumors—capecitabine, ixabepilone, and eribulin mesylate—but gemcitabine is also frequently used in this setting, and other drugs in the list are used occasionally. The benefits from treating patients whose tumors have become unresponsive to anthracyclines and taxane are small, but these drugs will palliate symptoms and may significantly improve the survival of patients with very advanced tumors when used appropriately (Figure 12.3).

In the past, the platinum compounds, cisplatin and carboplatin, have not been used to treat breast cancer. These drugs are cross-resistant with both the taxanes and anthracyclines, and in almost all phase II trials involving pretreated patients the response rates have been very low.[38] In contrast, they are very active as single agents in previously untreated patients, but randomized trials comparing them with other single agents or comparisons of platinum-containing combinations with non-platinum combinations have shown increased RR to platinum-containing combinations with no difference in either TTP or OS.[39] In light of the excess toxicity associated with the drugs, they have no role in the management of most breast cancer patients. This is now being reassessed for patients with HER2 positive and triple negative tumors, two groups where they *might* play a unique role.

DIFFICULT JUDGMENT CALLS

Selecting a Single Agent or Drug Combination

Most clinical trials and a meta-analysis of these trials have demonstrated that drug combinations are more effective than single agents both as first-line therapy and for more advanced disease. Combinations have significantly higher RRs and CBRs and are associated with longer TTP and OS.[40–42] Combinations are also significantly more toxic. Trials comparing combinations with a planned sequence of single agents are limited in number and size, but the largest of such trials suggests that a combination may not have a clear advantage.[43] In this trial, 739 patients with metastatic breast cancer previously untreated with chemotherapy were randomized to a combination of doxorubicin and paclitaxel or either drug alone with crossover to the other at the time of first progression. Although the RR and first TTP were significantly higher with the combination, there were no QofL or OS differences between the three study arms. Breast cancer oncologists in the United States and Europe have concluded that ". . . there is no compelling evidence that combination regimens are superior to sequential single agents."[42,44] Patients who are very symptomatic with evidence of rapid progression but a good performance status may be best served by combination therapy, especially as their first form of chemotherapy, since it increases their chance of an immediate response; sequential single agents may be compatible with a better quality of life in all others.

The most commonly used combination regimens are shown in Table 12.8.

Discontinuing a Regimen

Once chemotherapy is begun, it is usually continued until disease progression. This policy is supported by a meta-analysis of clinical trials in which patients were randomized to discontinue chemotherapy after 3–6 months or to continue until disease progression.[45] Patients randomized to receive prolonged courses had substantially and significantly longer PFS and a modest but still significantly longer OS. Quality of life was formally assessed in only one of these trials, and the longer duration of treatment was associated with better QofL. Nonetheless, in light of the relatively small survival advantage from prolonged chemotherapy, patients with stable disease, few symptoms from their cancer, and substantial chemotherapy-related toxicity may be better served by discontinuing chemotherapy when a plateau in benefit has been reached.

Dose Response

In preclinical cancer models and in the management of the hematological malignancies, there is unequivocal evidence of a marked increase in tumor response with increased dose of these drugs. There is some evidence of a threshold effect in dosing cytotoxic therapies used to treat breast cancer—that is, there are doses below which the response rate falls off quickly. However, it has not been shown that escalating doses, including very high doses requiring autologous marrow support, provide clinically meaningful benefit for patients with metastases. In general, doses demonstrated to have benefit in clinical trials should be used and reduced only to the extent necessary to achieve acceptable degrees of toxicity.

TRIPLE NEGATIVE BREAST CANCER (TNBC): ER–/PR–/HER2–

Triple negative or basal-like cancers are increasingly being recognized as distinct entities with a more aggressive biology (see Chapter 7). All of the clinical trials cited earlier include patients with triple negative tumors, along with multiple other types. Analysis of the TNBC subset in some of these trials, as well as in phase II trials specifically designed for TNBC, suggests that these tumors are very responsive to all of the commonly used chemotherapy agents, but the patients relapse and die after relatively short intervals in spite of their response.[46]

Table 12.8 Drug Combinations Commonly Used to Treat Metastatic Breast Cancer

Regimen	Cycle Length (Weeks)	Anthracyclines	Cyclophosphamide (C)	5-Fluorouracil (F)	Methotrexate (M)	Microtubule Targeted Drugs	Capecitabine (X)	Gemcitabine (G)
		Doxorubicin* (A)				Paclitaxel** (T or P)		
CMF	4		100 po d1–14	600 IV d1 & d8	40 IV d1 & d8			
AC	3	60 IV d1	600 IV d1					
FAC (iv)	3	50 IV d1	500 IV d1	500 IV d1 & d8				
CAF (oral)	4	30 IV d1 & 8	100 po d1–14	500 IV d1 & 8				
AT or AP	3	60 IV d1				125–200 IV d1		
GT	3					175 IV d1		1250 IV d1 & d8
						Docetaxel (T or D)		
		Epirubicin* (E)				Ixabepilone (I)		
AT or AD	3	50 IV d1				75 IV d1		
TX	3					75 IV d1	950 po bid d 1–14	
IX	3					40 IV d1	2000 po d1–14	
EC	3	75 IV d1	600 IV d1					
FEC (iv)	4	50 IV d1	400 IV d1	500 IV d1				
FEC (Oral)	4	60 IV d1 & 8	75 po d1–14	500 IV d1 & 8				

Note: There are several variations of some of these regimens. (See Chapter 10 for additional combinations used in the adjuvant setting. See Table 12.7 for toxicities associated with each drug)

* Cumulative doses of doxorubicin > 500 mg/m² and epirubicin > 900 mg/m² are associated with high incidence of cardiomyopathy.

** Paclitaxel regimens developed prior to recognition that weekly doses are more effective.

A = doxorubicin; C = cyclophosphamide; F = 5-Fluorouracil.

There are no clinical trial data that support treating TNBC differently from any other form of metastatic breast cancer. Combinations are not clearly better than sequential single agents. However, BRCA1/2 germline and somatic mutations occur in 11%–39% of these tumors, and since BRCA1/2 genes are important for DNA repair, it has been hypothesized that they might be particularly sensitive to agents that damage DNA. Platinums and PARP (poly(ADP-ribose) polymerase) inhibitors both fall into this category.

Multiple small trials using cisplatin and carboplatin alone or in various combinations suggest that these compounds may be more effective than they are in non-TNBCs,[47] but the evidence is not sufficiently robust to conclude that these regimens should be used preferentially over standard regimens used to treat other types of metastatic breast cancer. Seven PARP inhibitors are under development, and some have shown activity in breast cancers with BRCA1/2 mutations, but a randomized trial failed to demonstrate any benefit over chemotherapy alone. They, too, seem unlikely to benefit unselected TNBC patients, but both the PARP inhibitors and platinum drugs may have value in TNBC patients with tumors that have a documented BRCA1/2 mutation.[46]

ANTI-HER2 AGENTS FOR HER2+ BREAST CANCERS

The development of agents that specifically target the EGFR tyrosine kinase receptors (EGFR, HER1–4, or ERBB1–4) have revolutionized the management of both early and metastatic breast cancer and provided proof of concept for using targeted agents for all types of cancer (see Chapter 7). Conventionally treated HER2+ breast cancers are among the most lethal, but with the use of anti-HER2 drugs they have relatively favorable prognoses. Trastuzumab was the first of these agents approved by the FDA. Three more have subsequently been approved: lapatinib, pertuzumab, and ado-trastuzumab emtansine (see Table 12.9). Four more are in advanced stages of development: afatinib, neratinib, ertumaxomab and MM-111. Each differs in specific target and/or composition, and there is evidence that using several of them together is advantageous.

The anti-HER2 drugs are effective only in patients with tumors that have a 3+ staining intensity in an immunohistochemical (IHC) assay or are FISH positive (see Chapter 7). Generally the value obtained at the time the primary tumor was diagnosed is used, but gain or loss of HER2 over the patient's disease course has been reported.

These drugs are generally very well tolerated, with flu-like symptoms, mild diarrhea, and nausea being the most common side effects. Cardiotoxicity, manifest as heart failure or an asymptomatic fall in LVEF, has been studied most carefully with trastuzumab where the incidence ranges from 3%–7% for trastuzumab alone to 27% for trastuzumab given concurrently with cumulative doxorubicin doses > 300 mg/m^2. The newer agents seem to be less cardiotoxic. Following discontinuation of trastuzumab and the use of appropriate heart failure drugs, cardiac function returns to normal in most patients. The risk of cardiotoxicity increases in patients with underlying cardiac disease, prior exposure to an anthracycline, or age > 50, but these are not absolute contraindications. A baseline determination of LVEF should always be performed; physicians commonly monitor LVEF at intervals of 3, 6, and 9 months of initiation

Table 12.9 FDA Approved Anti-HER2 Drugs and Combination of These Drugs With Other Systemic Therapies

Category Drug	Target	Route/Dose	Route/Dose of Other Agents Often Used in Combination	Toxicity to Anti-HER2 Drug; Comments
Monoclonal Antibody				
Trastuzumab (Herceptin®)	HER2, external domain	IV loading 8mg/kg over 90 minutes, then 6 mg/kg q 3 wks	IV paclitaxel 175 mg/m^2 q 3 wks	Mild flu-like symptoms with fever and rigors in 15%–20% of patients; Less often fatigue, headache, nausea. Most serious is cardiotoxicity (see text).
Pertuzumab (Perjeta®)	HER2, external domain but different epitope than trastuzumab	IV loading 840 mg over 60 minutes, then 420 mg q 3 wks	IV docetaxel 75 mg/m^2 q 3 wks	Mild diarrhea in ~ 45% of patients, grade 3/4 in 3%. (Probably less cardiotoxicity than trastuzumab.)
Ado-trastuzumab emtansine (T-DM1 or Kadcyla®)	HER2, external domain. Conjugated with maytansine (DM1)	IV infusion 3.6 mg/kg q 3 wks		< 10% grade 3/4 hypokalemia, thrombocytopenia (potentially severe,—avoid antiplatelet drugs), fatigue, liver toxicity. (Probably less cardiotoxicity than trastuzumab.)
Tyrosine Kinase Inhibitor				
Lapatinib (Tykerb®)	HER1 & HER2, internal domain	PO 1250–1500 (5 or 6 tabs) daily	PO capecitabine 1000 mg mg/m^2 BID d 1–14 q 3 wks For ER+ tumors, letrozole 2.5 mg daily	Mild diarrhea in ~ 40% and grade 3 in < 10%; rash and nausea less frequent. (Very low incidence of cardiotoxicity.)

Note: Unlike combinations of chemotherapy, the dose schedules of these drugs and the chemotherapy agents do not usually need to be adjusted when combined because the two drug classes do not have overlapping toxicities that are life-threatening.

of treatment. Concurrent use of these agents with doxorubicin or epirubicin is usually avoided.

ANTI-HER2 AGENTS IN PATIENTS WITHOUT PRIOR CHEMOTHERAPY FOR METASTASES (FIRST LINE)

Trastuzumab, alone or in combination with paclitaxel, is the treatment most frequently used first line for HER2+ tumors. When combined with either paclitaxel or an anthracycline and compared to the same cytotoxics drugs without trastuzumab, the respective RRs to the trastuzumab and non-trastuzumab regimens were 50% and 32% ($p < 0.001$), median TTP 7.4 and 4.6 months ($p < 0.001$), and median OS 25.1 and 20.3 months ($p < 0.046$).[48] Similar results have been obtained combining trastuzumab with vinorelbine or docetaxel instead of paclitaxel.[49] In preclinical studies, trastuzumab treatment increases sensitivity to a number of drugs including carboplatin, cyclophosphamide, docetaxel, and vinorelbine. In a phase II trial, the RR to a combination of trastuzumab plus cisplatin in heavily pretreated patients was 24.3%; the expected response rate to cisplatin alone in this group of patients was < 5%. In previously untreated patients, the value of adding carboplatin is unclear; in one randomized trial its addition to trastuzumab and paclitaxel improved RR and PFS,[50] while in another carboplatin added nothing to a combination of trastuzumab and docetaxel.[51]

Using several anti-HER2 agents concomitantly may be even more effective than trastuzumab alone. Most patients with HER2+ metastatic breast cancer eventually develop resistance to trastuzumab. It is plausible that this is due at least in part to signaling through other receptors, including HER1, HER3, and HER4, and that targeting several receptors or several HER2 epitopes will be more effective than trastuzumab alone. This was proven to be the case in the CLEOPATRA trial, which randomized 808 patients who had not received chemotherapy or biologic therapy for metastases to treatment with trastuzumab and docetaxel or the same plus pertuzumab. The RRs to the pertuzumab and the non-pertuzumab combination were 80% and 70%, respectively ($p < 0.001$), the median PFS was 18.5 and 12.4 months ($p < 0.001$), and the OS median has not been reached for the pertuzumab arm and is 37.6 months for non-pertuzumab ($p = 0.0008$). The incidence of diarrhea, rash, stomatitis, febrile neutropenia, and dry skin was at least 5% greater among patients on the pertuzumab arm. It is likely that dual targeted therapy with these two agents will now become standard first-line therapy for HER2+ patients. It has been shown in the neoadjuvant setting that a combination of trastuzumab plus lapatinib may be similarly synergistic (see Chapter 11).

Lapatinib is also an active agent as first-line therapy for HER2+ metastatic breast cancer, but direct comparisons between trastuzumab and lapatinib combinations favor trastuzumab. (This is true in the neoadjuvant setting, as well; see Chapter 11.) An interim analysis of a study in which 636 patients with HER2+ breast cancers not previously treated with chemotherapy or anti-HER2 agents for metastases were randomized to trastuzumab or lapatinib, each with either paclitaxel or docetaxel, showed a significantly longer PFS and greater cardiotoxicity for patients receiving trastuzumab and a higher frequency of other side effects, including rash and diarrhea, for the lapatinib arm.[52]

Anti-HER2 agents used without chemotherapy are very active and less toxic than when combined with chemotherapy. There are no randomized trials comparing an anti-HER2 agent plus chemotherapy with the same anti-HER2 agent alone, but cross-trial comparisons suggest that the combinations are more effective.[53] When used alone, trastuzumab has been reported to induce a RR of 19%–34% and a CBR of 33%–48%; for lapatinib alone, the RR and CBR have been reported to be 24% and 31%.[53]

Combining anti-HER agents without chemotherapy also increases efficacy. Pertuzumab as a single agent was not very active, but in combination with trastuzumab induced an RR and CBR of 24% and 50%. A combination of lapatinib plus trastuzumab is more effective than lapatinib alone. In 296 trastuzumab refractory patients, the PFS was 27% better for those randomized to receive both drugs, and the CBR was twice as large (24.7%) compared to lapatinib alone (12.4%, $p = 0.01$).[53]

Sometimes an anti-HER2 agent is used alone as initial treatment with chemotherapy being added at the time of first progression, but randomized trials have shown that starting out with both treatments results in a significantly better PFS.[49] However, for patients who want to avoid the toxicities of the cytotoxic drugs, trastuzumab alone, lapatinib alone, a combination of pertuzumab and trastuzumab, or a combination of lapatinib and trastuzumab are all reasonable options.

Trastuzumab is administered either with an initial dose of 4 mg/kg over 90 minutes followed by a weekly dose of 2 mg/kg, or an initial dose of 8 mg/kg followed by a 3-weekly dose of 6 mg/kg. Sometimes patients are converted from one to the other schedule midway through their course of treatment. Lapatinib has been given daily at either 1,500 mg once or 500 mg twice.

TREATING HER2+ TUMORS AFTER PROGRESSION ON TRASTUZUMAB PLUS CHEMOTHERAPY

Once started on anti-HER2 therapy, patients with metastatic breast cancer generally continue it for the remainder of their lives.

Three options exist for tumors that progress while on trastuzumab plus chemotherapy: continue the trastuzumab and change the chemotherapy; change the anti-HER2 treatment to lapatinib plus the same chemotherapy or ado-trastuzumab emtansine without chemotherapy; or change both chemotherapy and the anti-HER2 agent. There are very few data to support continuing the same anti-HER2 treatment, but a single small, randomized trial plus indirect comparisons between studies suggests that RR and PFS are significantly improved by continuing administration of trastuzumab when a new chemotherapy is started.[49]

Lapatinib was specifically approved as second-line therapy after trastuzumab failure based on a trial in which 399 women who had progressed after trastuzumab and chemotherapy were randomized to lapatinib plus capecitabine or capecitabine alone. The RRs were, respectively, 22% and 14% ($p = 0.09$), the CBRs 27% and 18%, median PFSs 8.8 and 4.4 months ($p < 0.001$), and OSs 18.9 and 16.2 months ($p = 0.21$).

Ado-trastuzumab emtansine (T-DM1) is trastuzumab linked to maytansine, a cytotoxin with limited efficacy and excessive toxicity when used alone to treat cancer. This new drug may be the most effective second-line treatment. In the EMILIA trial, 991 patients who had progressive disease while receiving trastuzumab and a taxane were randomized to ado-trastuzumab or lapatinib plus capecitabine. The RRs were, respectively, 44% and 31% ($p = 0.0002$), median duration of response 12.6 and 6.5 months ($p < 0.001$), median PFS 9.6 and 6.4 months ($p < 0.001$), and median OS 30.9 and 25.1 months ($p = 0.0006$).[54]

HER2+/ER+ TUMORS

This subset constitutes a large percentage of the HER2 population. Only 10% of HR+ (ER+ and/or PR+) tumors are also HER2+, but 50% of HER2+ tumors are also HR+.[55] Preclinical studies have demonstrated molecular cross-talk between the HER2 and ER pathways and synergy between agents that inhibit signaling in each of the pathways (see Chapter 7).

The optimal treatment of HER2+/ER+ tumors is unknown. Endocrine therapy is less effective in tumors that are ER+/HER2+ than tumors that are ER+/HER2–, and randomized clinical trials have shown an advantage for adding anti-HER2 therapy to endocrine therapy. For example, combinations of anastrozole plus trastuzumab and letrozole plus lapatinib resulted in a significantly better RR, CBR, and PFS but no difference in OS compared to anastrozole or letrozole alone.[55] For older patients and those with more indolent disease, an anti-HER2/AI combination may be sufficient, at least as first-line therapy.

However, combining an anti-HER2 drug, chemotherapy and endocrine therapy may be preferable for younger patients and those with more rapidly growing disease. Indirect comparisons suggest that an anti-HER2 drug/chemotherapy combination is more effective than anti-HER2/endocrine therapy for ER+/HER2+ tumors.[55] No randomized trials have evaluated the relative benefit of adding endocrine therapy to an anti-HER2/chemotherapy combination, but indirect comparisons also show that a combination of chemotherapy plus trastuzumab plus endocrine therapy results in longer PFS and OS than chemotherapy plus trastuzumab without endocrine therapy.[55] This was true whether the endocrine therapy was administered concomitantly or in sequence with the trastuzumab/chemotherapy.

NEWER TARGETED AGENTS: EVEROLIMUS, SORAFENIB, BEVACIZUMAB, PALBOCICLIB

The most important systemic therapies for breast cancer have specific targets: ER and HER2. Many new targets have been identified over the past 2 decades, and a large number of agents that are in or are about to enter clinical trials have been developed for these targets.[56] Many are receptor tyrosine kinases (RTK), like HER2/*neu*, and signal transduction pathways connected to these RTKs. The PI3K/AKT/mTOR pathway is the most frequently mutated in breast cancer and is the target for the largest number of drugs, but agents are also being developed to modify the behavior of SRC, CDK, and the MAPK/MEK pathways. These new, targeted drugs frequently have only modest effects when used alone, but add value when given with established endocrine or chemotherapy. A prototype drug is an mTOR inhibitor, everolimus or Afinitor®, which does not, by itself, induce tumor regression, but which in combination with an AI or tamoxifen will increase RR, PFS, and OS (see Table 12.3). The FDA has very recently approved the use of an inhibitor of cyclin-dependent kinases 4/6 (palbociclib or

Ibrance®) to be used in combination with letrozole for postmenopausal women with ER+/HER2– metastatic breast cancer that has not previously been treated with endocrine therapy. The multikinase and anti-angiogenic drug sorafenib, which is already approved for the treatment of renal and hepatocellular cancer, has been shown to have some activity in breast cancer and is in a large phase III trial.[57] The most studied (and most controversial) target is VEGF (vascular endothelial growth factor).

In preclinical breast cancer models, angiogenesis has been shown to correlate with metastatic potential, and higher microvessel density in breast cancer histology is associated with increased likelihood of recurrence and mortality. In preclinical models and in other tumor types, inhibition of VEGF has been shown to alter tumor behavior and in some settings significantly improve survival. For this reason, anti-VEGF drugs, especially bevacizumab (Avastin®), have been extensively evaluated for breast cancer.

Five studies randomized 1,784 patients who had not previously received chemotherapy for metastatic disease either to chemotherapy plus bevacizumab or the same chemotherapy alone. The regimens studied were paclitaxel 90 mg/m^2 weekly ± bevacizumab 10 mg/kg every 2 weeks; docetaxel 100 mg/m^2 every 3 weeks ± bevacizumab 7.5 mg/kg every 3 weeks; docetaxel 100 mg/m^2 every 3 weeks ± bevacizumab 15 mg/kg every 3 weeks; capecitabine 1,000 mg/m^2 twice daily days 1–14 of a 3-week cycle ± bevacizumab 15 mg/kg every 3 weeks; or one of several doxorubicin-containing regimens ± bevacizumab 15 mg/kg every 3 weeks.[58] In each of these trials, bevacizumab was associated with a significant increase in PFS and RR, and a meta-analysis of all 5 demonstrated a 33% reduction in recurrence rate and an increase in response rate (RR) from 33.3% to 49.7% ($p < 0.0001$ for both outcomes).[58] The median increase in PFS from adding bevacizumab was between 0.9 and 2.9 months in four of the trials and 5.5 months in a trial considered an outlier.[59] Bevacizumab also significantly increased the frequency of SAEs (serious adverse events, such as death or hospitalization) by 41% and of grade III/IV AEs by 77%.[58] Most of the SAEs and AEs were those commonly associated with the cytotoxic drugs. Toxicities associated specifically with bevacizumab are hypertension, proteinuria, bleeding, congestive heart failure, left ventricular systolic dysfunction, and cardiomyopathy. All of these were increased among the bevacizumab-treated patients; hypertension, proteinuria, and bleeding ≥ grade 3 were increased by 15-, 11-, and 3-fold, respectively.[60] In a more recent single arm study of 2,251 patients, the incidence of grade ≥ 3 hypertension, proteinuria, and bleeding were 4.4%, 1.7%, and 1.4%, respectively.[61] In a randomized comparison of paclitaxel and capecitabine, each with bevacizumab, there was a higher response rate to the paclitaxel regimen (44% vs. 27%, $p < 0.0001$) and a longer PFS (11.0 vs. 8.1 months, $p = 0.0052$).[62] Formal comparison of QofL showed no difference between the treatment arms in the two trials that evaluated this endpoint. Each of the trials individually and the meta-analysis *failed* to show a survival advantage from adding bevacizumab.

The pooled results of three trials in which 691 patients who had previously been treated with chemotherapy for metastases were randomized to chemotherapy ± bevacizumab also demonstrated an improvement in response rate from 17.7% to 31.7% ($p = 0.000068$) and a 15% reduction in recurrences ($p = 0.03$).[58] The median increase in PFS was 2.1 and –0.7 months in the 2 largest studies. No survival benefits were observed in individual trials or the meta-analysis of these patients receiving bevacizumab as second-line therapy.

Bevacizumab was given an accelerated approval by the FDA that was later withdrawn because no survival benefit was observed, and many oncologists feel that the small improvements in PFS are outweighed by increased toxicity.[59] In Europe the drug is approved in combination with paclitaxel or capecitabine, but only in previously untreated patients. These contradictory actions by the regulatory agencies reflect confusion among oncologists regarding the use of bevacizumab. It seems inappropriate to routinely use this drug for all patients receiving chemotherapy, and it may be contradicted in elderly patients and those with history of bleeding, thrombotic disorders, hemoptysis, cerebral vascular accident, significant cardiac disease (ischemic or congestive heart failure), or GI perforation because they may experience greater than average toxicity.[63] There appears to be little or no benefit in patients with prior chemotherapy for metastases. No subgroups have been defined that clearly benefit more or less than other groups, but there is a trend toward greater effects in patients who have previously received chemotherapy in the adjuvant setting and those with ER negative tumors.[58] Patients with triple negative do not benefit more than others. Taken together, the evidence suggests that bevacizumab might reasonably be added to paclitaxel and given to patients who have had no prior chemotherapy for metastases, have had adjuvant chemotherapy, are ER negative, and for whom obtaining a good response is important enough to justify the added toxicity (see following section on "visceral crisis").

"VISCERAL CRISIS"

"Visceral crisis" is an old concept developed prior to the discovery of tumor markers such as ER, HER2, Ki-67, and genomic profiles that enable a more refined determination of the likelihood that a patient will benefit from a particular treatment. This category was originally defined as those with "lymphangetic lung metastases, bone marrow replacement, carcinomatous meningitis, or significant liver metastases."[64] These patients were thought to have rapidly progressive disease that was unlikely to be responsive to endocrine therapy. In fact, they were unlikely to respond to any form of therapy. Most clinical trials specifically exclude them. As a result, there is limited information about outcomes following treatment of these patients. This term should no longer be applied to any group of patients and should not be the basis of a treatment decision.

Hormone receptor positive (ER+) patients with liver, lung, or other visceral metastases are as likely to respond to endocrine therapy as patients *with a similar level of ER positivity* who do not have visceral metastases. Most randomized trials that compared endocrine and chemotherapy enrolled patients without knowledge of their ER status or included patients with a wide range of ER values.[65] The RRs based on an intent-to-treat analysis of these studies were always higher for patients randomized to chemotherapy, but in subset analyses the relative effects of endocrine and chemotherapy were the same in those with and without visceral involvement. Differences in RRs did not translate into differences in OS. No attempt has been made to compare the relative efficacy of these two modalities in patients with high ER values (with or without visceral involvement), and it is plausible that in this group of patients endocrine therapy would result in a greater benefit than chemotherapy.

There are no data to support the commonly held belief that patients respond to chemotherapy "faster" than to endocrine therapy. This idea is likely an artifact of the higher likelihood of responding to chemotherapy. An ER+ patient who fails to respond to a 3–6 month trial of endocrine therapy and then responds to chemotherapy will certainly have a longer time to response than the same patient treated immediately with chemotherapy, but this does not support the conclusion that the chemotherapy actually induces response more quickly.

Patients who are very symptomatic with a high likelihood that critical organ function will be soon compromised by tumor progression should always be given the treatment most likely to induce a response. (This assumes that the patient agrees that toxicity is of secondary concern to tumor response.) This might be a patient with very abnormal liver function tests, widespread liver metastases, and a short disease-free interval. If that patient had a low ER level, the treatment of choice would likely be combination chemotherapy (plus an anti-HER2 regimen if HER2+). For other patients, long-term quality of life should remain an important or even the most important determinant of therapeutic choice. In general, ER+ patients should receive endocrine therapy and ER– patients with slower growing tumors (e.g., those with a DFI > 1 year) and normal organ function should receive single agent chemotherapy (each with an anti-HER2 drug if the tumor is HER2+).

BONE METASTASES

Breast cancer metastasizes to the bone more often than to any other organ, and these are the greatest source of pain and serious dysfunction for breast cancer patients (see Chapter 4). The pain is often sudden in onset, even when multiple bones are involved, but just as often subtle pain will wax and wane for weeks or even months. Even quite severe pain may subside after a few days. A normal X-ray is insufficient to rule out metastases. In a patient who has ever had breast cancer, bone pain should always be investigated early with a bone or a PET/CT scan. Multiple modalities are required for the proper management of pain and dysfunction from bone metastases in breast cancer patients.

Most physicians will initially control pain with a non-steroidal anti-inflammatory drug (NSAID) alone or combined with an opioid.[66] Severe bone pain requires relatively large doses of strong opioids, but large doses of opioids reduce patient activity, thus exacerbating bone loss. Patients with spinal cord compression should also receive corticosteroids, and those with hypercalcemia should receive bisphosphonates, calcitonin, gallium nitrate, or mithramycin in addition to analgesics. All forms of analgesia control pain for only a limited period of time unless the underlying disease process is successfully treated. Patients with disease limited to bone are likely to have prolonged survival even without treatment, so the use of analgesia alone is not recommended.

RADIOTHERAPY FOR BONE METASTASES

Radiation therapy provides the most certain and durable form of pain relief. Some evidence of symptom relief is often apparent within 24 hours of the first dose, suggesting that the effect of radiotherapy is not entirely dependent on tumor response. It is possible that this early pain relief is due to radiotherapy destroying osteoclasts. The median time from the start of treatment to pain relief ranges from 2 to 4 weeks.[67] The duration of response is also quite variable. Many patients will have no further pain in the irradiated lesion for the remainder of their lives (often 2–5 years). Pain relief lasting 6–12 months is common, but the median duration in various trials is 11–24 weeks.

About 60% of patients will have some pain relief and 25% will have complete pain relief from radiation to bone lesions.[68] The pathological fracture rate after radiotherapy is about 3%. In a meta-analysis of randomized trials, pain relief was not related to the dose of radiotherapy or fractionation schedule used.[68] There were more pathological fractures and spinal cord compressions after a single compared with multiple doses, but these differences are small and not statistically significant. However, the frequency of retreatment was 2.5-fold higher among patients randomized to a single fraction arm ($p < 0.00001$), and multiple fractions resulted in significantly greater bone remineralization in the one study that looked at this.

The major toxicity from external beam radiotherapy is marrow suppression, which may be prolonged. Because of the relatively short duration of benefit from radiotherapy in many patients and the tendency of breast cancer metastases to continuously appear in other bony sites throughout the axial skeleton, radiotherapy must be administered repeatedly if it is the only means used to manage the disease. This will make the administration of cytotoxic agents, most of which also cause marrow suppression, extremely difficult. Radiation effects on soft tissue and viscera in the radiation field may cause time-limited toxicity. Neural tissue is more sensitive to radiation, and long-lasting damage may occur; this limits the doses that can be used to treat vertebral metastases. "Pain flare" is a 2-point or greater increase in bone pain that occurs *transiently* while the patient is receiving or within 10 days after completion of radiation therapy. This occurs in more than 50% of breast cancer patients and requires a transient increase in analgesia.[69]

Bone-seeking radionuclides have also been used to treat pain from bone metastases. Two agents, strontium-89 and samarium-153, have been approved in both the United States and Europe and one, rhenium-189, has a more limited approval in a few countries outside the United States. These agents are usually administered as a single intravenous dose. In studies involving predominantly prostate cancer patients and a few breast cancer patients, these agents have been shown to reduce pain in the majority of patients treated for durations of 3–6 months. The agents can be re-administered. They cause marrow suppression, and patients may experience flare (see earlier discussion). However, the evidence is too limited to draw conclusions regarding the relative effectiveness of these drugs in breast cancer or to define situations where they should be used.[70]

In a patient with multiple lesions, it is reasonable to initiate systemic therapy first and add radiotherapy later to areas that do not respond completely. If the primary purpose is to prevent impending fractures, then surgery should be considered as well.

SURGERY AND RADIOTHERAPY FOR FRACTURES OR IMPENDING FRACTURES

Fractures, especially in the spine, pelvis, and femurs, occur frequently and, in contrast to traumatic fractures, do not heal well or quickly because of tumor growth, the effects of treatment (radiation, chemotherapy), and the generalized debility of the patient. Whenever possible, pathological fractures should be treated with open reduction and internal fixation with the goal of providing pain-free movement. Radiation therapy with multiple fraction dosage is generally administered postoperatively.

Both an orthopedic surgeon and a radiotherapist should see all patients with an impending fracture. The challenge is defining "impending fracture." Objective scoring systems have been developed, but it is not clear that these are superior to simpler, conventional definitions of risk. The factor most predictive of fracture is > 30 mm involvement of the axial cortex and circumferential cortex obliteration of > 50%.[71] Osteolytic lesions that do not penetrate the cortex generally do not need surgical intervention. Post-radiotherapy pain is not helpful in identifying bones that will fracture. Patients often have increased susceptibility to fracture following radiotherapy alone because pain relief leads to increased activity before adequate recalcification has taken place. Thus, if a lesion is deemed to be an impending fracture, both surgery and radiotherapy are indicated.

Surgical treatments of the spine are particularly challenging because they often necessitate prolonged recovery in a patient with a limited lifespan. However, the complications of vertebral collapse—spinal compression and/or permanent compromise of one or multiple nerve roots, kyphosis, and scoliosis—seriously compromise the patient's mobility and independence, so surgery should never be ruled out too quickly, especially in patients without visceral involvement. Percutaneous vertebroplasty, in which polymethylmethacrylate (PMMA) is injected into a collapsed vertebrae, and kyphoplasty, in which the vertebrae is re-expanded with a small balloon, *might* be helpful, but randomized trials evaluating vertebroplasty in *non-cancer* patients have not been shown it to be superior to a sham procedure.[72]

Aggressive pain relief using opioids coupled with radiotherapy may fail to relive pain in as many as 20%–30% of patients.[73] Often this is because the pain is due to the destruction of bone and skeletal structures rather than tumor progression, and in this situation the use of orthotics, such as back braces, will be more effective than either analgesia or further anticancer treatment.

BONE TARGETED THERAPY: BISPHOSPHONATES AND DENOSUMAB

Drugs specifically targeting bone resorption have had a major impact on the treatment of bone metastases. Bisphosphonates have a high affinity for calcium at sites of active bone metabolism and decrease the affinity of osteoclasts for bone (see Figure 4.5 in Chapter 4), In addition, bisphosphonates enter intracellular vesicles within the osteoclast and cause osteoclast apoptosis. There is preclinical evidence that these agents have direct anti-tumor effects, too.[74] Monoclonal antibodies to RANKL (denosumab) block binding of the ligand to its receptor, RANK. This prevents the formation and activation of osteoclasts (Figure 4.5).

Bisphosphonates will reduce pain in ~ 60% of patients with painful bone metastases and decrease analgesic use in ~ 40%.[75] The first evidence of reduced pain appears gradually over the first month of treatment. In addition, these agents significantly reduce the frequency of skeletal related events (SREs such as fractures, spinal cord compression, and hypercalcemia) and generally increase the time to the first new SRE or to more severe pain.[76]

There is no evidence from clinical studies that bisphosphonates benefit patients without bone metastases. In randomized trials they neither reduced the overall incidence of bone metastases or prolonged patient survival.[76] Indirect comparisons suggest that zoledronic acid (ZA), the most potent of these agents, is the most effective, but in a randomized comparison of ZA and pamidronate in 1,130 breast cancer patients, 43% and 45% of the ZA and pamidronate patients, respectively, developed an SRE (p = NS).[77] The results of an unplanned (and therefore less valid) subgroup analysis of 528 patients who had at least one lytic lesion were more favorable for ZA (p = 0.058) and the difference in the median time to the first SRE was 310 days for ZA and 174 for pamidronate (p = 0.013). When both the first and subsequent SREs (including hypercalcemia) were included in a multi-event analysis, there was a 20% reduction in risk for ZA compared to pamidronate (p = 0.037). These unconfirmed observations have led many oncologists to choose ZA as their first choice bisphosphonate.

Three of four bisphosphonates commonly used to treat breast cancer are administered intravenously every 3–4 weeks. Denosumab is given subcutaneously every 4 weeks (see Table 12.10). These drugs are generally well tolerated. The most common adverse events are fever and generalized myalgias/arthralgias that may start a day or two after drug administration and may continue for a week or more. The first episode may not be with the first dose, but the symptoms usually abate with additional courses. In a similar fashion, patients may experience bone pain, and occasionally this can be incapacitating and require strong analgesics. Hypocalcemia occurs in a small percentage of patients and with increased frequency among those with a low creatinine clearance. Renal toxicity is more likely to occur with more rapid infusions, in those who already have abnormal renal function, and after many treatment cycles. For this reason, creatinine is monitored and infusion times strictly adhered to. There is an

Table 12.10 Bone Targeted Agents for the Management of Breast Cancer Patients With Bone Metastases

Drug	Administered	Dosage	Cycle Length
Bisphosphonates[a]			
Zoledronic Acid (Zometa)	Intravenously	4 mg IV over 15+ minutes	3–4 weeks[b]
Ibandronate (Boniva)[c]	Oral or Intravenously	50 mg 6 mg	Daily 3–4 weeks
Pamidronate (Aredia)	Intravenously	90 mg IV over 2+ hours	4 weeks
Clodronate[d]	Oral	1600 mg	Daily
RANKL INHIBITOR			
Denosumab (Xgeva)	Subcutaneously	120 mg	4 weeks

[a] Bisphosphonates are listed in order from most to least potent

[b] There are no established guidelines to choose between 3 and 4 weeks; trials evaluating longer intervals are underway.

[c] Approved by the FDA to treat osteoporosis but not bone metastases in the United States

[d] Not approved by the FDA for use in the United States

increased incidence of subtronchanteric fractures with minimal or no trauma. Patients may complain of pain for weeks to months before the fracture is diagnosed. The fractures may be bilateral and often heal poorly. In a large case control study, the overall incidence was 0.35%, but in those treated for 3–5 years the risk was increased by about 60% and for > 5 years 2.7-fold.[78]

Safety has been demonstrated for up to 5 years of bisphosphonate use. Two years is usually the minimum duration recommended, and they should be continued in spite of the appearance of new bone metastases and/or an SRE because they reduce the frequency and prolong the time to secondary events.

The toxicities from denosumab are mild and similar to those of the bisphosphonates.[79] In a direct comparison with ZA, there was significantly less fever, arthralgias, and bone pain with denosumab, but the frequency of hypocalcemia was a little higher. Renal toxicity was higher with ZA (8.5% vs. 4.9% for denosumab), especially in those with a baseline creatinine clearance ≤ 20% (20% vs. 5.9%). Adverse events lead 12.3% of denosumab and 9.6% of ZA patients to discontinue treatment.

Osteonecrosis of the jaw (ONJ) is an uncommon but serious complication of both bisphosphonate and denosumab therapy. Patients usually present with jaw pain. ONJ is defined as exposed bone in the maxillofacial or mandibular bones that does not heal for 8 weeks. Most patients have a history of a dental extraction, poor oral hygiene, or use of a dental appliance.[79] Patients should have a base-line dental evaluation before starting bone-modifying therapies, should avoid open dental procedures while on them, and should wait 14–21 days before starting therapy to allow wound healing if invasive dental procedures are required. The incidence of ONJ increases with longer use, but it may occur as early as 6 months after starting treatment. There was no significant difference in the incidence for patients randomized to ZA (1.4%) or denosumab (2.0%) ($p = 0.39$).[79]

A bisphosphonate or denosumab should be started as soon as bone metastases are diagnosed and continued indefinitely, but with careful monitoring following the guidelines in Box 12.1.[80,81] The newer agents are more powerful and appear to be more effective than older, but there is no consensus on whether denosumab or zoledronic acid should be used preferentially. When a patient repeatedly fails one bisphosphonate, another—especially a stronger one—may be effective.

HYPERCALCEMIA

Hypercalcemia that is severe (≥ 14 mg/dL) or symptomatic is a medical emergency. Isotonic saline should be started immediately and the patient made euvolemic.[82] Four mg of zoledronic acid should be administered intravenously over no less than 15 minutes. Another 4 mg can be administered as retreatment after a minimum of 7 days. Calcitonin can also be used, but this is useful for only 48 hours.

PLEURAL EFFUSIONS

Pleural effusions occur in ~ 10% of breast cancer patients, may present as cough or dyspnea, are often an incidental finding on chest X-ray with or without pleural nodules in otherwise asymptomatic patients, and may persist in a patient responding to systemic therapy at other sites. If an effusion is symptomatic, the treatment of choice is pleurodesis with talc, doxycycline, or other sclerosing agents, and this is most effective

Box 12.1 Recommended Use of Bone-Modifying Agents (BMA) for Patients With Metastatic Breast Cancer

- Initiate treatment with a BMA at the first onset of bone pain
  - A BMA is not recommended for patients without documented bone metastases, including those with abnormalities only on a bone scan
- No single BMA is recommended over others.
  - However, the evidence for zoledronic acid, pamidronate, and denosumab are the most compelling. Adhere to the dose schedules, and especially the infusion times, shown in Table 12.10.
  - Denosumab might be preferable for elderly patients with decreased creatinine clearance, those receiving a nephrotoxic drug such as cisplatin, and those who are not already receiving intravenous therapies.[a]
  - Alendronate might also be a better option for patients where potential renal toxicity is an issue.
- Monitor creatinine level with each dose of an intravenous bisphosphonate.
- Monitor calcium level in patients with creatinine clearance < 30 mL/min.
- Continue BMA until substantial decline in patient's performance status, even in the face of an SRE or new bone metastases since they may decrease secondary SREs.
- Perform dental exam and preventative dentistry or hygiene before starting and avoid invasive dental procedures during therapy.
- Give daily supplements of
  - Elemental calcium: 1200–1500 mg for postmenopausal and 1200 mg for premenopausal women.
  - Vitamin D3 400–2000 units depending in part on evidence of deficiency.
- Biochemical markers of bone turnover predict patients most likely to experience SREs, but they should not be used for monitoring since their clinical utility has not been demonstrated in proper trials.
  - Promising markers of bone formation that may prove useful in the future include bone-specific alkaline phosphatase (BALP), osteocalcin, and propeptide of type I collagen (PINP).
  - Promising markers of bone resorption include C-terminal propeptide of type I collagen (CTX) and N-terminal propeptide of type I collagen (NTX).
- Whenever possible, participate in comparative effectiveness trials.

Recommendations are ASCO Clinical Practice Guidelines except where otherwise noted. From Van Poznak CH, Temin S, Yee GC, et al. American Society of Clinical Oncology executive summary of the clinical practice guideline update on the role of bone-modifying agents in metastatic breast cancer. J Clin Oncol. 2011;29:1221–7.
[a] *Fournier (2010).*

if the fluid is totally removed so that the pleural surfaces appose. In many cases this requires placement of a pleural catheter and leaving it in place for several days. Multiple thoracenteses may create many small pockets of fluid surrounded by scar tissue, making it more difficult to completely drain fluid through a catheter. The use of a definitive procedure early on is recommended.

CNS METASTASES

Most patients with CNS metastases, especially those who are symptomatic, are immediately placed on steroids and anti-seizure medications. Symptoms may then subside over a few days.

More definitive therapy depends, in part, on the number of lesions. For those with 1 to 3 or 4 brain lesions, surgery should be used, alone or with whole brain radiotherapy. In randomized trials of patients with a solitary lesion, the median survival was 4–6 months after whole brain radiotherapy (WBRT) alone and 10 months after surgical excision followed by WBRT.[83] Two modest-sized randomized trials comparing stereotactic radiosurgery (SRS) alone with SRS plus WBRT failed to demonstrate a survival advantage for adding WBRT. However, patients treated with SRS alone had more frequent intracranial relapses. Patients treated with SFS plus WBRT *may* have had greater decrease in cognitive function, but the results from trials are not consistent on this point.

All patients with > 3 or 4 lesions should have WBRT as their primary treatment, but there is no evidence that prophylactic WBRT is ever indicated for breast cancer patients.

There are scattered reports of individual lesions responding to endocrine treatment, chemotherapy, or anti-HER2 agents, but these are inconsistent. There is no established role for systemic therapy as the primary treatment of brain metastases. Most of these agents do not cross the blood brain barrier (BBB). The BBB is often disrupted by tumor or treatment, such as WBRT, but this seems to be variable from one patient to another.[83] Patients with HER2+ tumors and CNS metastases should receive anti-HER2 agents and chemotherapy in addition to WBRT. In comparisons across trials, the median survival in HER2+ patients with brain metastases not treated with trastuzumab is 2–9 months, but with trastuzumab (and usually with chemotherapy as well) 9–25 months.[83] It is not clear whether this is only because of the effect of systemic therapy on extra-cranial disease, or whether trastuzumab crosses the disrupted BBB in a sufficient number of patients to directly affect the CNS metastases, too. The latter is suggested by the fact that the median time to the appearance of CNS metastases was 2.1 months in HER2+ patients not receiving trastuzumab and 13.1 months in those who did. Although lapatinib by itself does not induce regression of brain metastases, a combination of lapatinib and capecitabine induced an objective CNS response in 67% of 43 evaluable patients who had not had previous treatment of the CNS metastases with radiation therapy. This needs further evaluation before it is accepted as standard treatment.

Leptomeningeal metastases have a dire prognosis. After spreading to meninges via hematogenous, lymphatic, or direct spread, the cancer cells grow and spread in the cerebral spinal fluid. Treatment is usually repeated intrathecal administration of methotrexate, thiotepa, or cytarabine either in a liposomal (DepoCyte®) or non-liposomal formulation. For patients whose disease is controlled at other sites, an Ommaya reservoir may be used. Radiation therapy is also used. Metastases to the meninges in HER2+ patients have been reported to respond to trastuzumab alone, trastuzumab plus capecitabine, and to intrathecal trastuzumab given 20 mg weekly as a single agent or in combination with chemotherapies such as methotrexate or thiotepa.[84]

BREAST CANCER IN MEN

Male breast cancer is generally treated the same as that in women, but since 90% of tumors are ER+, endocrine therapy is used more often and for longer durations. Tamoxifen has largely replaced orchiectomy as the treatment of choice. These tumors respond to AIs, but AIs have not been shown to be superior. Other additive hormonal therapies induce responses, and when the male breast cancer patients stop responding to endocrine treatment, their tumors respond to the same cytotoxic agents used for women.

OVERALL APPROACH TO THE PATIENT: ADVICE, SUPPORT

The management of metastatic breast cancer is complex and requires input from many specialists. The most common judgments errors are to (a) underestimate the life expectancy of the patient and her likely need for many different types of therapy over a period of years, (b) initially over-treat with multiple toxic treatments even though "throwing the book" at the patient does not necessarily improve survival, or (c) under-treat in the mistaken idea that quality of life is related more to the avoidance of treatment than controlling the underlying disease. These errors occur primarily because inexperienced physicians do not understand the natural history of this disease (see Chapter 4 on Natural History and Biology).

Formal surveys of patient attitudes indicates that in retrospect many wish they had received more complete information on their prognosis earlier in the course of their disease, but the needs of individual patients are almost as varied as the nature and course of the disease. Some patients fare better with less and others with more information. The patient is best served if her caregivers first listen carefully to ascertain her particular needs. All patients share the need for hope and the assurance that they will not be abandoned.[85] Participation in clinical trials is an important source of hope for some patients, but this should be considered early in a patient's course when symptoms are limited since she will become ineligible for many studies after she has been extensively treated.

Patients are optimally managed in multidisciplinary clinics that provide all modalities of standard therapy, clinical trials, alternative therapies (or information on how to access alternative therapies), support groups, exercise programs, and, most important, nurses who have specialized in the care of patients with breast cancer.

REFERENCES

1. Smerage J, Barlow W, Hayes D, et al. SWOG S0500: a randomized phase III trial to test the strategy of changing therapy versus maintaining therapy for metastatic breast cancer patients who have elevated circulating tumor cell (CTC) levels at first follow-up assessment. *Cancer Res.* 2013;73:S5–07.

2. Bruce J, Carter DC, Fraser J. Patterns of recurrent disease in breast cancer. *Lancet.* 1970;1:433–5.

3. Hellman S, Weichselbaum RR. Oligometastases. *J Clin Oncol.* 1995;13:8–10.

4. Tait CR, Waterworth A, Loncaster J, et al. The oligometastatic state in breast cancer: hypothesis or reality. *Breast.* 2005;14:87–93.

5. Schmoor C, Sauerbrei W, Bastert G, et al. Role of isolated locoregional recurrence of breast cancer: results of four prospective studies. *J Clin Oncol.* 2000;18:1696–708.

6. Howell SJ. Advances in the treatment of luminal breast cancer. *Curr Opin Obstet Gynecol.* 2013;25:49–54.

7. Stoll B. Rechallenging breast cancer with tamoxifen therapy. *Clin Oncol.* 1983;9:347–51.

8. Crump M, Sawka CA, DeBoer G, et al. An individual patient-based meta-analysis of tamoxifen versus ovarian ablation as first line endocrine therapy for premenopausal women with metastatic breast cancer. *Br Cancer Res Treat.* 1997;44:201–10.

9. Ellis MJ, Gao F, Dehdashti F, et al. Lower-dose vs high-dose oral estradiol therapy of hormone receptor-positive, aromatase inhibitor-resistant advanced breast cancer: a phase 2 randomized study. *JAMA.* 2009;302:774–80.

10. Ingle JN. Estrogen as therapy for breast cancer. *Breast Cancer Res.* 2002;4:133–6.

11. Dowsett M, Nicholson RI, Pietras RJ. Biological characteristics of the pure antiestrogen fulvestrant: overcoming endocrine resistance. *Br Cancer Res Treat.* 2005;93 Suppl 1:S11–8.

12. Di Leo A, Jerusalem G, Petruzelka L, et al. Results of the CONFIRM phase III trial comparing fulvestrant 250 mg with fulvestrant 500 mg in postmenopausal women with estrogen receptor-positive advanced breast cancer. *J Clin Oncol.* 2010;28:4594–600.

13. Santen RJ, Song RX, Masamura S, et al. Adaptation to estradiol deprivation causes up-regulation of growth factor pathways and hypersensitivity to estradiol in breast cancer cells. *Adv Exp Med Biol.* 2008;630:19–34.

14. Masamura S, Santner SJ, Heitjan DF, et al. Estrogen deprivation causes estradiol hypersensitivity in human breast cancer cells. *J Clin Endocrinol Metab.* 1995;80:2918–25.

15. Gibson L, Lawrence D, Dawson C, et al. Aromatase inhibitors for treatment of advanced breast cancer in postmenopausal women. *Cochrane Database Syst Rev.* 2009:CD003370.

16. Xu HB, Liu YJ, Li L. Aromatase inhibitor versus tamoxifen in postmenopausal woman with advanced breast cancer: a literature-based meta-analysis. *Clin Breast Cancer.* 2011;11:246–51.

17. Goss PE, Ingle JN, Pritchard KI, et al. Exemestane versus anastrozole in postmenopausal women with early breast cancer: NCIC CTG MA.27—a randomized controlled phase III trial. *J Clin Oncol.* 2013;31:1398–404.

18. Nabholtz JM, Bonneterre J, Buzdar A, et al. Anastrozole (Arimidex) versus tamoxifen as first-line therapy for advanced breast cancer in postmenopausal women: survival analysis and updated safety results. *Eur J Cancer.* 2003;39:1684–9.

19. Mouridsen H, Gershanovich M, Sun Y, et al. Phase III study of letrozole versus tamoxifen as first-line therapy of advanced breast cancer in postmenopausal women: analysis of

survival and update of efficacy from the International Letrozole Breast Cancer Group. *J Clin Oncol.* 2003;21:2101–9.

20. Paridaens RJ, Dirix LY, Beex LV, et al. Phase III study comparing exemestane with tamoxifen as first-line hormonal treatment of metastatic breast cancer in postmenopausal women: the European Organisation for Research and Treatment of Cancer Breast Cancer Cooperative Group. *J Clin Oncol.* 2008;26:4883–90.

21. Robertson JF, Lindemann JP, Llombart-Cussac A, et al. Fulvestrant 500 mg versus anastrozole 1 mg for the first-line treatment of advanced breast cancer: follow-up analysis from the randomized 'FIRST' study. *Br Cancer Res Treat.* 2012;136:503–11.

22. Mehta RS, Barlow WE, Albain KS, et al. Combination anastrozole and fulvestrant in metastatic breast cancer. *N Engl J Med.* 2012;367:435–44.

23. Bergh J, Jonsson PE, Lidbrink EK, et al. FACT: an open-label randomized phase III study of fulvestrant and anastrozole in combination compared with anastrozole alone as first-line therapy for patients with receptor-positive postmenopausal breast cancer. *J Clin Oncol.* 2012;30:1919–25.

24. Baselga J, Campone M, Piccart M, et al. Everolimus in postmenopausal hormone-receptor-positive advanced breast cancer. *N Engl J Med.* 2012;366:520–9.

25. Bachelot T, Bourgier C, Cropet C, et al. Randomized phase II trial of everolimus in combination with tamoxifen in patients with hormone receptor-positive, human epidermal growth factor receptor 2-negative metastatic breast cancer with prior exposure to aromatase inhibitors: a GINECO study. *J Clin Oncol.* 2012;30:2718–24.

26. Johnston SR, Kilburn LS, Ellis P, et al. Fulvestrant plus anastrozole or placebo versus exemestane alone after progression on non-steroidal aromatase inhibitors in postmenopausal patients with hormone-receptor-positive locally advanced or metastatic breast cancer (SoFEA): a composite, multicentre, phase 3 randomised trial. *Lancet Oncol.* 2013;14:989–98.

27. Chia S, Gradishar W, Mauriac L, et al. Double-blind, randomized placebo controlled trial of fulvestrant compared with exemestane after prior nonsteroidal aromatase inhibitor therapy in postmenopausal women with hormone receptor-positive, advanced breast cancer: results from EFECT. *J Clin Oncol.* 2008;26:1664–70.

28. Buzdar AU, Jonat W, Howell A, et al. Anastrozole versus megestrol acetate in the treatment of postmenopausal women with advanced breast carcinoma: results of a survival update based on a combined analysis of data from two mature phase III trials. Arimidex Study Group [published erratum appears in *Cancer* 1999 Feb 15;85(4):1010]. *Cancer.* 1998;83:1142–52.

29. Klijn JG, Blamey RW, Boccardo F, et al. Combined tamoxifen and luteinizing hormone-releasing hormone (LHRH) agonist versus LHRH agonist alone in premenopausal advanced breast cancer: a meta-analysis of four randomized trials. *J Clin Oncol.* 2001;19:343–53.

30. Lee CK, Gebski VJ, Coates AS, et al. Trade-offs in quality of life and survival with chemotherapy for advanced breast cancer: mature results of a randomized trial comparing single-agent mitoxantrone with combination cyclophosphamide, methotrexate, 5-fluorouracil and prednisone. *Springerplus.* 2013;2:391.

31. Piccart-Gebhart MJ, Burzykowski T, Buyse M, et al. Taxanes alone or in combination with anthracyclines as first-line therapy of patients with metastatic breast cancer. *J Clin Oncol.* 2008;26:1980–6.

32. Oostendorp LJ, Stalmeier PF, Donders AR, et al. Efficacy and safety of palliative chemotherapy for patients with advanced breast cancer pretreated with anthracyclines and taxanes: a systematic review. *Lancet Oncol.* 2011;12:1053–61.

33. Cortes J, O'Shaughnessy J, Loesch D, et al. Eribulin monotherapy versus treatment of physician's choice in patients with metastatic breast cancer (EMBRACE): a phase 3 open-label randomised study. *Lancet.* 2011;377:914–23.

34. Kiely BE, Soon YY, Tattersall MH, et al. How long have I got? Estimating typical, best-case, and worst-case scenarios for patients starting first-line chemotherapy for metastatic breast cancer: a systematic review of recent randomized trials. *J Clin Oncol.* 2011;29:456–63.

35. Buzdar AU, Xu B, Digumarti R, et al. Randomized phase II non-inferiority study (NO16853) of two different doses of capecitabine in combination with docetaxel for locally advanced/metastatic breast cancer. *Ann Oncol.* 2012;23:589–97.

36. Seidman AD, Berry D, Cirrincione C, et al. Randomized phase III trial of weekly compared with every-3-weeks paclitaxel for metastatic breast cancer, with trastuzumab for all HER-2 overexpressors and random assignment to trastuzumab or not in HER-2 nonoverexpressors: final results of Cancer and Leukemia Group B protocol 9840. *J Clin Oncol.* 2008;26:1642–9.

37. A'Hern RP, Smith IE, Ebbs SR. Chemotherapy and survival in advanced breast cancer: the inclusion of doxorubicin in Cooper type regimens. *Br J Cancer.* 1993;67:801–5.

38. Shamseddine AI, Farhat FS. Platinum-based compounds for the treatment of metastatic breast cancer. *Chemotherapy.* 2011;57:468–87.

39. Carrick S, Ghersi D, Wilcken N, et al. Platinum containing regimens for metastatic breast cancer. *Cochrane Database Syst Rev.* 2004:CD003374.

40. Fossati R, Confalonieri C, Torri V, et al. Cytotoxic and hormonal treatment for metastatic breast cancer: a systematic review of published randomized trials involving 31,510 women [see comments]. *J Clin Oncol.* 1998;16:3439–60.

41. Carrick S, Parker S, Thornton CE, et al. Single agent versus combination chemotherapy for metastatic breast cancer. *Cochrane Database Syst Rev.* 2009:CD003372.

42. Cardoso F, Bedard PL, Winer EP, et al. International guidelines for management of metastatic breast cancer: combination vs sequential single-agent chemotherapy. *J Nat Cancer Inst.* 2009;101:1174–81.

43. Sledge GW, Neuberg D, Bernardo P, et al. Phase III trial of doxorubicin, paclitaxel, and the combination of doxorubicin and paclitaxel as front-line chemotherapy for metastatic breast cancer: an Intergroup trial (E1193). *J Clin Oncol.* 2003;21:588–92.

44. National Comprehensive Cancer Network. NCCN clinical practice guidelines in oncology: breast cancer. Version 1.2014. (Accessed December 27, 2013, at http://www.nccn.org/professionals/physician_gls/PDF/breast.pdf.)

45. Gennari A, Stockler M, Puntoni M, et al. Duration of chemotherapy for metastatic breast cancer: a systematic review and meta-analysis of randomized clinical trials. *J Clin Oncol.* 2011;29:2144–9.

46. Gelmon K, Dent R, Mackey JR, et al. Targeting triple-negative breast cancer: optimising therapeutic outcomes. *Ann Oncol.* 2012;23:2223–34.

47. Isakoff SJ, Goss PE, Mayer EL, et al. TBCRC009: A multicenter phase II study of cisplatin or carboplatin for metastatic triple-negative breast cancer and evaluation of p63/p73 as a biomarker of response. *J Clin Oncol.* 2011; 29 1025.

48. Slamon DJ, Leyland-Jones B, Shak S, et al. Use of chemotherapy plus a monoclonal antibody against HER2 for metastatic breast cancer that overexpresses HER2. *N Engl J Med.* 2001;344:783–92.

49. Nielsen DL, Kumler I, Palshof JA, et al. Efficacy of HER2-targeted therapy in metastatic breast cancer: monoclonal antibodies and tyrosine kinase inhibitors. *Breast.* 2013;22:1–12.

50. Robert N, Leyland-Jones B, Asmar L, et al. Randomized phase III study of trastuzumab, paclitaxel, and carboplatin compared with trastuzumab and paclitaxel in women with HER-2-overexpressing metastatic breast cancer. *J Clin Oncol.* 2006;24:2786–92.

51. Valero V, Forbes J, Pegram MD, et al. Multicenter phase III randomized trial comparing docetaxel and trastuzumab with docetaxel, carboplatin, and trastuzumab as first-line chemotherapy for patients with HER2-gene-amplified metastatic breast cancer (BCIRG 007 study): two highly active therapeutic regimens. *J Clin Oncol.* 2011;29:149–56.

52. Gelmon KA, Boyle F, Kaufman B, et al. Open-label phase III randomized controlled trial comparing taxane-based chemotherapy (Tax) with lapatinib (L) or trastuzumab (T) as first-line therapy for women with HER2+ metastatic breast cancer: Interim analysis (IA) of NCIC CTG MA.31/GSK EGF 108919. *J Clin Oncol.* 2012;30:LBA671.

53. Constantinidou A, Smith I. Is there a case for anti-HER2 therapy without chemotherapy in early breast cancer? *Breast.* 2011;20 Suppl 3:S158–61.

54. KADCYLA™(ado-trastuzumab emtansine) for injection, for intravenous use [package insert]. San Francisco, CA: Genentech; 2013.

55. Mehta A, Tripathy D. Co-targeting estrogen receptor and HER2 pathways in breast cancer. *Breast.* 2014;23:2–9.

56. Zardavas D, Baselga J, Piccart M. Emerging targeted agents in metastatic breast cancer. *Nature Rev: Clin Oncol.* 2013;10:191–210.

57. Gradishar WJ. Sorafenib in locally advanced or metastatic breast cancer. *Expert Opin Invest Drugs.* 2012;21:1177–91.

58. Wagner AD, Thomssen C, Haerting J, et al. Vascular-endothelial-growth-factor (VEGF) targeting therapies for endocrine refractory or resistant metastatic breast cancer. *Cochrane Database Syst Rev.* 2012;7:CD008941.

59. Lyman GH, Burstein HJ, Buzdar AU, et al. Making genuine progress against metastatic breast cancer. *J Clin Oncol.* 2012;30:3448–51.

60. Wagner AD, Thomssen C, Haerting J, et al. Vascular endothelial growth factor (VEGF)-targeting therapies for endocrine-refractory or -resistant metastatic breast cancer (MBC): preliminary results of a systematic review and meta-analysis. *J Clin Oncol.* 2011;29:e11564.

61. Smith IE, Pierga JY, Biganzoli L, et al. First-line bevacizumab plus taxane-based chemotherapy for locally recurrent or metastatic breast cancer: safety and efficacy in an open-label study in 2,251 patients. *Ann Oncol.* 2011;22:595–602.

62. Lang I, Brodowicz T, Ryvo L, et al. Bevacizumab plus paclitaxel versus bevacizumab plus capecitabine as first-line treatment for HER2-negative metastatic breast cancer: interim efficacy results of the randomised, open-label, non-inferiority, phase 3 TURANDOT trial. *Lancet Oncol.* 2013;14:125–33.

63. Hershman DL, Wright JD, Lim E, et al. Contraindicated use of bevacizumab and toxicity in elderly patients with cancer. *J Clin Oncol.* 2013;31:3592–9.

64. Barrios CH, Sampaio C, Vinholes J, et al. What is the role of chemotherapy in estrogen receptor-positive, advanced breast cancer? *Ann Oncol.* 2009;20:1157–62.

65. Wilcken N, Hornbuckle J, Ghersi D. Chemotherapy alone versus endocrine therapy alone for metastatic breast cancer. *Cochrane Database Syst Rev.* 2003:CD002747.

66. Mercadante S. Malignant bone pain: pathophysiology and treatment. *Pain.* 1997;69:1–18.

67. Wu JS, Wong R, Johnston M, et al. Meta-analysis of dose-fractionation radiotherapy trials for the palliation of painful bone metastases. *Int J Radiat Oncol Biol Phys.* 2003;55:594–605.

68. Chow E, Harris K, Fan G, et al. Palliative radiotherapy trials for bone metastases: a systematic review. *J Clin Oncol.* 2007;25:1423–36.

69. Hird A, Chow E, Zhang L, et al. Determining the incidence of pain flare following palliative radiotherapy for symptomatic bone metastases: results from three canadian cancer centers. *Int J Radiat Oncol Biol Phys.* 2009;75:193–7.

70. Christensen MH, Petersen LJ. Radionuclide treatment of painful bone metastases in patients with breast cancer: a systematic review. *Cancer Treat Rev.* 2012;38:164–71.

71. Van der Linden YM, Dijkstra PD, Kroon HM, et al. Comparative analysis of risk factors for pathological fracture with femoral metastases. *J Bone Joint Surg Br.* 2004;86:566–73.

72. Weinstein JN. Balancing science and informed choice in decisions about vertebroplasty. *N Engl J Med.* 2009;361:619–21.

73. Mercadante S, Fulfaro F. Management of painful bone metastases. *Curr Opin Oncol.* 2007;19:308–14.

74. Neville-Webbe HL, Gnant M, Coleman RE. Potential anticancer properties of bisphosphonates. *Sem Oncol.* 2010;37 Suppl 1:S53–65.

75. Carteni G, Bordonaro R, Giotta F, et al. Efficacy and safety of zoledronic acid in patients with breast cancer metastatic to bone: a multicenter clinical trial. *Oncologist.* 2006;11:841–8.

76. Wong MH, Stockler MR, Pavlakis N. Bisphosphonates and other bone agents for breast cancer. *Cochrane Database Syst Rev.* 2012;2:CD003474.

77. Rosen LS, Gordon DH, Dugan W, Jr., et al. Zoledronic acid is superior to pamidronate for the treatment of bone metastases in breast carcinoma patients with at least one osteolytic lesion. *Cancer.* 2004;100:36–43.

78. Park-Wyllie LY, Mamdani MM, Juurlink DN, et al. Bisphosphonate use and the risk of subtrochanteric or femoral shaft fractures in older women. *JAMA.* 2011;305:783–9.

79. Stopeck AT, Lipton A, Body JJ, et al. Denosumab compared with zoledronic acid for the treatment of bone metastases in patients with advanced breast cancer: a randomized, double-blind study. *J Clin Oncol.* 2010;28:5132–9.

80. Van Poznak CH, Temin S, Yee GC, et al. American Society of Clinical Oncology executive summary of the clinical practice guideline update on the role of bone-modifying agents in metastatic breast cancer. *J Clin Oncol.* 2011;29:1221–7.

81. Fornier MN. Denosumab: second chapter in controlling bone metastases or a new book? *J Clin Oncol.* 2010;28:5127–31.

82. Irvin W, Jr., Muss HB, Mayer DK. Symptom management in metastatic breast cancer. *Oncologist.* 2011;16:1203–14.

83. Mehta AI, Brufsky AM, Sampson JH. Therapeutic approaches for HER2-positive brain metastases: circumventing the blood-brain barrier. *Cancer Treat Rev.* 2013;39:261–9.

84. Lueck H-J, Luebbe K, Bischoff J, et al. A randomized phase III study to determine the efficacy of capecitabine in addition to a taxane and bevacizumab as first-line therapy in patients with metastatic breast cancer. *J Clin Oncol.* 2013;31:1082.

85. van Vliet LM, van der Wall E, Plum NM, et al. Explicit prognostic information and reassurance about nonabandonment when entering palliative breast cancer care: findings from a scripted video-vignette study. *J Clin Oncol.* 2013;31:3242–9.

INDEX

Page numbers followed by "b", "f", and "t" indicate boxes, figures, and tables.

Made in the USA
Lexington, KY
30 June 2016